Periodontology and Periodontics: Case Studies

Periodontology and Periodontics: Case Studies

Editor: Georgia Reid

AMERICAN
MEDICAL PUBLISHERS
www.americanmedicalpublishers.com

AMERICAN
MEDICAL PUBLISHERS
www.americanmedicalpublishers.com

Cataloging-in-Publication Data

Periodontology and periodontics: case studies / edited by Georgia Reid.
p. cm.
Includes bibliographical references and index.
ISBN 979-8-88740-653-4
1. Periodontitis. 2. Periodontal disease. 3. Periodontal disease--Diagnosis.
4. Periodontal disease--Treatment. 5. Dental therapeutics. I. Reid, Georgia.
RK450.P4 P47 2023
617.601--dc23

American Medical Publishers,
41 Flatbush Avenue,
1st Floor, New York,
NY 11217, USA

ISBN 979-8-88740-653-4 (Hardback)

Contents

Preface IX

Chapter 1 **Treatment of Miller Class I Gingival Recession with using Nonpedicle Adipose Tissue after Bichectomy Surgical Technique: A Case Report** 1
Carmen Lucia Mueller Storrer, Leonardo Luiz Muller, Janes Francio Pissaia, Carla Frehner Andrade, Claudia Roberta Tenório Trevisani and Tatiana Miranda Deliberador

Chapter 2 **Periodontitis and Intra-Oral Plasmacytosis in a Noonan's Syndrome Patient** 6
Hadeel Alqatami, Khalid N. Said, Adham A. Ammar and Hani Nazzal

Chapter 3 **Emphysema after Sinus Grafting: Importance of Patient's Information, Early Diagnosis and Management** 11
Marc El Hage, Nathalie Nurdin, Mark Bischof and Rabah Nedir

Chapter 4 **Prevention of Periodontal Pocket Formation after Mandibular Third Molar Extraction using Dentin Autologous Graft: A Split Mouth Case Report** 16
Alberto De Biase, Giulia Mazzucchi, Dario Di Nardo, Marco Lollobrigida, Giorgio Serafini and Luca Testarelli

Chapter 5 **Laterally Positioned Flap with Subepithelial Connective Tissue Graft Modified One-Stage Procedure for the Treatment of Deep Isolated Gingival Recessions in Mandibular Incisors** 23
Alvaro Francisco Bosco, Juliano Milanezi de Almeida, Belén Retamal-Valdes, Renata Tavares, Jessica M. Latimer, Diego Messina, Matheus Henke, Laura Gantes Rodrigues Dias and Thiago Marchi Martins

Chapter 6 **Multidisciplinary Oral Rehabilitation of a Severely Compromised Dentition** 32
Carlo Maiorana, Dario Andreoni, Paola Polacco and Pier Paolo Poli

Chapter 7 **Metastatic Carcinoma of the Breast Presenting as Gingival Swelling in the Maxilla: A Case Report** 39
Arun Sadasivan, K. Rakul Nambiar, Deepu George Mathew, Elizabeth Koshi, Roshni Ramesh and Ashna Mariya Benny

Chapter 8 **Combined Surgical and Restorative Procedures to Treat Maxillary Canine with Gingival Recession and Cervical Wear** 48
Dler Ali Khursheed and Faraedon Mostafa Zardawi

Chapter 9 **A Rare Case of Plasma Cell Gingivitis with Cheilitis** 53
Yashodeep Chauhan, Shaleen Khetarpal, Madhu Singh Ratre and Manish Varma

Chapter 10 **A Journey toward Immediate Denture: Overcoming Bitter Reality with Psychotherapy** 58
R. Varsha, P. S. Manoharan, Vigneshvar Chandrasekaran and K. Savitha

Chapter 11 **Morphological and Molecular Characterization of Human Gingival Tissue Overlying Multiple Oral Exostoses** 62
Luca Francetti, Claudia Dellavia, Stefano Corbella, Nicolò Cavalli, Claudia Moscheni, Elena Canciani and Nicoletta Gagliano

Chapter 12 **A Successful Esthetic Approach of Gingival Depigmentation using Microneedling Technique and Ascorbic Acid (Vitamin C)** 72
Diana Mostafa and Shaden M. Alotaibi

Chapter 13 **A Modified Bilaminar Technique with the use of a Fibrin- Fibronectin System for a Single Gingival Recession: A Case Report with a Follow-Up of 3 Years** 79
Michele Perelli, Paolo Giacomo Arduino, Mario Semenza, Roberto Abundo and Hector Sarmiento

Chapter 14 **Necrotizing Ulcerative Gingivitis, a Rare Manifestation as a Sequel of Drug-Induced Gingival Overgrowth: A Case Report** 85
Marah Damdoum, Sudhir Rama Varma, Mohamed A. Jaber and Manjusha Nambiar

Chapter 15 **Bone Regeneration in Vertical Osseous Defect in Periodontitis Patients using Bovine Colostrum** 92
P. L. Ravishankar, Preethikaa Guruprasath, Padmaja Vangipuram, Jasmine Vaidya, G. Visithiriyan, A. Thirumal Raj, Shilpa Bhandi, Shankargouda Patil and Snehashish Ghosh

Chapter 16 **Lateral Periodontal Cyst Treated with Enucleation and Guided Bone Regeneration: A Report of a Case and a Review of Pertinent Literature** 97
Sundar Ramalingam, Yasser Fahad Alrayyes, Khalid Buayjan Almutairi and Ibrahim O. Bello

Chapter 17 **The Gingival Oral Lichen Planus: A Periodontal-Oral Medicine Approach** 105
Abdulhameed Alsarraf, Kunj Mehta and Nabil Khzam

Chapter 18 **Customized Titanium Mesh for Guided Bone Regeneration in the Posterior Mandible in a Patient Previously Treated with Bisphosphonates** 108
Johannes Müller and Rüdiger Junker

Chapter 19 **Palatal Obturator after Maxillectomy following Squamous Cell Carcinoma** 123
Karim Chebbi, Khaoula Bouaziz, Oumaima Tayari, Azza Berkaoui, Mohamed Ali Bouzidi and Jamila Jaouadi

Chapter 20 **Adenoid (Acantholytic) Squamous Cell Carcinoma of Mandibular Gingiva** 129
T. Raut, S. Keshwar, M. R. Jaisani and A. Shrestha

Chapter 21 **Ligneous Periodontitis in a Patient with Type 1 Plasminogen Deficiency: A Case Report and Review of the Literature** 133
Arun Sadasivan, Roshni Ramesh and Deepu George Mathew

Chapter 22 **Proliferative Verrucous Leukoplakia of the Gingiva: An Early Lesion Refractory to Surgical Excision** 141
Dhanushka Leuke Bandara, Primali Rukmal Jayasooriya and Ruwan Duminda Jayasinghe

Chapter 23 **The Creeping Attachment Induced Technique (CAIT) in Natural and Restored Teeth: Case Reports with 24 Months of Follow-Up** 145
Michele Perelli, Roberto Abundo, Giuseppe Corrente and Paolo Giacomo Arduino

Chapter 24 **Actinomycosis as a Rare Local Manifestation of Severe Periodontitis** 151
Moody Kaldas, André Barghorn and Patrick R. Schmidlin

Chapter 25 **Symptomatic Apical Periodontitis of the Mandibular First Molar with the Accessory Canal in the Furcation Area Mimicking Furcation Perforation** 158
Alexei Bolyachin, Zurab Khabadze, Oleg Mordanov, Magomed Gasbanov and Takhir Teberdiev

Chapter 26 **Combined Periodontal and Endodontic Management of Palatal Radicular Groove with Platelet-Rich Fibrin and Biodentine®** 163
Arjun Hari Rijal, Bhageshwar Dhami and Pratistha Ghimire

Chapter 27 **Severe, Treatment-Refractory Periodontitis and Vitamin D Deficiency: A Multidisciplinary Case Report** 171
Figliuzzi Michele Mario, Parentela Luca, Aiello Domenico and Altilia Simone

Chapter 28 **Periodontal Manifestation in a Patient with Kindler Syndrome** 180
Aysegul Sari and Salih Celik

Chapter 29 **Resolution of Abfraction-Associated Gingival Fenestration Utilizing Connective Tissue Grafting** 184
Braydon Haskell, J. Kobi Stern, Jordan Ghiassi, Andrew Kurialacherry, Sadja Gaud-Quintana and Mark E. Peacock

Chapter 30 **Restoring Teeth with an Advanced Lithium Disilicate Ceramic: A Case Report and 1-Year Follow-Up** 188
Felicitas Hölken and Helmut Dietrich

Permissions

List of Contributors

Index

Preface

This book has been an outcome of determined endeavour from a group of educationists in the field. The primary objective was to involve a broad spectrum of professionals from diverse cultural background involved in the field for developing new researches. The book not only targets students but also scholars pursuing higher research for further enhancement of the theoretical and practical applications of the subject.

Periodontology, also known as periodontics, is a dental specialty that focuses on the prevention, diagnosis, and treatment of diseases and conditions that affect the supporting structures of the teeth, including the gums, periodontal ligament and the alveolar bone. Some of the key aspects of periodontology and periodontics include the diagnosis and treatment of periodontal diseases, periodontal surgery and treatment of gum recession. A few of the gum diseases treated within this field are gingivitis and periodontitis. There are also numerous surgical procedures carried out within this field of dentistry such as flap surgery, dental implant placement and bone grafts. This book unfolds the innovative aspects of periodontology, which will be crucial for the progress of this field in the future. It will also provide interesting topics for research which interested readers can take up. Periodontists and students actively engaged in this field will find this book full of crucial and unexplored concepts.

It was an honour to edit such a profound book and also a challenging task to compile and examine all the relevant data for accuracy and originality. I wish to acknowledge the efforts of the contributors for submitting such brilliant and diverse chapters in the field and for endlessly working for the completion of the book. Last, but not the least; I thank my family for being a constant source of support in all my research endeavours.

Editor

1

Treatment of Miller Class I Gingival Recession with using Nonpedicle Adipose Tissue after Bichectomy Surgical Technique: A Case Report

Carmen Lucia Mueller Storrer, Leonardo Luiz Muller, Janes Francio Pissaia, Carla Frehner Andrade, Claudia Roberta Tenório Trevisani, and Tatiana Miranda Deliberador

School of Health Science, Universidade Positivo, Curitiba, Paraná, Brazil

Correspondence should be addressed to Carmen Lucia Mueller Storrer; carmen.storrer@gmail.com and Tatiana Miranda Deliberador; tdeliberador@gmail.com

Academic Editor: Giuseppe Alessandro Scardina

Gingival recession is an oral health problem that affects a large part of the population. Several treatments are suggested in the current literature; among them is the use of buccal fat pad grafting. The objective of this case report is to describe the treatment of a Miller Class I gingival recession using a nonpedicled buccal fat pad graft immediately after performing the surgery for buccal fat pad removal (bichectomy technique). First, bilateral surgical removal of the buccal fat pad was performed with the main objective of eliminating oral mucosa biting. The recipient site was prepared to receive a portion of the fat pad that was cut and macerated in a size that was sufficient to cover the recession. The patient was followed up at 15, 30, 60, and 365 days postsurgery, and the results showed an elimination of the oral mucosa biting and complete coverage of the gingival recession. It was concluded that the nonpedicled buccal fat pad graft is another option for the treatment of Miller Class I recessions.

1. Introduction

Gingival recession is the apical displacement of the gingival tissue in relation to the cementoenamel junction resulting in the root surface being exposed to the oral environment [1]. This exposure may lead to dentin sensitivity, pain, risk of root caries, abrasion, and erosion lesions, in addition to not being esthetic. Its etiology is associated with several factors such as biofilm accumulation, chemical and mechanical trauma, orthodontic treatment, quantity and quality of keratinized gingiva, and occlusal trauma [2–4].

Success in the treatment of gingival recessions is directly related to its severity. In Miller Class I and Class II recessions, there is no interproximal tissue loss; thus, complete root coverage is feasible [5].

Different surgical techniques such as free gingival graft, flap repositioning, and connective tissue graft have been used in the treatment of gingival recessions. Treatments with pedicled buccal fat pad grafts are also described in the literature with satisfactory results regarding root coverage, clinical attachment level, and keratinized tissue gain [6, 7]. However, the use of nonpedicled buccal fat pad grafts is still poorly described [8].

Currently, the surgical technique of buccal fat pad removal/bichectomy technique (removal of part of the buccal adipose tissue) has been frequently performed in dentistry with the main objective of eliminating oral mucosa biting. In a systematic review of 8 of the 220 articles found, it was concluded that the bichectomy technique has an initial favorable outcome regarding facial aesthetics with a low rate of

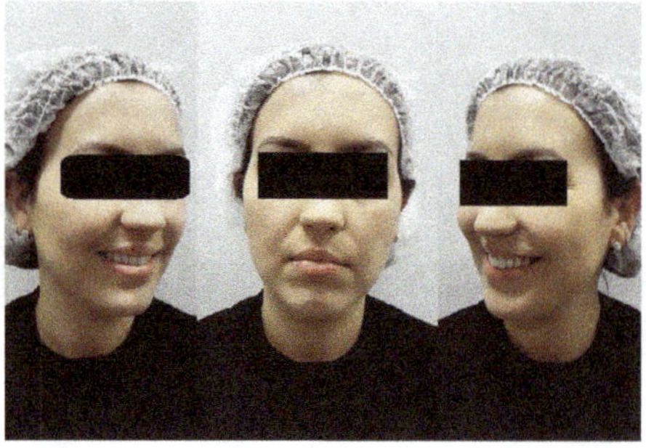

FIGURE 1: The clinical exam confirmed the face rounded and the indication for Bichectomy technique.

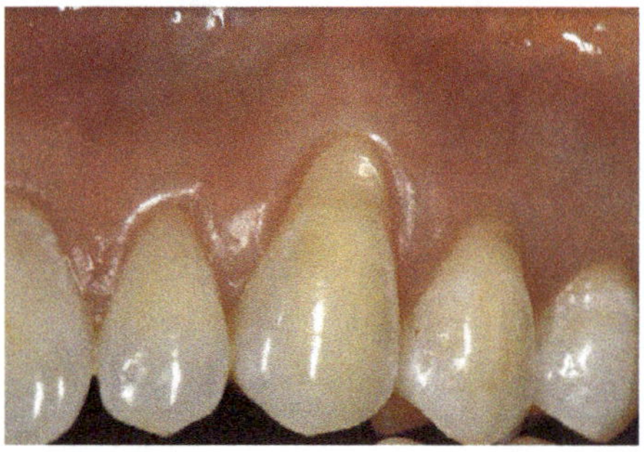

FIGURE 2: Miller Class I gingival recession on the maxillary left canine (recipient site).

complications, but there is a lack of randomized clinical trials to evaluate long-term outcomes [9].

The objective of this case report is to describe the treatment of a Miller Class I gingival recession using a nonpedicled buccal fat pad graft immediately after performing the surgery for buccal fat pad removal.

2. Case History

Prior to the surgical intervention, the patient was informed about the surgical procedure and signed an ethical consent form.

The patient, a young female, presented to the Dentistry Clinic reporting a lack of gingival symmetry between the maxillary left and right canines and with the desire to eliminate oral mucosa biting. The clinical exam confirmed the face rounded (Figure 1) and cheek biting and revealed a Miller Class I gingival recession on the maxillary left canine (Figure 2). The removal of the Bichat fat pad was suggested to the patient with the objective of eliminating the oral mucosa biting and using the tissue for the root coverage.

The surgical procedure was initiated by harvesting the buccal fat pad. The incision location is at the vestibule fundus, at the distal caries of the second molar with a 30 mm distance from the vestibule and above the Parotid duct (Figure 3). The incision is made, initially, by perforating the alveolar mucosa, buccinator muscle, and connective tissue capsule that surrounds the Bichat buccal fat pad. Then, the incision is extended about 1.5 cm until it reaches the mesial caries of the first molar (Figure 4). A curved hemostat was used to enlarge the tissues. The buccal extension of the

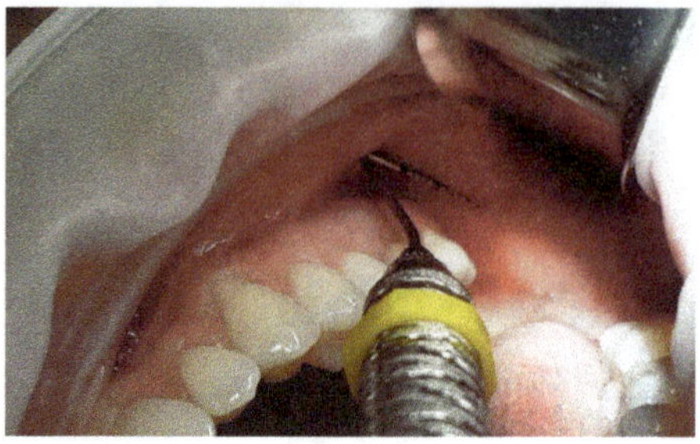

FIGURE 3: The incision location in donor site: vestibule fundus, at the distal caries of the second molar with a 30 mm distance from the vestibule and above the parotid duct.

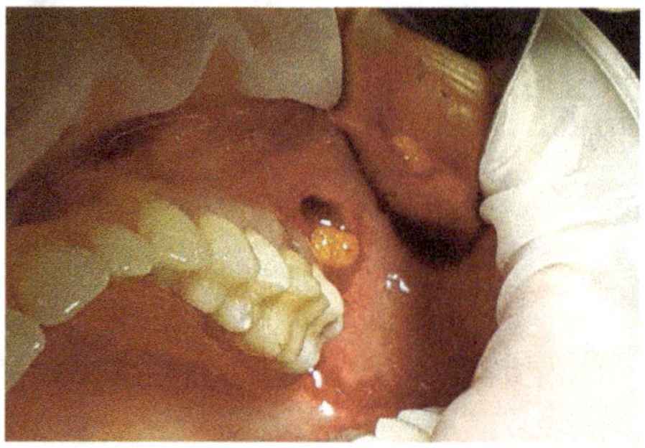

FIGURE 4: Extension of the incision: from the distal caries of the second molar to the mesial caries of the first molar.

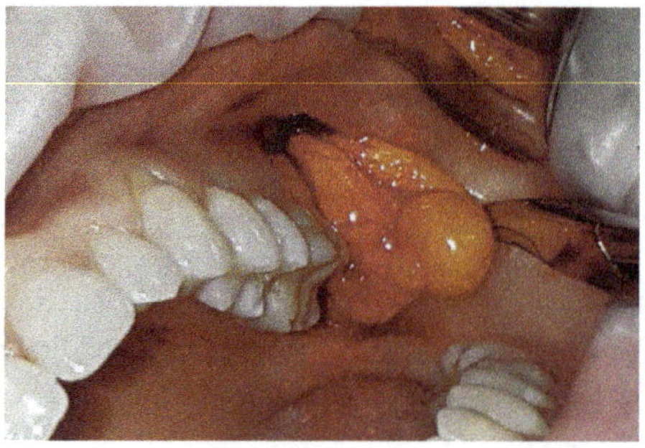

FIGURE 5: Removal of the buccal extension of the Bichat ball.

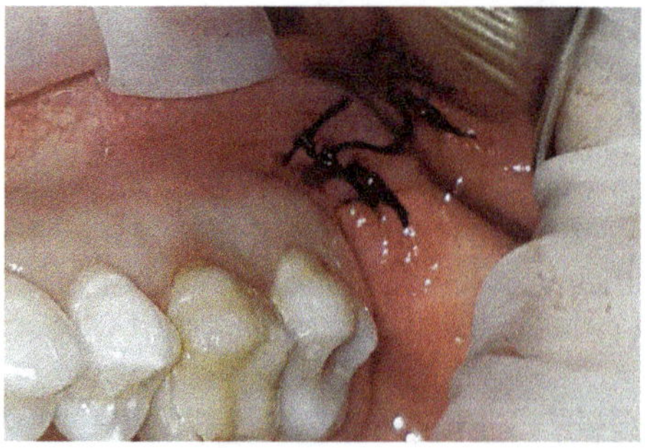

FIGURE 6: Simple suture in donor site with 4.0 silk thread.

Bichat ball is completely removed by careful circular movements (Figure 5). 4 ml of buccal fat pad was removed. The donor site was immediately sutured with a 4.0 silk thread (braided black silk, Technofio, Goiania, GO, Brazil) with a simple suture (Figure 6).

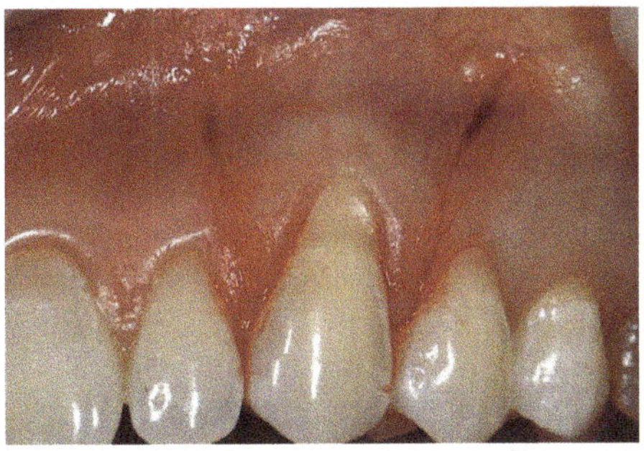

FIGURE 7: Preparation of the recipient site: with an intrasulcular incision and two diverging vertical incisions up to the alveolar mucosa.

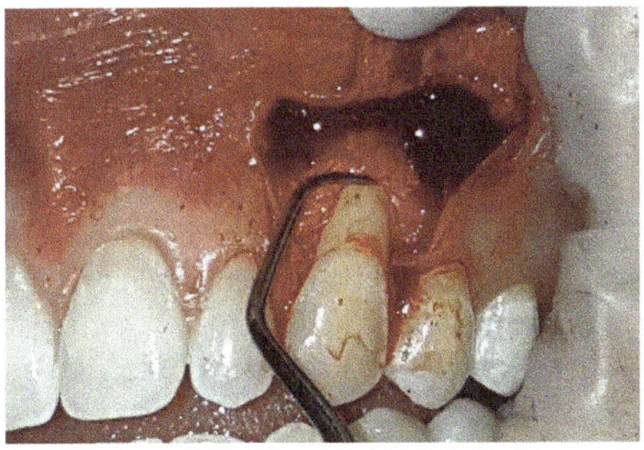

FIGURE 8: Scaled and planned with 5-6 Gracey curettes in canine root prior to receiving graft of adipose tissue.

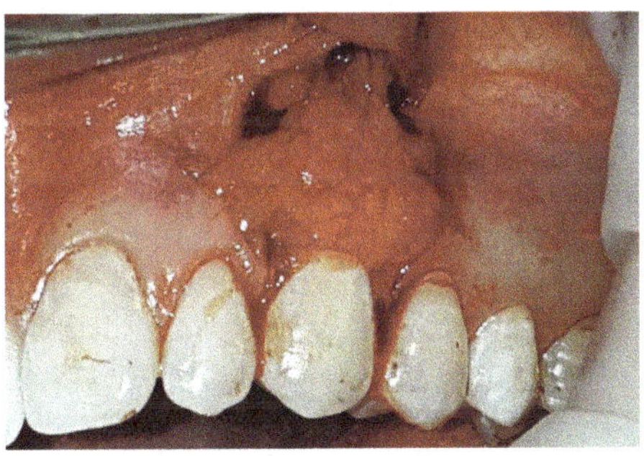

FIGURE 9: Macerated portion of the buccal fat pad cover of the recipient site.

The preparation of the recipient site (gingival recession on the maxillary left canine) was performed with an intrasulcular incision and two divergent vertical incisions toward the vestibule bottom (Figure 7). A partial thickness flap was then raised, and a periosteal releasing incision was made so the flap could be loosened and slid to cover the graft. The canine root was then scaled and planned with 5-6 Gracey curettes (Figure 8) (Hu-Friedy, Chicago, IL, USA) and irrigated with sterile saline solution. A portion of the buccal fat pad was cut into a size that was sufficient to cover the recipient site, its surface was macerated with a scalpel blade, and the graft was positioned (Figure 9). The graft was stabilized with an X suture using a 5.0 resorbable suture thread (polyglycolic acid suture, Technofio, Goiania, GO, Brazil), and the flap was then coronally positioned and anchored with simple and suspension sutures (Figure 10).

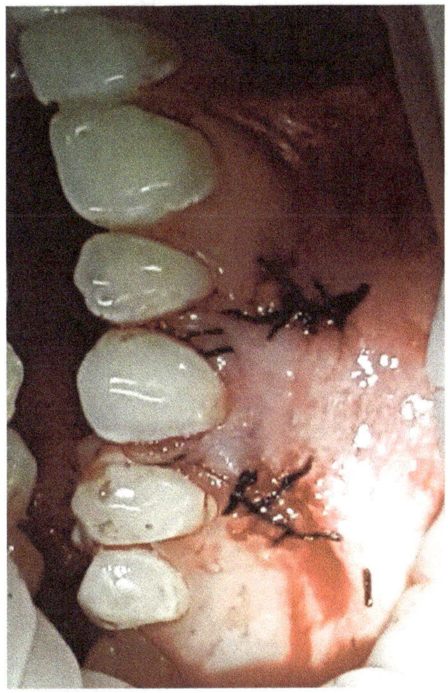

FIGURE 10: Flap coronally positioned and anchored with simple and suspension sutures.

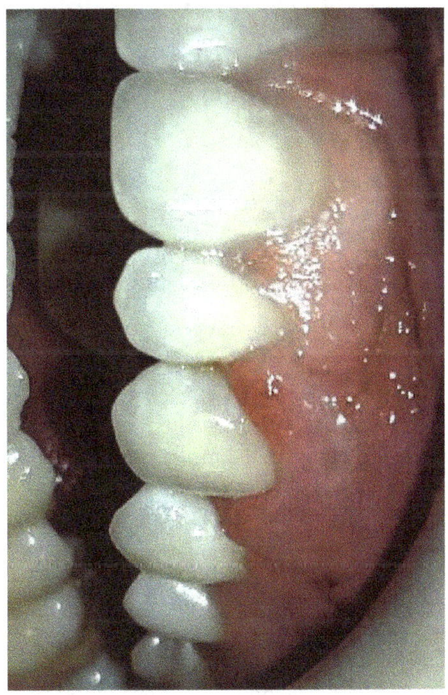

FIGURE 11: Removal of sutures 15 days postoperatively.

As postoperative medications, amoxicillin 500 mg (8/8 h for 07 days) and ibuprofen 400 mg (8/8 h for 03 days) were prescribed. The patient was instructed to rinse the surgical site with 0.12% 58 chlorhexidine digluconate solution twice a day, for 1 week. The suture was removed 15 days postsurgery (Figure 11), and follow-up visits were scheduled at 30 (Figure 12), 60 (Figure 13), and 365 (Figure 14) days.

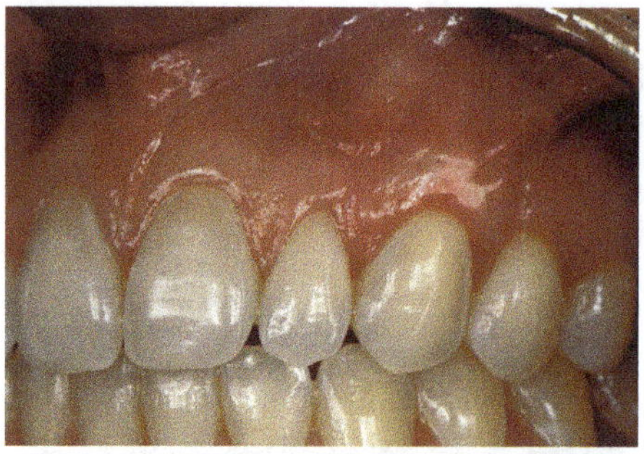

FIGURE 12: 30-day postoperative follow-up.

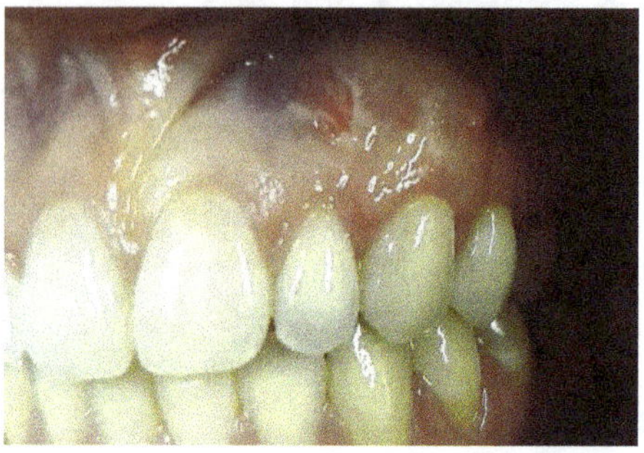

FIGURE 13: 60-day postoperative follow-up.

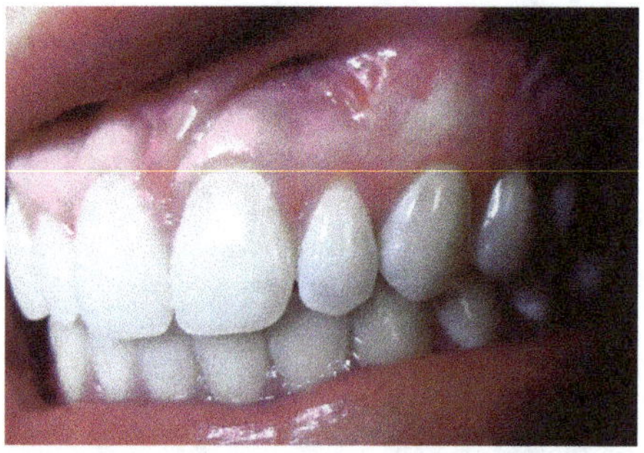

FIGURE 14: 1-year postoperative follow-up.

The patient reported that the oral mucosa biting was completely eliminated and that she was satisfied with the esthetic and functional results of the buccal fat pad removal surgery. Additionally, she was satisfied with the root coverage of the maxillary left canine, which favored smile esthetics and reduced dentin sensitivity.

3. Discussion

The free gingival graft technique presents good results in the treatment of gingival recessions. However, it is not recommended in esthetic areas, since the color discrepancy is unfavorable [7]. Root coverage using subepithelial connective tissue graft is considered the gold standard when compared to the other surgical techniques, as it provides satisfactory root coverage, gain in clinical attachment level, and keratinized tissue, resulting in therapeutic and esthetic success [10]. However, the palatal donor site usually entails a pronounced postoperative pain, and therefore, different autogenous graft alternatives have been applied in the treatment of gingival recessions [11].

The results of the proposed treatment have been described as positive, and success has been attributed to the ease in harvesting the buccal fat graft through a fast surgical technique with low donor site morbidity and a low rate of complications [12]. The positive results are also attributed to the rich vascular supply that guarantees maintaining the vitality of the graft and the presence of stem cells that aid in tissue regeneration and differentiation of the grafted adipose tissue into stratified squamous epithelium and dense connective tissue [13]. There is a report of long-term maintenance of the graft structure and volume since the buccal fat pad does not undergo lipolysis [14].

El Haddad et al. [7] reported the therapy with pedicled buccal fat pad grafting in a maxillary first molar with the buccal root surface almost completely exposed, presenting grade III mobility and Class II furcation involvement. One month after treatment, there was an average gain of 8 mm in root coverage and gained keratinized tissues with excellent matching of color and texture were observed. In 2010, Kumari et al. [15] used the same technique to cover a Miller Class III defect in a maxillary right molar and obtained a 4 mm gain in the attachment level. Agarwal [6] also applied the technique in a maxillary molar with class IV gingival recession and obtained clinical attachment level and keratinized tissue gain. Ercan et al. [12] described two clinical cases, where the first one showed a gain of 7 mm in the attachment level, reducing the gingival recession to 4 mm. Panda et al. [16] performed a subepithelial graft using the pedicled buccal fat pad and buccal flap advancement for root coverage of a Miller Class III gingival recession exhibiting a 7 mm attachment loss and obtained keratinized tissue gain—which was initially absent—in addition to a gain of 4 mm in the attachment level.

In 2015, Deliberador et al. [8] conducted a split-mouth randomized controlled trial to analyze the transplant efficiency of a nonpedicled buccal fat pad graft for the treatment of Miller Class I and Class II gingival recessions and compared the results with those of a subepithelial connective tissue graft. The authors concluded that the use of a buccal fat pad graft can be considered a predictable alternative, as no significant statistical differences were observed between the two techniques with respect to the esthetic results, gain in clinical attachment level, gain in keratinized tissue, and root coverage; thus, both therapies were considered to be clinically successful.

In the present case report, a nonpedicled buccal fat pad graft was performed with flap advancement, resulting in complete root coverage, with maintenance of the extension of the keratinized tissue width, normal color and texture characteristics, and a small increase in gingival volume. The results were maintained after one year of follow-up suggesting that the technique is safe and effective, in agreement with a previously performed study [8].

4. Conclusion

Nonpedicled buccal fat pad graft is an effective technique in the treatment of Miller Class I gingival recessions and may be considered a treatment option. The technique is safe and easy to perform, presents excellent esthetic and therapeutic results, and can also be applied in areas distant from the donor site or even in the lower arch.

Additional Points

Key Messages. The aim of this case report is to address the treatment of a Miller Class I gingival recession using a non-pedicled buccal fat pad graft after buccal fat pad removal surgery (bichectomy technique).

Consent

The authors certify that they have obtained all appropriate patient consent forms. In the form, the patient has given her consent for her images and other clinical information to be reported in the journal. The patient understands that her name will not be published and due efforts will be made to conceal identity, but anonymity cannot be guaranteed.

References

[1] F. Cairo, "Periodontal plastic surgery of gingival recessions at single and multiple teeth," *Periodontology 2000*, vol. 75, no. 1, pp. 296–316, 2017.

[2] K. F. G. Yared, E. G. Zenobio, and W. Pacheco, "A etiologia multifatorial da recessão periodontal," *Revista Dental Press de Ortodontia e Ortopedia Facial*, vol. 11, no. 6, pp. 45–51, 2006.

[3] M. G. Marini, S. L. A. Greghi, E. Passanezi, and A. C. P. Sant'ana, "Gingival recession: prevalence, extension and severity in adults," *Journal of Applied Oral Science*, vol. 12, no. 3, pp. 250–255, 2004.

[4] G. Serino, J. L. Wennström, J. Lindhe, and L. Eneroth, "The prevalence and distribution of gingival recession in subjects with a high standard of oral hygiene," *Journal of Clinical Periodontology*, vol. 21, no. 1, pp. 57–63, 1994.

[5] A. P. Yadav, A. Kulloli, S. Shetty, S. S. Ligade, S. S. Martande, and M. J. Gholkar, "Sub-epithelial connective tissue graft for the management of Miller's class I and class II isolated gingival recession defect: a systematic review of the factors influencing the outcome," *Journal of Investigative and Clinical Dentistry*, vol. 9, no. 3, article e12325, 2018.

[6] C. Agarwal, G. V. Gayathri, and D. S. Mehta, "An innovative technique for root coverage using pedicled buccal fat pad," *Contemporary Clinical Dentistry*, vol. 5, no. 3, pp. 386–388, 2014.

[7] A. S. El Haddad, M. Y. A. Razzak, and M. El Shall, "Use of pedicled buccal fat pad in root coverage of severe gingival recession defect," *Journal of Periodontology*, vol. 79, no. 7, pp. 1271–1279, 2008.

[8] T. M. Deliberador, C. T. Trevisani, C. L. M. Storrer et al., "Non-pedicled buccal fat pad grafts to treatment for class I and II gingival recessions: a clinical trial," *Brazilian Dental Journal*, vol. 26, no. 6, pp. 572–579, 2015.

[9] L. B. Moura, J. R. Spin, R. Spin-Neto, and V. A. Pereira-Filho, "Buccal fat pad removal to improve facial aesthetics: an established technique?," *Medicina Oral, Patología Oral y Cirugía Bucal*, vol. 23, no. 4, pp. e478–e484, 2018.

[10] L. Chambrone, D. Chambrone, F. E. Pustiglioni, L. A. Chambrone, and L. A. Lima, "Can subepithelial connective tissue grafts be considered the gold standard procedure in the treatment of Miller class I and II recession-type defects?," *Journal of Dentistry*, vol. 36, no. 9, pp. 659–671, 2008.

[11] S. El-Haddad and M. El-Shall, "Two-Year Clinical Evaluation of Pedicled Buccal Fat Pad Alone and with Emdogain for Root Coverage of Severe Gingival Recession Defects: A Case Series," *The International journal of periodontics & restorative dentistry*, vol. 37, no. 6, pp. 901–901, 2017.

[12] E. Ercan, C. Çandirli, C. Uysal, B. C. Uzun, and E. Yenilmez, "Treatment of severe gingival recession using pedicled buccal fat pad: histological and clinical findings," *Clinical and Experimental Health Sciences*, vol. 6, no. 4, pp. 191–194, 2016.

[13] E. Farré-Guasch, C. Martí-Pagè, F. Hernádez-Alfaro, J. Klein-Nulend, and N. Casals, "Buccal fat pad, an oral access source of human adipose stem cells with potential for osteochondral tissue engineering: an in vitro study," *Tissue Engineering Part C: Methods*, vol. 16, no. 5, pp. 1083–1094, 2010.

[14] P. W. Poeschl, A. Baumann, G. Russmueller, E. Poeschl, C. Klug, and R. Ewers, "Closure of oroantral communications with Bichat's buccal fat pad," *Journal of Oral and Maxillofacial Surgery*, vol. 67, no. 7, pp. 1460–1466, 2009.

[15] B. N. Kumari, R. Thiagarajan, V. Narayanan, P. Devadoss, B. Mammen, and P. Emmadi, "A new technique for root coverage using buccal fat pad–a short case report," *Quintessence International*, vol. 41, no. 7, pp. 547–549, 2010.

[16] S. Panda, M. D. Fabrro, A. Satpathy, and A. C. Das, "Pedicled buccal fat pad graft for root coverage in severe gingival recession defect," *Journal of Indian Society of Periodontology*, vol. 20, no. 2, pp. 216–219, 2016.

2

Periodontitis and Intra-Oral Plasmacytosis in a Noonan's Syndrome Patient

Hadeel Alqatami,[1] Khalid N. Said,[2,3] Adham A. Ammar,[4] and Hani Nazzal[1,3]

[1]*Pediatric Dental Department, Hamad Dental Centre, Doha, Qatar*
[2]*Department of Dentistry, Oral Health Institute, Al Wakra Hospital, Hamad Medical Corporation, Doha, Qatar*
[3]*College of Dental Medicine, Qatar University, Doha, Qatar*
[4]*Surrey and Sussex Health care Trust, Surrey, UK*

Correspondence should be addressed to Hani Nazzal; haninazzal@hotmail.com

Academic Editor: Wen Lin Chai

A 13-year-old female patient with Noonan's syndrome, intra-oral periodontitis, and associated periodontal lesions is presented in this case report. The patient suffered early onset severe molar pattern periodontitis and recurrent intra-oral inflammatory lesions, pyogenic granuloma, and plasmacytosis, which were excised and controlled using a strict oral hygiene protocol based on long-term use of chlorhexidine-based products as auxiliary aid to regular home care and brushing.

1. Introduction

Noonan syndrome (NS) is an autosomal dominant disorder characterized by a spectrum of congenital heart defects, webbed neck, unusual chest deformity, mild mental deficiencies, short stature, facial deformities, and bleeding tendencies [1] (OMIM #163950).

Several oral manifestations have been associated with this syndrome including high arched palate, malocclusion, micrognathia, numerical tooth anomalies, mandibular cysts resembling cherubism, extensive caries, periodontal diseases, and giant cell lesions [1, 2].

The following case describes the dental and periodontal management of a 13-year-old female patient with a combination of severe periodontitis in localized molar pattern, pyogenic granuloma, and plasmacytosis lesions.

2. Case Report

The patient was referred by her cardiologist to the Pediatric Dental Department at Hamad Medical Corporation, Doha, Qatar, for the management of gingival bleeding. Medically, the patient presented in with NS heterozygous *SOS1*, *MTO1*, and *MYPNS* genes, hypertrophic cardiomyopathy with myomectomy and mitral valve repair in 2017, short stature, scoliosis with congenital tethering of spinal cord, and transient synovitis. The patient was prescribed $\beta 1$ blocker, aspirin, Lasix, iron supplement, and growth hormone (Norditropin®).

Dentally, the patient presented with high cariogenic diet, which involved regular consumption of PediaSure® dietary supplements and high plaque accumulation on her teeth secondary to poor oral hygiene practice. Periodontally, the patient presented with edematous gingivae with erythema and enlargement associated with bleeding on probing (Figure 1), localized severe angular periodontal bone loss mesial to teeth #3 and #14 associated with deep probing depth of 5 mm, bleeding on probing, furcation involvement, and severe clinical attachment loss. A class 2 mobility was observed with tooth #3, whereas a moderate bone loss was observed interproximally between teeth #13 and #14.

In addition, the patient presented with localized, soft, and bluish red soft tissue enlargement interproximally (mainly palatally) between teeth #7, #8, and #9. Other clinical findings include an impacted tooth #6 with an associated

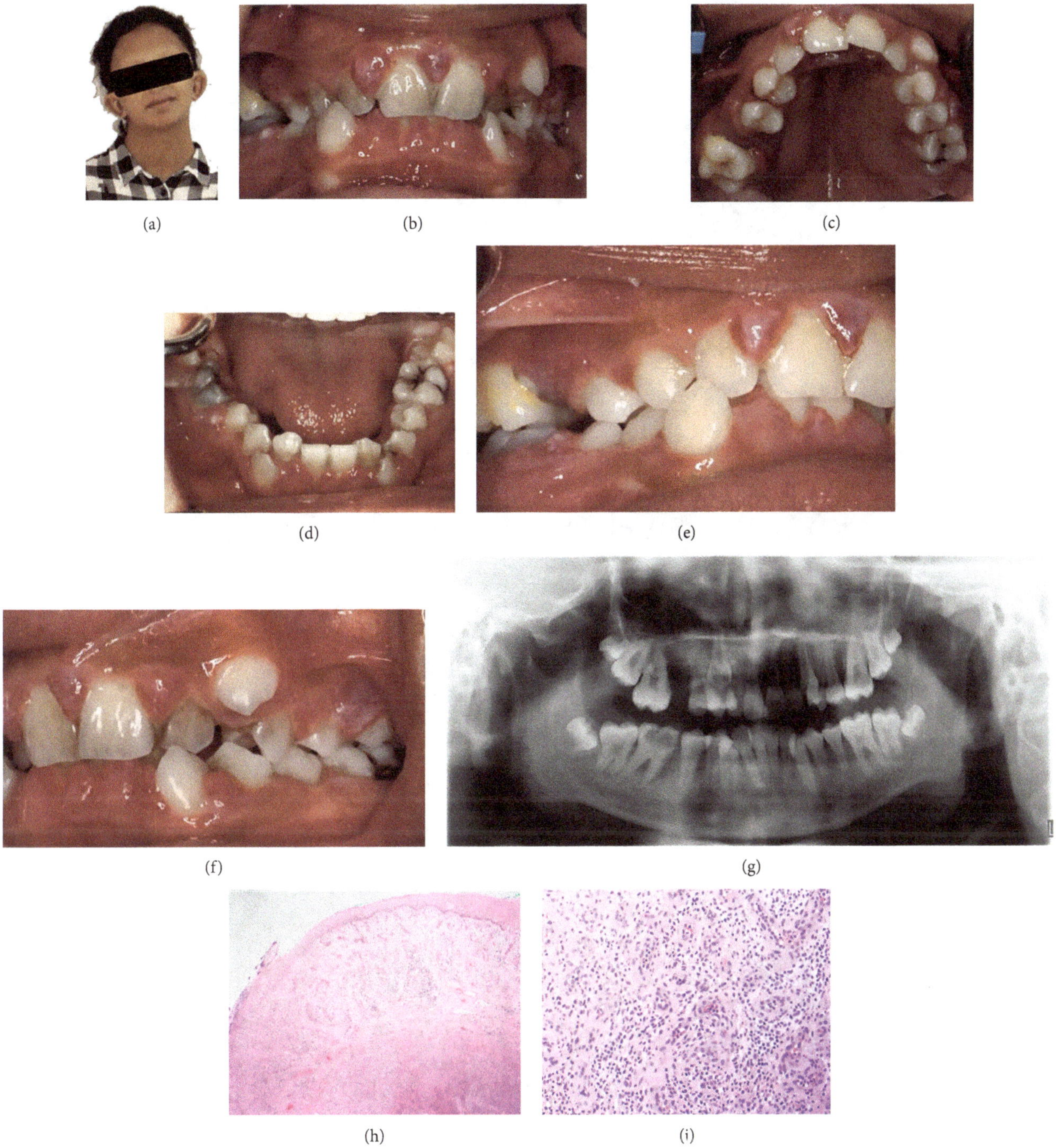

Figure 1: (a) Extra-oral frontal view at presentation. (b)–(f) Intra-oral views at presentation. (g) Orthopantomogram at presentation. (h) and (i) Hematoxylin & eosin stained images of first excisional biopsy of gingival lesion palatal to teeth #8 and #9. (h) Photomicrograph depicting surface squamous mucosa exhibiting focal ulceration, and underlying submucosal proliferation of capillary sized blood vessels with lobular arrangement (×40). (i) High power view showing proliferation of capillaries admixed with numerous mononuclear and polymorphonuclear inflammatory cells (×200).

supplemental premolar tooth, space loss, crowding in both arches, high arched palate, micrognathia, and taurodontism of teeth #2 and #15. Clinical and radiographic findings are summarized in Figure 1.

Communication with the patient's physician ruled out an associated hemorrhagic tendency, whereas antibiotic prophylaxis against infective endocarditis was recommended and carried out during all future invasive treatments. An interdisciplinary treatment plan was developed and performed (Figure 2), whereby the patient underwent an intensive home preventive care, regular scaling with selective root planning of deep periodontal pockets, restoration of the

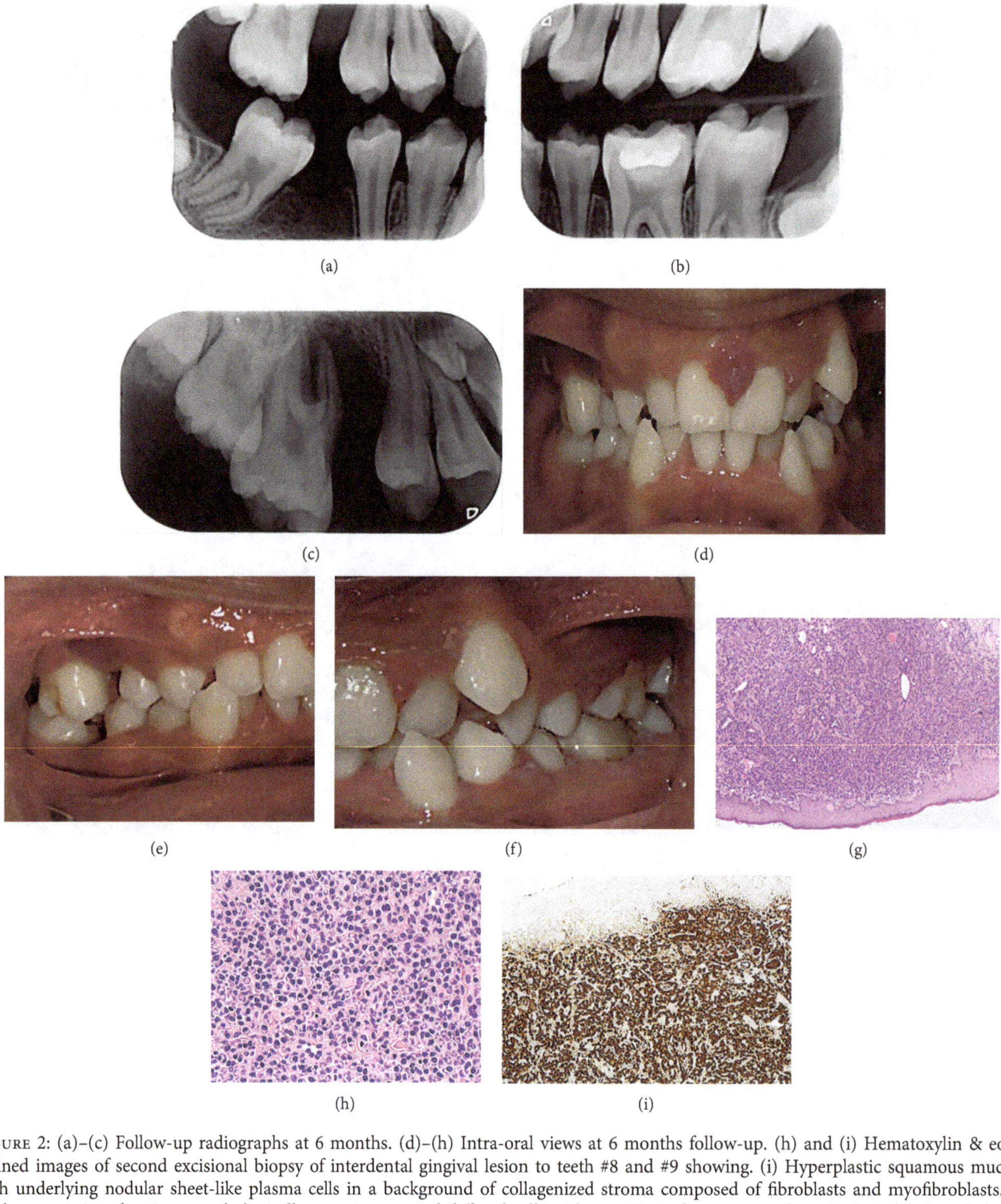

FIGURE 2: (a)–(c) Follow-up radiographs at 6 months. (d)–(h) Intra-oral views at 6 months follow-up. (h) and (i) Hematoxylin & eosin stained images of second excisional biopsy of interdental gingival lesion to teeth #8 and #9 showing. (i) Hyperplastic squamous mucosa with underlying nodular sheet-like plasma cells in a background of collagenized stroma composed of fibroblasts and myofibroblasts. (j) High power view showing morphologically monotonous and diffused cells with no mitotic figures or nuclear atypia indicative of plasma cell infiltrate. (k) Immunostains for kappa and lambda showing a strong diffused positivity with no light chain restriction. Findings were indicative of polyclonality of the lesion.

carious teeth #14 and #19, and extraction of the unrestorable tooth #30. An excisional biopsy of the interdental soft tissue masses at the maxillary incisor region was performed. The histopathological assessment showed proliferation of capillaries admixed with numerous mononuclear and polymorphonuclear inflammatory cells consistent with pyogenic granuloma (Figure 1). Orthodontic intervention was delayed until the periodontal disease status is controlled.

Up to 6 months recall, the initial treatment plan was found to be partially successful in improving the patient's oral health with initial resolution of gingival edema and erythema, and the periodontal and gingival lesions associated

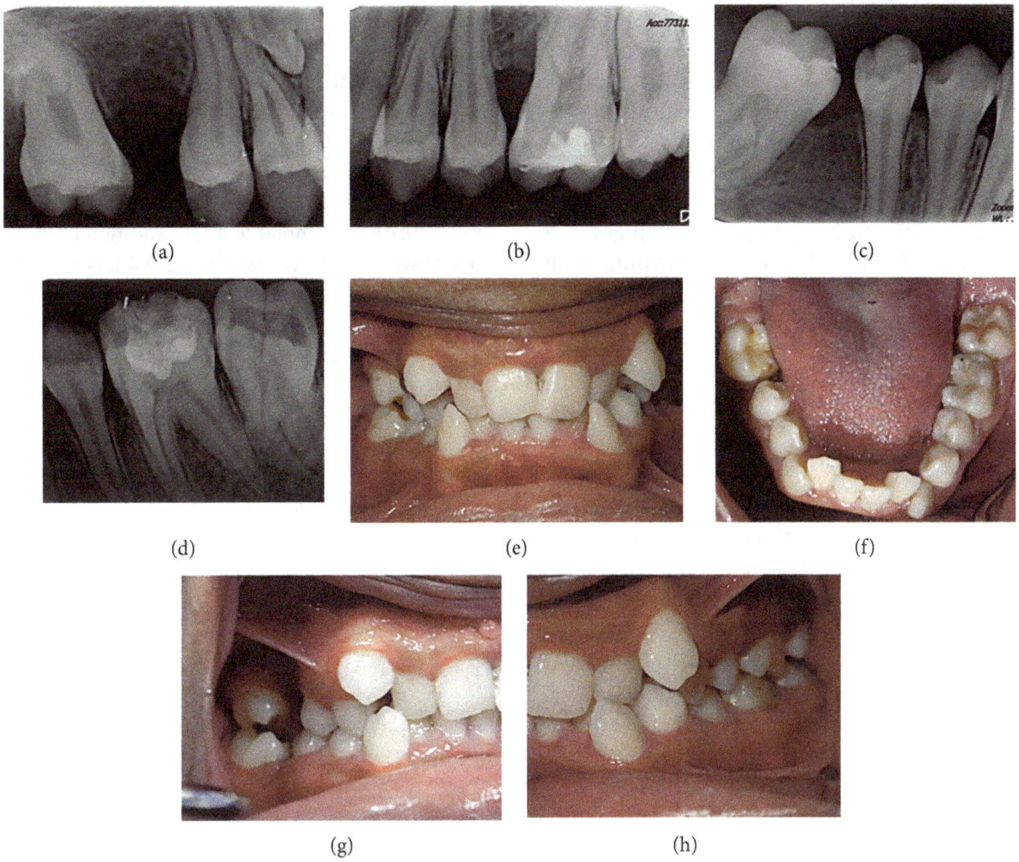

FIGURE 3: Periapical radiographs and intra-oral images taken at 6 months recall from second excisional biopsy (no recurrence was observed up to 12 months).

with tooth #3 (Figure 2). In addition, the interdental masses adjacent to teeth #8 and #9 had recurred.

A second treatment phase included extraction of tooth #3 as a result of the severe bone loss, severe mobility, and possible associated periodontic–endodontic lesion. In addition, a second excisional biopsy of the recurrent lesions between teeth #8 and #9 along with a labial frenoplasty, which aimed at releasing the aberrant low attachment maxillary labial frenum thought to contribute to the recurrent lesion, was performed. The second histopathological assessment showed evidence of hyperplastic squamous mucosa with underlying nodular sheet-like plasma cells in a background of collagenized stroma composed of fibroblasts and myofibroblasts, and morphologically monotonous and diffused cells with no mitotic figures or nuclear atypia indicative of plasma cell infiltrate (Figure 2). In addition, immunostains for kappa and lambda showed a strong diffused positivity with no light chain restriction (Figure 2). The histopathological findings, therefore, were indicative of intra-oral plasmacytosis.

The patient's home care plan was modified by introducing twice daily tooth brushing using chlorhexidine 0.12% toothpaste and the application of chlorhexidine 0.2% spray to the site of recurrent lesions before bedtime and in the morning, daily, during the healing process. The patient was maintained on the chlorhexidine 0.12% toothpaste thereafter. This approach led to total resolution of inflammation signs and prevented the recurrence of the lesion between teeth #8 and #9 up to 12 months post-operatively (Figure 3).

3. Discussion

Although the patient presented with several characteristics in line with NS, this case report focuses on the diagnosis and management of the gingival masses and periodontitis lesions in patients with NS.

The incidence of periodontitis in children is low and usually is linked to the presence of a systemic diseases, such as severe systemic immune alterations or associated with hereditary disorders, such as Papillon–Lefèvre syndrome [3]. Among adolescents and young adults, the incidence of molar-incisor pattern of periodontitis, historically known as localized juvenile periodontitis, remains low at less than 0.5% [4]. Nevertheless, the devastating health, nutrition, and psychological effects, associated with pathologic migration of teeth and early loss of dentition, are high.

The patient presented with a combination of localized molar pattern of severe periodontitis, which is generally rare in children and infrequently reported in patients with NS [1, 5, 6]. Torres-Carmona et al. [5] reported the presence of severe periodontitis in a 15- and 18-year-old NS patients with molar-incisor pattern of alveolar bone destruction. Similar findings were observed in this case, where severe periodontitis was associated with advanced bone loss and clinical attachment loss mesial to teeth #3, #14, and #30.

The patient also presented with two distinct gingival masses that showed histopathological presentations of pyogenic granuloma and intra-oral plasmacytosis.

Pyogenic granuloma is considered a reactive tumor like lesion developed in response to different stimuli, such as low grade local irritation, trauma, hormone changes, and certain drugs [7]. This condition is prevalent in young adult females as a possible result of the vascular effects of female hormonal changes [7]. Oral lesions usually involve the anterior maxillary interdental gingiva with predilection to affect the facial aspects. The poor oral hygiene with associated supra and subgingival plaque and calculus coupled with hormonal changes might have contributed to the development of these lesions in this patient.

Mucous membrane plasmacytosis is a rare, benign disorder where plasma cells infiltrate the mucous membranes including the buccal mucosa, palate, gingiva, lips, and tongue [8]. Different terms have been used to describe this condition, such as atypical/idiopathic/allergic gingivostomatitis, plasmacytosis circumorificialis, plasmacytosis mucosae, plasma cell-gingivitis, plasmacytosis of the gingival, plasma-cell cheilitis, and plasma-cell orificial mucositis [8]. Currently, variants of the term plasma-cell orificial mucositis, such as mucous membrane plasmacytosis and plasma-cell mucositis, have been used in the majority of cases [8]. Different treatments of this condition, such as corticosteroids, antibiotics, liquid nitrogen, CO_2 laser, electrocoagulation, excision of the tissue, and radiation therapy, have been reported in the literature [8]. None of these treatment modalities has been shown to be more superior [8].

In the presented case, a combination of good home care supplemented with chlorhexidine toothpaste and spray, regular scaling/root debridement, and extraction of the teeth with questionable long-term prognosis were successful in controlling the periodontal condition, whereas surgical excision and long-term use of chlorhexidine toothpaste/spray appeared effective in resolving the gingival pathological lesions for 12 months. Patients with NS present with multiple physical disabilities and some with mental complications that may limit their ability to effectively maintain oral health; therefore, the use of additional oral hygiene adjuncts is helpful in improving their oral hygiene.

Careful review of the patient especially with regard to the recurrence of the intra-oral plasmacytosis is essential. Despite the good prognosis associated with intra-oral plasmacytosis, few studies have demonstrated progression into the larynx occasionally causing airway obstruction [8].

Interestingly, the patient has mutations in *SOS1* gene, which has been linked to the development of gingival fibromatosis, which is a rare hereditary disease characterized by progressive slow enlargement of interdental and attached gingiva [9]. Although not observed in this case, further investigations are needed to understand the possible correlation between the *SOS1* gene and the tendency to develop mucosal lesions, such as gingival plasmacytosis.

On reflection, microbiological sampling of the infected periodontal pockets in order to assess the microbial flora associated with the severe periodontal tissue destruction could have helped in the management of any persistent lesions in the future.

This case, in addition to previously published reports on NS, highlights the risk of severe periodontitis in young age, leading to premature loss of molar teeth, in addition to the high inflammatory systemic burden associated with periodontitis. Given the nature of the syndrome, most patients suffer from malnutrition, which is worsened by presence of intra-oral swelling and infections. Therefore, careful gingival, periodontal, and soft tissue assessments and frequent recalls in the hygiene or periodontal clinics are recommended in such patients. Long-term use of chlorhexidine toothpaste and other preparations may play a role in prevention of recurrence of intra-oral plasmacytosis. However, further studies are required to confirm this observation.

References

[1] A. W. Sugar, A. Ezsias, A. L. Bloom, and W. E. Morcos, "Orthognathic surgery in a patient with Noonan's syndrome," *Journal of Oral and Maxillofacial Surgery*, vol. 52, no. 4, pp. 421–425, 1994.

[2] I. Hwang, Y. Lee, D. Sim, and Y. Mah, "Oral features in a child with Noonan syndrome: a case report," *Journal of the Korean Academy of Pediatric Dentistry*, vol. 45, no. 1, pp. 115–122, 2018.

[3] J. Meyle and J. R. Gonzáles, "Influences of systemic diseases on periodontitis in children and adolescents," *Periodontology 2000*, vol. 2001, no. 26, pp. 92–112, 2000.

[4] M. M. Nassar, O. Afifi, and R. D. Deprez, "The prevalence of localized juvenile periodontitis in Saudi subjects," *Journal of Periodontology*, vol. 65, no. 7, pp. 698–701, 1994.

[5] M. A. Torres-Carmona, M. L. Arenas-Sordo, D. Saavedra-Ontiveros, and M. C. Sánchez-Guerrero, "Periodontal disease in Noonan's syndrome," *Boletín Médico del Hospital Infantil de México*, vol. 48, no. 4, pp. 271–274, 1991.

[6] O. Ortega Ade, O. Guaré Rde, N. S. Kawaji, and A. L. Ciamponi, "Orofacial aspects in Noonan syndrome: 2 case report," *Journal of Dentistry for Children*, vol. 75, no. 1, pp. 85–90, 2008.

[7] H. Jafarzadeh, M. Sanatkhani, and N. Mohtasham, "Oral pyogenic granuloma: a review," *Journal of Oral Science*, vol. 48, no. 4, pp. 167–175, 2006.

[8] R. Bharti and D. R. Smith, "Mucous membrane plasmacytosis: a case report and review of the literature," *Dermatology Online Journal*, vol. 9, no. 5, p. 15, 2003.

[9] K. Gawron, K. Łazarz-Bartyzel, J. Potempa, and M. Chomyszyn-Gajewska, "Gingival fibromatosis: clinical, molecular and therapeutic issues," *Orphanet Journal of Rare Diseases*, vol. 11, no. 1, p. 9, 2016.

3

Emphysema after Sinus Grafting: Importance of Patient's Information, Early Diagnosis and Management

Marc El Hage,[1] **Nathalie Nurdin**,[2] **Mark Bischof**,[1] **and Rabah Nedir**[2]

[1]*Ardentis Clinique Dentaire Lausanne, Swiss Dental Clinics Group, Voie du Chariot 6, 1003 Lausanne, Switzerland*
[2]*Ardentis Clinique Dentaire Vevey, Swiss Dental Clinics Group, Rue du Collège 3, 1800 Vevey, Switzerland*

Correspondence should be addressed to Marc El Hage; publications@ardentis.ch

Academic Editor: Daniel Torres-Lagares

The sinus elevation procedure is a safe and predictable technique that allows the placement of implants in atrophic posterior maxillae. However, some recommendations have to be followed by the patient to ensure reliable healing. It is particularly important to avoid inducing trauma in the region concerned and through the sinuses. This report describes a rare complication that occurred after the grafting of a sinus, which was attributed to a violent sneeze a few hours after the intervention. The diagnosis of emphysema following air entry was confirmed by the suddenness of the swelling and associated crepitation, and by the radiographic observation of a delimited radiolucent zone in the grafted sinus. The immediate diagnosis and subsequent management prevented further adverse events. This case report supports the need for complete comprehensive instruction of patients after oral surgery, swift diagnosis, and management of emphysema.

1. Introduction

Sinus grafting is often necessary when the residual bone height under the sinus is not sufficient to rehabilitate maxillary sites with implant-supported prostheses. Implants can be placed simultaneously with grafting or during additional surgery after allowing for a healing period of the grafted region. After each surgical procedure, patients are informed of possible complications. The parameters that may compromise the healing are also described, such as smoking, poor oral hygiene, and behaviors that may cause trauma to the surgical site.

Emphysema induced by the introduction of air through tissues during a dental procedure is not common. It can be associated with the following treatments: crown removal and subgingival curettage, tooth extraction, orthodontic miniscrew placement, class-V resin fillings, tooth preparation, and root canal treatment [1]. The use of high-speed handpieces and air/water syringes can induce this complication [2]. The entry of air through the tissues generally results in facial or cervicofacial swelling that appears immediately after the dental intervention. Crepitation may accompany clinical palpation of the swelling region due to the air entrapped in the tissues. Emphysema can extend to the neck and thorax, and lead to severe complications when a large amount of air reaches the mediastinum and the pleural space [2, 3].

This report describes a case of emphysema that occurred after the grafting of a sinus as the first step of implant treatment to rehabilitate a missing single tooth in the maxillary molar region. The complication was related to the forced entry of air via the maxillary sinus after a violent sneeze. The immediate diagnosis of emphysema and subsequent management prevented further adverse events.

2. Case Presentation

2.1. Initial Patient Assessment. In November 2013, a 28-year-old Caucasian man visited the office for the replacement of the upper right first molar, which had been lost some years previously. The patient presented good oral hygiene and was not a smoker. During the clinical examination, the patient did not report any pain in the region of the maxillary sinuses. Bitewing radiography showed an extremely low residual bone height at the site of the upper right first molar.

The upper right second molar was subject to endodontic root canal treatment (Figure 1). The general medical and dental history did not reveal any particular problem or symptoms related to maxillary sinusitis.

After discussion, the patient chose to receive an implant with a single crown rather than a fixed prosthesis of three units supported by the maxillary right second premolar and molar. Cone-beam computerized tomography (CBCT; Model CS 9300, Carestream Health, Inc., Rochester, New-York, USA) performed before surgery did not demonstrate the presence of a septum at the former position of the upper right first molar. The residual bone height was 1.0 mm (Figure 2).

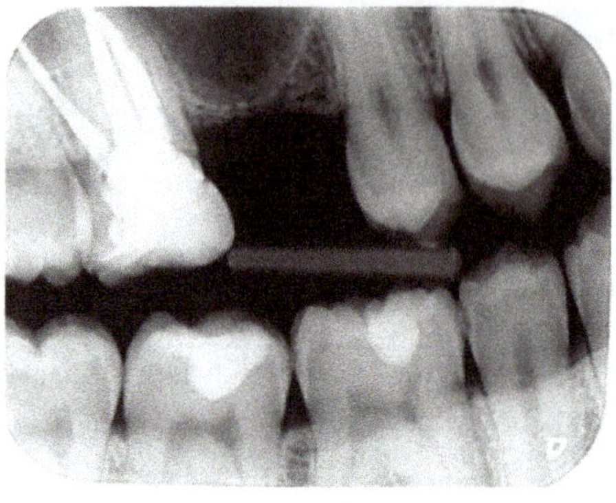

FIGURE 1: Bitewing radiography. Initial situation.

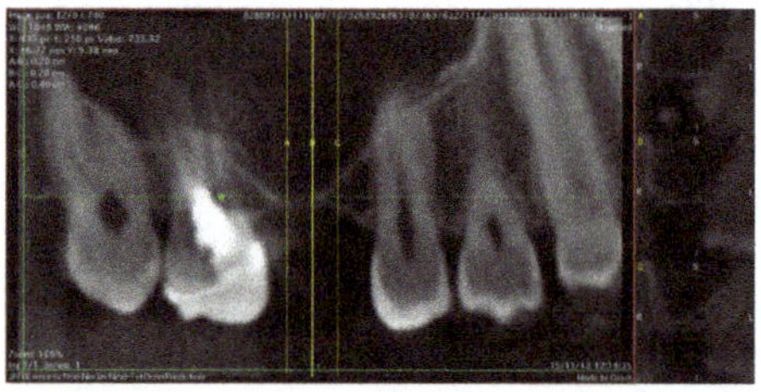

FIGURE 2: CBCT. Initial situation.

2.2. Sinus Grafting. Lateral sinus floor augmentation with a xenograft was conducted. Antibiotic prophylaxis was started within 1 hour before the surgery (Dalacin® C, Pfizer SA, Zürich, Switzerland, 300 mg) and was administered for 5 days (300 mg, 3 times per day). Local anaesthetic (Ubistesin™, 3 M ESPE AG, Germany) was infiltrated at the vestibular and palatal areas of the sites of the upper right second premolar to the second molar. A mucoperiosteal access flap was created with a crestal incision and two vertical incisions in order to expose the lateral wall of the maxillary sinus. A bony lateral window was obtained with a piezoelectric device. To decrease the risk of perforation, the Schneiderian membrane was carefully elevated using flat-head ultrasonic inserts. After its complete elevation, the membrane was reflected to obtain a space large enough for the grafting material. No perforation of the membrane was clinically observable immediately after its elevation. The integrity of the membrane was controlled by using the Valsalva maneuver. A mixture of deproteinized bovine bone material (Bio-Oss®, Geistlich AG, Wolhusen, Switzerland) and the patient's blood collected at the surgical site were then inserted. The lateral window was covered with two layers of a resorbable porcine collagen membrane (Bio-Gide®, Geistlich Pharma AG, Switzerland). The flap was closed without tension using nonresorbable polyamide sutures (Suturamid® 4.0, B. Braun Aesculap, Sempach, Switzerland). Postoperative examination was carried out with a panoramic radiograph (Figure 3), which validated the insertion of the graft in the space created under the nonperforated membrane. Standard postoperative recommendations were made, including not blowing the nose during the healing period and avoiding traumatic behaviors that may have deleterious effects on the treated region.

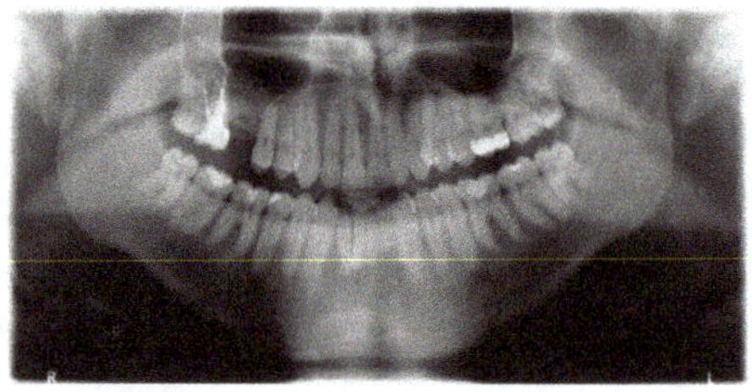

FIGURE 3: Panoramic radiograph taken immediately after sinus grafting.

One day after surgery, the patient came to the clinic and requested an examination. A few hours after the procedure, he had sneezed violently while keeping his mouth closed. He had immediately felt the swelling of the genian region with a simultaneous sound of cracking. The clinical examination confirmed unilateral tumefaction of the right genian region accompanied with crepitation on palpation (Figure 4). CBCT was performed in order to check the integrity of the Schneiderian membrane and the stability of the grafting material under the sinus, without spreading inside the sinus. However, it did reveal a delimited radiolucent zone inside the grafted region (Figure 5). The diagnosis of emphysema by air entry was thus made. Treatment with metronidazole (Flagyl® 500 mg, Sanofi-Aventis SA, Vernier, Switzerland, 500 mg, 3 times per day for 7 days) was then introduced in addition to the existing antibiotic medication. Examinations were made two and ten days afterwards (at suture removal). The grafted site healed completely without any symptoms of further complications.

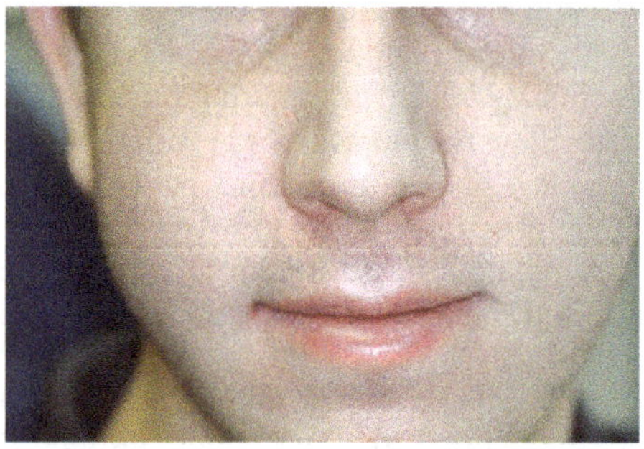

FIGURE 4: Photograph taken one day after the sinus grafting showing the unilateral tumefaction in the right genian region.

2.3. Implant Placement. Ten months after sinus grafting, the implant was placed. First, preoperative panoramic radiography

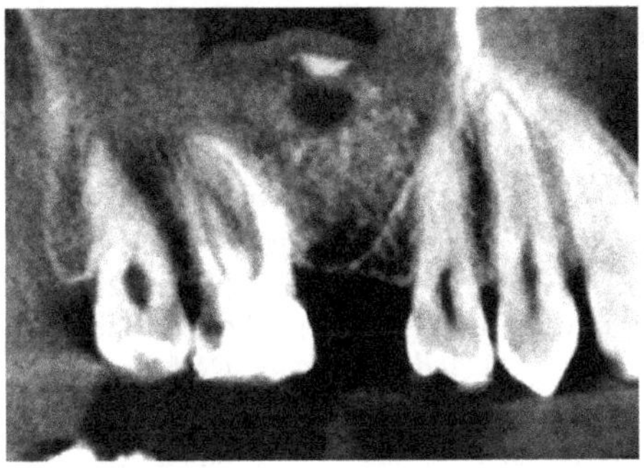

FIGURE 5: CBCT obtained one day after the sinus grafting. A delimited radiolucent zone can be observed in the grafted region.

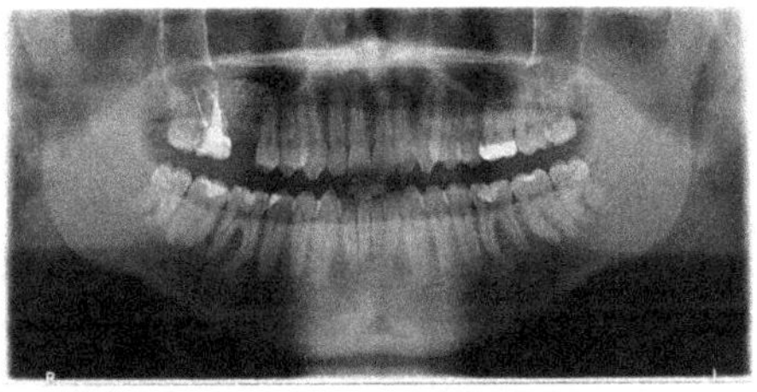

FIGURE 6: Panoramic radiograph. Preoperative situation before implant placement.

was performed to examine the graft (Figure 6). A radiographic bone height of 14 mm was measured at the site to be implanted.

The implant bed was prepared according to the manufacturer's instructions, followed by the insertion of a Standard Plus Regular Neck implant with a SLActive® surface (diameter: 4.1 mm, length: 10 mm; Straumann AG, Basel, Switzerland). A periapical radiograph was obtained immediately after implant placement (Figure 7). The sutures were removed after 10 days. Healing was uneventful.

2.4. Prosthetic Restauration and Follow-Up. Ten weeks after surgery, the abutment was tightened with a torque of 15 Ncm. A ceramo-metal crown was cemented and functionally loaded. The clinical and radiographic examination after one year showed a stable situation and the implant in function (Figure 8).

3. Discussion

In oral implantology, the standard clinical practice used to treat the presented case required a sinus augmentation procedure with graft insertion and delayed implant placement [4]. With such an atrophic site, a lateral approach with the use of grafting material and delayed implant placement was recommended [5]. The main intraoperative concerns with the lateral window approach are perforation of the Schneiderian membrane, graft migration, haemorrhagic accident, and postoperative acute or chronic sinus infection, bleeding, wound dehiscence, exposure of the barrier membrane, and graft loss [6, 7].

Prevalence of damages to the Schneiderian membrane during a sinus elevation and grafting was estimated about 10 to 50%. Most damages are 1- to 3-mm tears and regenerate spontaneously. When tears and lacerations are detected, the sinus

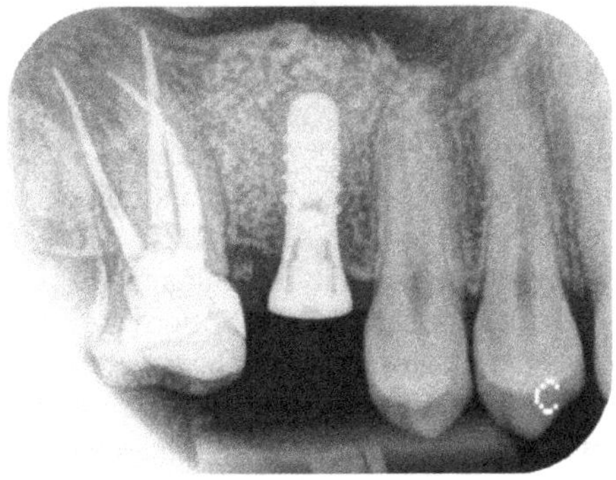

FIGURE 7: Periapical radiograph obtained immediately after implant placement.

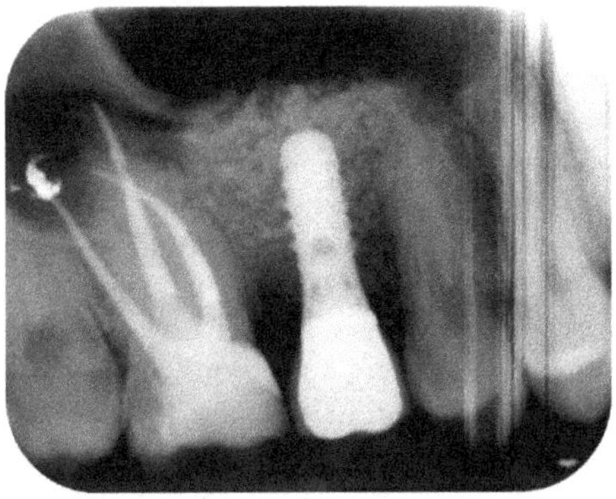

FIGURE 8: Periapical radiograph obtained one year after implant placement.

membrane can be protected with biological resorbable membranes [7–9]. Such complications may compromise the outcomes of the inserted graft by resulting contamination and infection. The sinus graft infection is considered a major complication requiring urgent treatment, based on the risk of infection which could spread throughout the graft and sinus cavity or the adjacent anatomical structures. It is rare between 1 and 4% [8] and occurred more frequently in patients with a history of sinusitis [10]. Various treatments were proposed such as systemic antibiotics, endoscopy of the sinus, surgical exploration, rinsing, and/or curettage of the affected maxillary sinuses to totally remove inserted biomaterials and inflammatory tissue [11].

In the present article, no perforation of the membrane was clinically observable immediately after its elevation. The integrity of the membrane was controlled by using the Valsalva maneuver.

Introduction of air and consequent emphysema are known and described in the literature. Emphysema is considered an early adverse event, and this acute complication needs emergency treatment [1]. This report presents a rare and minor case of emphysema after sinus grafting due to a strong sneeze with a closed mouth. The positive pressure created by the sneeze led to the spread of air through the soft tissues and consequent facial swelling. Keeping the mouth closed increased the internal antral pressure. The medical history of the patient was noncontributory, without sinus-related problems. The CBCT taken one-day later has not shown opacity of the sinus and thickening of the Schneiderian membrane, usually observable when the sinus is affected. No oroantral communication was detectable. Therefore, the risk of graft infection was discarded. Emphysema was then quickly diagnosed, which was confirmed by the presence of a delimited radiolucent zone in the grafted region and the crepitation on palpation. The swelling was localized. Therefore, treatment covering specifically anaerobic microorganisms in combination with the initial antibiotic prescription was administered. This treatment and close monitoring of the patient were sufficient to resolve the complication. The event did not compromise the placement of the implant. The implant procedure and management of its complication have led to a successful outcome over one year of follow-up.

Emphysema is more common after dental procedures involving the maxilla or posterior region than after those involving the mandible or anterior region [1]. In the majority of cases of subcutaneous emphysema, a diffuse swelling is observable. A conservative management is carried out, and an antibiotic therapy is indicated in order to prevent soft tissue abscessation. Spontaneous resolution is then expected; the emphysema is likely to decrease within 4 to 7 days [12].

The complete history of the patient is of primary importance to the diagnosis. A rapid swelling may be also *inter alia* the sign of allergic reaction. Clinical palpation is the first action required to evaluate the area concerned. Crepitation and/or an air bubble consistency under finger pressure is often felt by the patient. Symptoms of fever and nausea may indicate infection. A history of periodontal disease may be a contributory factor for further severe complications [13]. The use of CBCT is needed to detect and evaluate the spread of air. Rapid diagnosis and strict follow-up of the patient avoid further potentially fatal complications such as venous air embolism and/or soft tissue infections [2, 3, 14, 15].

Most cases of emphysema caused by intrusion of air after dental surgery are iatrogenic, for example, due to the use of rotary surgical tools or air syringes during the procedure [16]. Cases due to the postoperative behavior of the patient following maxillary sinus floor grafting are rare. Sakakibara et al., Farina et al., and Sevilla Heras et al. described sinus elevation and sudden facial swelling that appeared after the patients blew their nose roughly or sneezed [17–19]. These cases were not severe, although the swelling extended to the peri-orbital and orbital regions [18, 19].

4. Conclusions

Subcutaneous emphysema resulting from the entry of air can occur as a complication of a sinus grafting procedure in an atrophic posterior maxilla. The causes for such a complication include sneezing while the mouth closed. This case report supports the need to provide complete comprehensive instructions to patients after oral surgery and more specifically sinus grafting. It also indicates the importance of an immediate diagnosis. The swift management of emphysema is vital to avoid potentially serious adverse events. It should include the use of CT to evaluate the location and importance of air-filled spaces.

References

[1] C. H. Jeong, S. Yoon, S. W. Chung, J. Y. Kim, K. H. Park, and J. K. Huh, "Subcutaneous emphysema related to dental procedures," *Journal of the Korean Association of Oral and Maxillofacial Surgeons*, vol. 44, no. 5, pp. 212–219, 2018.

[2] W. S. McKenzie and M. Rosenberg, "Iatrogenic subcutaneous emphysema of dental and surgical origin: a literature review," *Journal of Oral and Maxillofacial Surgery*, vol. 67, no. 6, pp. 1265–1268, 2009.

[3] G. Greenstein, J. Cavallaro, G. Romanos, and D. Tarnow, "Clinical recommendations for avoiding and managing surgical complications associated with implant dentistry: a review," *Journal of Periodontology*, vol. 79, no. 8, pp. 1317–1329, 2008.

[4] O. T. Jensen, L. B. Shulman, M. S. Block, and V. J. Lacono, "Report of the sinus consensus conference of 1996," *International Journal of Oral and Maxillofacial Implants*, vol. 13, Supplement, pp. 11–32, 1998.

[5] R. Nedir, N. Nurdin, P. Khoury, M. el Hage, S. Abi Najm, and M. Bischof, "Paradigm shift in the management of the atrophic posterior maxilla," *Case Reports in Dentistry*, vol. 2014, Article ID 486949, 7 pages, 2014.

[6] P. Boffano and T. Forouzanfar, "Current concepts on complications associated with sinus augmentation procedures," *Journal of Craniofacial Surgery*, vol. 25, no. 2, pp. e210–e212, 2014.

[7] D. Schwartz-Arad, R. Herzberg, and E. Dolev, "The prevalence of surgical complications of the sinus graft procedure and their impact on implant survival," *Journal of Periodontology*, vol. 75, no. 4, pp. 511–516, 2004.

[8] J. C. Moreno Vazquez, A. S. Gonzalez de Rivera, H. S. Gil, and R. S. Mifsut, "Complication rate in 200 consecutive sinus lift procedures: guidelines for prevention and treatment," *Journal of Oral and Maxillofacial Surgery*, vol. 72, no. 5, pp. 892–901, 2014.

[9] L. Schwarz, V. Schiebel, M. Hof, C. Ulm, G. Watzek, and B. Pommer, "Risk factors of membrane perforation and postoperative complications in sinus floor elevation surgery: review of 407 augmentation procedures," *Journal of Oral and Maxillofacial Surgery*, vol. 73, no. 7, pp. 1275–1282, 2015.

[10] M. Chiapasco, G. Felisati, M. Zaniboni, C. Pipolo, R. Borloni, and P. Lozza, "The treatment of sinusitis following maxillary sinus grafting with the association of functional endoscopic sinus surgery (FESS) and an intra-oral approach," *Clinical Oral Implants Research*, vol. 24, no. 6, pp. 623–629, 2013.

[11] A. Scarano, A. Cholakis, and A. Piattelli, "Histologic evaluation of sinus grafting materials after peri-implantitis-induced failure: a case series," *The International Journal of Oral & Maxillofacial Implants*, vol. 32, no. 2, pp. e36–e75, 2017.

[12] L. R. Eversole, *Clinical Outline of Oral Pathology: Diagnosis and Treatment. Third Edition*, BC Decker Inc., Hamilton, Ontario, USA, 2002.

[13] S.-W. Lee, Y.-H. Huh, and M.-S. Cha, "Iatrogenic subcutaneous cervicofacial emphysema with pneumomediastinum after class V restoration," *Journal of the Korean Association of Oral and Maxillofacial Surgeons*, vol. 43, no. 1, pp. 49–52, 2017.

[14] J. M. Davies and L. A. Campbell, "Fatal air embolism during dental implant surgery: a report of three cases," *Canadian Journal of Anaesthesia*, vol. 37, no. 1, p. 112, 1990.

[15] J. Frühauf, R. Weinke, U. Pilger, H. Kerl, and R. R. Müllegger, "Soft tissue cervicofacial emphysema after dental treatment:

report of 2 cases with emphasis on the differential diagnosis of angioedema," *Archives of Dermatology*, vol. 141, no. 11, pp. 1437–1440, 2005.

[16] S. N. Heyman and I. Babayof, "Emphysematous complications in dentistry, 1960-1993: an illustrative case and review of the literature," *Quintessence International*, vol. 26, no. 8, pp. 535–543, 1995.

[17] A. Sakakibara, H. Suzuki, A. Yamashita et al., "Facial emphysema after sinus lift," *Journal of Surgical Case Reports*, vol. 2015, no. 6, article rjv067, 2015.

[18] R. Farina, A. Zaetta, L. Minenna, and L. Trombelli, "Orbital and periorbital emphysema following maxillary sinus floor elevation: a case report and literature review," *Journal of Oral and Maxillofacial Surgery*, vol. 74, no. 11, pp. 2192.e1–2192.e7, 2016.

[19] M. Sevilla Heras, L. Martorell Calatayud, R. Zaragozí Alonso, and M. Peñarrocha Diago, "Subcutaneous emphysema after a direct sinus lift: a case report," *Journal of Oral Science & Rehabilitation*, vol. 5, no. 2, pp. 8–13, 2019.

4

Prevention of Periodontal Pocket Formation after Mandibular Third Molar Extraction using Dentin Autologous Graft: A Split Mouth Case Report

Alberto De Biase, Giulia Mazzucchi, Dario Di Nardo, Marco Lollobrigida, Giorgio Serafini, and Luca Testarelli

Department of Oral and Maxillo-Facial Sciences, Sapienza University of Rome, Italy

Correspondence should be addressed to Dario Di Nardo; dario.dinardo@uniroma1.it

Academic Editor: Alberto C. B. Delbem

Surgical extraction of the third molar can often result in the development of a periodontal pocket distal to the second molar that could delay the healing, and the socket could be colonized by bacteria and lead to secondary abscesses, or it may cause mobility or hypersensitivity. The aim of this case report is to assess the efficacy of a dentin autograft in the prevention of periodontal dehiscences after the surgical extraction of the third molar, obtained by the immediate grinding of the extracted tooth. A healthy 18-year-old male patient underwent surgery of both impacted mandibular molars: right postextractive socket was filled with grinded dentin; then, the left one was filled with fibrin sponge. The patient was followed up for six months, and clinical and radiographic assessment were performed: measurements of plaque index (PI), bleeding on probing (BOP), gingival index (GI), clinical attachment level (CAL), and probing pocket depth (PPD) were done before surgery and repeated at 90 and 180 days after the extractions. Measurements made at six months after the surgery revealed that the grafted site was characterized by a minor depth of the pocket if compared with the nongrafted site, with no clinical/radiographic signs of complications.

1. Introduction

Surgical extraction of the third molar can often result in the development of a periodontal pocket distal to the second molar: this condition could delay the healing and the socket could be colonized by bacteria and lead to secondary abscesses or it may cause mobility, hypersensitivity, or the formation of a periodontal pocket. The formation of a dehiscence can be due to other factors like the adopted surgical technique (extractive procedures and suture), postoperative care of the wound, and occurrence of complications during and after the procedures (iatrogenic errors, infection, retraction, resorption or collapse of the flap, and foreign body reaction) [1–6].

The socket preservation technique is considered an effective procedure to preserve the alveolar bone from the postextractive physiological resorption [7, 8]. However, as like other surgical intervention, it can be affected by the same complications that could lead to a failure of the graft (exposition of the graft, infection, resorption, loss of grafted material, and adverse reaction to the grafted materials) [9]. Different types of grafts can be used for the scope: synthetic grafts, xenografts (from other species), allografts (from human donors), and autografts (from the patient itself). Each type of graft is characterized by different morbidity, risk of diseases transmission, grade of resorption, osteoinductivity, and osteogenicity. However, actually, only the autologous bone graft is characterized by nonimmunogenic and nonpathogenic properties, with osteoinductive, osteoconductive, and osteogenic properties, and it is widely considered the gold standard [10–12].

Socket preservation is usually performed with commercial products (e.g., NanoBone®, Artoss GmbH, Rostock, Germany; Geistlich Bio-Oss®, Geistlich Pharma AG, Wolhusen, Switzerland; and Laddec®, Biohorizons, Birmingham, AL, USA) that could be expensive, and for so, they are preferred to be used only when the positioning of an implant is expected or when aesthetic purposes are requested: autogenous tooth graft is considered to be an osteoconductive material, characterized by a high bone formation activity and biocompatibility [9, 13–15].

Since commercial alloplasts, allografts, and xenografts are considered safe for human purposes and their outcomes are mostly successful, the possibility of retrieving an effective and ready-to-use grafting material directly from a tooth that is going to be extracted could result advantageous for the patient and for the clinician in terms of saving time and reducing costs, with the same outcome of other products. The use of autologous dentin is obviously cheaper than other grafts and it is fully compatible with the patient tissues. Furthermore, it is immediately available and its amount usually corresponds exactly to the amount of graft needed to fill up the postextractive socket [16–18].

The aim of this case report is to assess the efficacy of a dentin autograft in the prevention of periodontal dehiscences after the surgical extraction of the third molar, obtained by the immediate grinding of the extracted tooth.

2. Case Presentation

An asymptomatic, generally and periodontally healthy 18-year-old male, nonsmoker and nonalcohol addicted patient needing the extraction of both mandibular third molars was enrolled for the case. A written informed consent was obtained prior to start the procedure. All the procedures were conducted according to the declaration of Helsinki, and the protocol was approved by the Policlinico Umberto I of Rome Ethical Committee (n. 5456/2019).

Prior to extractions, periapical radiographs of the interested third molars were taken, and the following periodontal indexes were recorded by a calibrated and blinded operator (G.S), at mesiobuccal, midbuccal, distobuccal, distolingual, midlingual, and mesiolingual sites of the bilateral mandibular second molars: plaque index (PI), bleeding on probing (BOP), gingival index (GI), clinical attachment level (CAL), and probing pocket depth (PPD) were recorded by the use of a PCP-15-UNC probe (Hu-Friedy, Leimen, Germany) (Table 1) [19, 20]. The registration of all those above-mentioned periodontal indexes was considered mandatory due to avoid invalid results caused by the shrinkage of the soft tissues during the healing. Measurements were repeated at 90 and 180 days after surgery by the same operator, and periapical radiographs were taken at every follow-up appointment. Since Rinn centrator was unable to reach a so posterior area, a rigid support for articulation paper was adopted to stabilize the radiographic film. The patient was instructed to keep the rigid support in contact and as much as possible parallel to the occlusal surface, and the radiograph was taken only after the operator's supervision due to standardizing the exam. To keep the irradiation as low as reasonably achievable (ALARA), the authors decided to not repeat the radiographic exam if small imperfections were present (Figures 1 and 2).

A 60 second 0.2% chlorexidine mouth rinse was administered before surgical procedures. Surgical interventions were

Table 1: Periodontal measurements of the second molar (mm), at different follow-up intervals.

Periodontal indexes		4.7 T1	4.7 T90	4.7 T180	3.7 T1	3.7 T90	3.7 T180
GI		1	1	0	0	0	1
PI	Buccal	1	0	0	2	1	1
	Lingual	2	2	2	2	2	2
PPD	Mesiobuccal	1	1	1	1	1	1
	Midbuccal	2	1	1	1	1	1
	Distobuccal	**4**	2	2	3	2	2
	Middistal	**4**	**4**	3	3	**4**	**4**
	Distolingual	**4**	3	2	3	**4**	**4**
	Midlingual	3	2	2	2	2	2
	Mesiolingual	3	3	2	3	2	2
BOP	Mesiobuccal	—	—	—	—	—	—
	Midbuccal	—	—	—	—	—	—
	Distobuccal	—	—	—	—	—	—
	Middistal	—	—	—	+	+	+
	Distolingual	+	+	—	—	—	+
	Midlingual	+	+	—	—	—	—
	Mesiolingual	+	+	—	—	—	—
CAL	Mesiobuccal	1	1	1	1	1	1
	Midbuccal	2	1	1	1	1	1
	Distobuccal	**4**	2	2	3	2	2
	Middistal	**4**	**4**	3	3	**4**	**4**
	Distolingual	**4**	3	2	3	**4**	**4**
	Midlingual	3	2	2	2	2	2
	Mesiolingual	3	3	2	3	2	2

all performed by the same skilled clinician (M.L). A full-thickness flap [21] was performed by the use of a Bard-Parker 15c scalpel, and the periostium was elevated by the use of a Molt elevator. Odontotomy was performed by the use of a multiblade cutter in tungsten carbide and mobilized by levers of different thickness, taking in considerations common recommendations to minimize the risk of intraoperational accidents [22].

Immediately after the extraction (Figure 1), the right molar's fragments were grinded for 3 seconds (300-1200 μm) by the use of the Smart Dentin Grinder™ (Kometa-Bio, Fort Lee, NJ, USA) and then immersed into a 0.5 M NaOH and 20% ethanol solution for 10 minutes, in order to dissolve all the organic remains from the tubules. The particulate was first dried with a sterile gauze, then rinsed two times (3 minutes each) with phosphate-buffered saline solution to remove all the NaOH and the ethanol [16, 23]. The right postextractive socket (test site) was filled with the grinded dentin; then, the left one (control site) was filled with a fibrin sponge.

Surgical flaps were stabilized with a 4.0 nylon suture (Ethilon, Johnson & Johnson, New Brunswick, NJ, USA), and both wounds were allowed to heal for first intention.

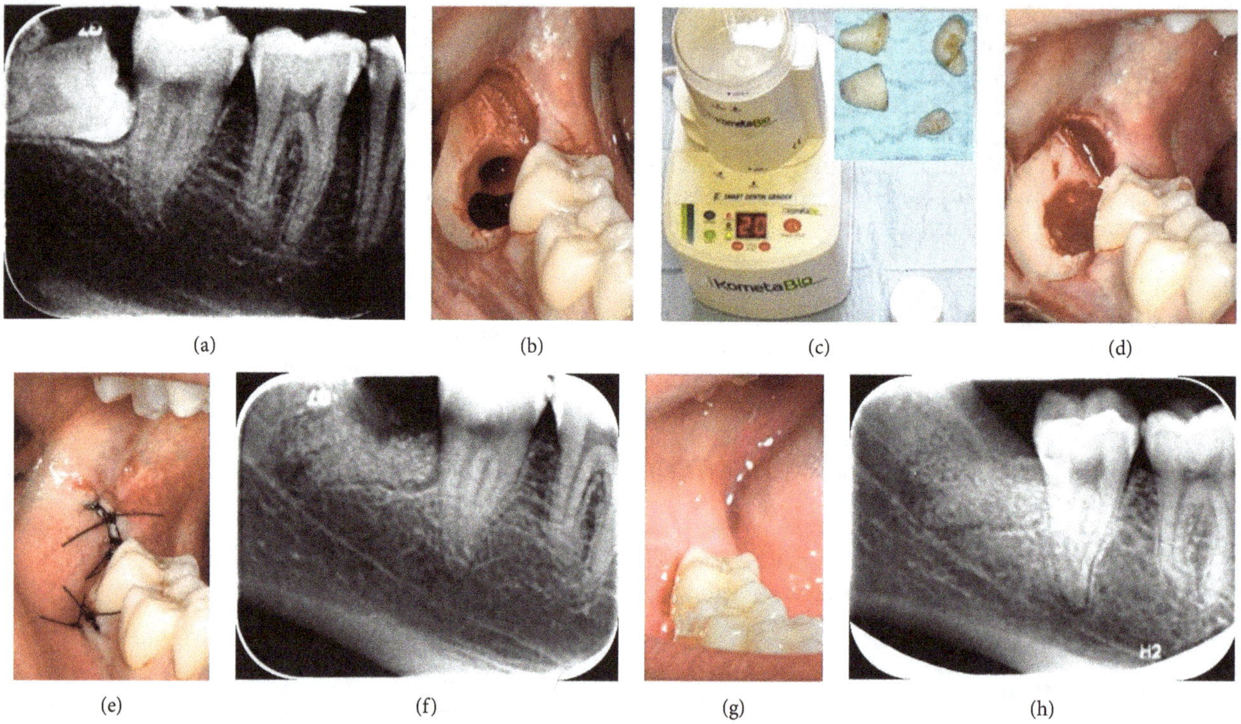

Figure 1: Presurgical periapical radiograph of the right third molar (test site) (a). Fresh post-extractive socket (b). The Smart Dentin Grinder™ (c) used for the test and the fragments of the tooth before being grinded (square). The dentin particulate filling the socket (d). The sutured wound (e). Periapical radiograph of the grafted socket taken after 15 days from the surgery (f). Soft (g) and hard (h) tissues healing at 180 days after surgery.

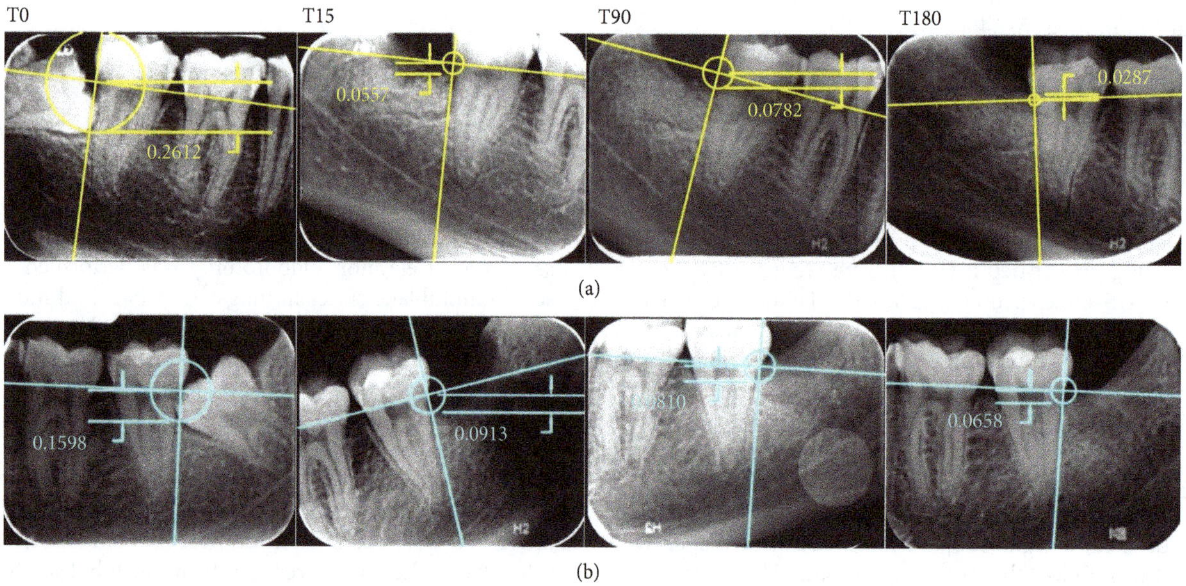

Figure 2: Periapical radiographs of the grafted site (a) and the control site (b) before surgery (T0) and after 15, 90, and 180 days. Since the positioning of the film in a so posterior area resulted difficult, a rigid support held by the patient was adopted instead of the Rinn centrator. Adjustments to tilted images were performed by the same software used for the measurements.

The patient was instructed to properly clean wounds with a soft surgical tooth brush and to not rinse or spit for the following 48 hours, to not practice sport for two weeks, and to avoid smoke or alcohol until suture removal.

Antibiotics were administered for 6 days (1 tablet of amoxicillin 875 mg + clavulanic acid 125 mg every 12 hours), and chlorhexidine digluconate 0.20% rinses were performed twice a day for two weeks.

Table 2: Radiographic measurements from CEJ to bone peak (mm) at different follow-up intervals.

Test site (right)				Control site (left)			
Day 0	Day 15	Day 90	Day 180	Day 0	Day 15	Day 90	Day 180
2.612	0.557	0.782	0.287	1.598	0.913	0.81	0.658

Analgesic drugs were administered orally after the intervention (nimesulide 100 mg) and prescribed to assume in case of pain every 10 hours.

Sutures were removed after 14 days, and periapical radiographs were taken in order to assess the conditions of the postextractive sockets. At 90 and 180 days, new periapical radiographs were taken, and periodontal parameters were reevaluated for both sites. A period of 180 days of follow-up was chosen since a period of 20-21 weeks is considered sufficient to obtain evidences about the status of the regenerated bone, as showed in many histological randomized controlled trials [24–27].

At the day of surgery, the distal pocket of the second molar measured 4 mm for both sites. After 3 months from the extraction, a reduction of pocket depth at the test site of 1 mm was observed, while the control test still measured 4 mm: no changes to these measurements were recorded after 6 months from the surgery (Table 1).

Differences between the postextractive sockets and changes occurred during the follow-up period were measured by the software AutoCAD 2017 (Autodesk, San Rafael, CA, USA) on periapical radiographs taken at different times and then validated by Invivo software (Anatomage Inc., San Jose, CA, USA) and 3D Endo Software (Dentsply Sirona, Charlotte, NC, USA) by a blinded operator (G.M). Measurements were performed from the CEJ to the bone peak distal to the second molar, on a line perpendicular to the one passing through the mesial and distal projection of the CEJ (Figure 2). Results of the measurements are reported in Table 2.

3. Discussion

Dental elements that are adjacent to an impacted or semi-impacted tooth are usually more predisposed to periodontal defects [28]. Obviously, it is not mandatory to perform socket preservation for every extracted third molar; however, it can be useful in those cases, like surgical extractions, where a great amount of bone can be lost, and this could lead to a periodontal defect which could lead to mobility or hypersensitivity of the second molar [29]. The amount of bone that could be retrieved during the osteotomy could be not enough for the dimension of the dehiscence: for so, it would be necessary additional bone or graft material to completely fill the postextractive socket. Other risk factors associated with the development of periodontal pocket distal to the second molar are considered the design of the flap, a preexistent bone defect, the age of the patient, and the distance between the adjacent teeth [30, 31].

The development of a periodontal defect distal to the second molar is not predictable, and it is considered a complication difficult to treat and that will not heal spontaneously. There is consensus that the best way to prevent distal defects is the early extraction of third molars [32–35], but when this condition is not applicable, the risk of bone loss should be always taken in consideration. Richardson and Dodson revealed that after 2 years from the extraction of impacted third molars, the 43.3% of the patients showed a PPD of ~7 mm [29].

Autologous dentin graft was investigated by Kim et al. by scanning electron microscopy, X-ray diffraction analysis, and calcium/phosphate dissolution test: results were compared with human bone and other heterologous, homologous, and allopastic grafting materials, revealing that the autologous dentin graft was the most similar to the human bone for structure and physico-chemical characteristics [36].

A study performed by the use of SEM-energy dispersive X-ray (SEM-EDX) measured the percentages of calcium ($23.42 \pm 0.34\%$) and phosphate ($9.51 \pm 0.11\%$) in the dentin of human extracted teeth and revealed a similarity with the bone [37]. Calvo-Guirado et al., in a study on beagle dogs, hystologically demonstrated the formation of new well-organized bone, with multiple osteons at 90 days after dentin autograft. Hystomorphometry revealed the presence of higher percentages of mature bone and less percentages of immature bone in the sites grafted with particulated dentin when compared with no-grafted sites at 90 days [23].

Calvo-Guirado et al. suggested the use of sound retained or redundant roots to preserve postextractive alveolar sockets: in an animal model, an effective osteointegration of dental implants was demonstrated histologically, with resorption of the grafted dental tissues and the formation of new vascularized bone [38].

Another advantage of the grinded tooth is that the volume of the particulate results to be 2-3 times greater than the volume of the entire tooth: furthermore, the presence of spaces between the particles and the presence of micro- and macropores could allow the infiltration of blood vessels and osteogenic cells [17].

In literature, it has been reported that human dental tissues contain different growth factors similar to the bone: IGF-II, BMP-2, and TGF-b are present in the dentin; TGF-b, IGF-1, and PDGF-BB are present in cementoblasts. It has been reported that such growth factors and type I collagen can be found also in the periodontal ligament, in association with VEGF and basic fibroblast growth factors. [39, 40] However, the use of NaOH and ethanol for the removal of the organic materials could incapacitate the action of such growth factors, and eventually, stem cells present in the pulpal tissues [17].

Results from this case report showed an enhanced reduction of bone loss in the grafted site if compared with the control one: when measuring the distance between the CEJ and the bone peak, the control site depth obtained a reduction of 0.94 mm instead of 2.32 mm of the grafted site. Clinical probing depth resulted to reduce of 1 mm in the grafted site

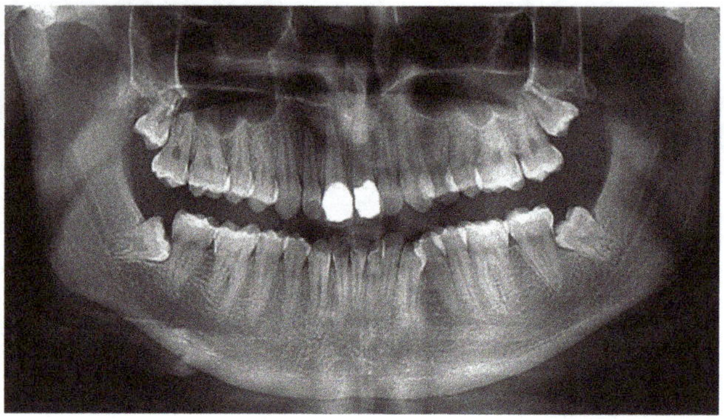

(a)

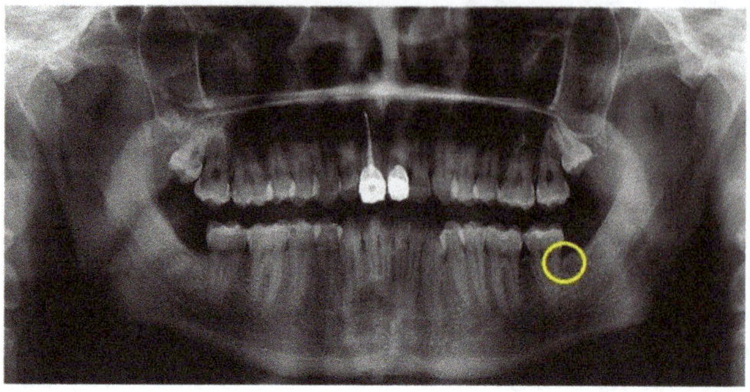

(b)

FIGURE 3: Panoramic radiographs of the patient before surgery (a) and after 6 months: left pocket (yellow circle) still resulted to be deeper than the grafted one (b). No signs of adverse reaction or bone resorption were present at the grafted site.

while no changes were recorded in the control site from the day of the surgery. Results can be explained by the presence of grafting material which avoided the apical migration of the soft tissues [14]. For what concerns the control site, it was filled with fibrin sponge, that is, a rapid resorbable material, which is unable to avoid soft tissue invasion of the post-extractive socket. Since the patient was informed on the possible complications of the surgical interventions and the possible adverse reaction or failure of the graft (swelling, pain, hemorrhage, dysfagia, alveolitis, displacement, and necessity of reintervention due to removing the graft), he was expected to experience any kind of adverse reactions, but he reported no discomfort even after 6 months from the surgery as like no hypersensitivity or pain at the sites of intervention. No hypersensitivity or mobility of the second molar was evidenced clinically. Furthermore, similarly to other hydroxyapatite grafting materials [41], no adverse reactions or delays in the healing were reported: this can suggest that the dentine autograft is safe, and it can be used effectively as bone substitute (Figure 3). Mazor et al. [42], in a study on grafts performed with autologous tooth particles, obtained with the Smart Dentin Grinder, revealed hystologically, that after three months, vital bone was in direct contact with the tooth particles, without evidence of inflammatory infiltrate. Since results of this case report are in line with other recent studies [16, 17, 23, 36–38, 43, 44], it can be concluded that the dentin autologous graft is a safe mean to preserve alveolar ridge, and its availability and low costs make it an affordable procedure if compared with the more expensive commercial materials. However, further studies are required, and the effectiveness of autologous dentine graft as a substrate for implant placement is still to be assessed.

Acknowledgments

The authors would like to thank KometaBio, Inc., Fort Lee, NJ, USA, for the Smart Dentin Grinder device.

References

[1] C. T. Lee, L. Hum, and Y. W. Chen, "The effect of regenerative periodontal therapy in preventing periodontal defects after the extraction of third molars: a systematic review and meta-analysis," *The Journal of the American Dental Association*, vol. 147, no. 9, pp. 709–719.e4, 2016.

[2] C. E. Nemcovsky, H. Libfeld, and Y. Zubery, "Effect of non-erupted 3rd molars on distal roots and supporting structures of approximal teeth. A radiographic survey of 202 cases," *Journal of Clinical Periodontology*, vol. 23, no. 9, pp. 810–815, 1996.

[3] V. Candotto, L. Oberti, F. Gabrione, A. Scarano, D. Rossi, and M. Romano, "Complication in third molar extractions," *Journal of Biological Regulators and Homeostatic Agents*, vol. 33, 3 Supplement 1, pp. 169–172, 2019.

[4] M. Coleman, A. McCormick, and D. M. Laskin, "The incidence of periodontal defects distal to the maxillary second molar after impacted third molar extraction," *Journal of Oral and Maxillofacial Surgery*, vol. 69, no. 2, pp. 319–321, 2011.

[5] G. Sammartino, M. Tia, T. Bucci, and H. L. Wang, "Prevention of mandibular third molar extraction-associated periodontal defects: a comparative study," *Journal of Periodontology*, vol. 80, no. 3, pp. 389–396, 2009.

[6] J. Montero and G. Mazzaglia, "Effect of removing an impacted mandibular third molar on the periodontal status of the mandibular second molar," *Journal of Oral and Maxillofacial Surgery*, vol. 69, no. 11, pp. 2691–2697, 2011.

[7] K. S. Hassan, H. F. Marei, and A. S. Alagl, "Does grafting of third molar extraction sockets enhance periodontal measures in 30- to 35-year-old patients?," *Journal of Oral and Maxillofacial Surgery*, vol. 70, no. 4, pp. 757–764, 2012.

[8] D. De Santis, S. Sinigaglia, P. Pancera et al., "An overview of socket preservation," *Journal of Biological Regulators and Homeostatic Agents*, vol. 33, Supplement 1, pp. 55–59, 2019.

[9] P. Gual-Vaques, C. Polis-Yanes, A. Estrugo-Devesa, R. Ayuso-Montero, A. Mari-Roig, and J. Lopez-Lopez, "Autogenous teeth used for bone grafting: a systematic review," *Medicina Oral, Patología Oral y Cirugía Bucal*, vol. 23, no. 1, pp. e112–e119, 2017.

[10] J. T. Mellonig, "Autogenous and allogeneic bone grafts in periodontal therapy," *Critical Reviews in Oral Biology and Medicine*, vol. 3, no. 4, pp. 333–352, 2016.

[11] G. Serafini, M. Lollobrigida, L. Fortunato et al., "Postextractive alveolar ridge preservation using L-PRF: clinical and

histological evaluation," *Case Reports in Dentistry*, vol. 2020, Article ID 5073519, 6 pages, 2020.

[12] G. Chiriac, M. Herten, F. Schwarz, D. Rothamel, and J. Becker, "Autogenous bone chips: influence of a new piezoelectric device (Piezosurgery) on chip morphology, cell viability and differentiation," *Journal of Clinical Periodontology*, vol. 32, no. 9, pp. 994–999, 2005.

[13] F. Al Yafi, B. Alchawaf, and K. Nelson, "What is the optimum for alveolar ridge preservation?," *Dental Clinics of North America*, vol. 63, no. 3, pp. 399–418, 2019.

[14] G. Mazzucchi, M. Lollobrigida, D. Laurito et al., "Microbiological and FE-SEM assessment of d-PTFE membrane exposed to oral environment after alveolar socket preservation managed with granular nc-HA," *The Journal of Contemporary Dental Practice*, vol. 21, no. 4, pp. 404–409, 2020.

[15] S. Das, R. Jhingran, V. K. Bains, R. Madan, R. Srivastava, and I. Rizvi, "Socket preservation by beta-tri-calcium phosphate with collagen compared to platelet-rich fibrin: a clinico-radiographic study," *Eur J Dent.*, vol. 10, no. 2, pp. 264–276, 2016.

[16] J. L. Calvo-Guirado, P. Cegarra Del Pino, L. Sapoznikov, R. A. Delgado Ruiz, M. Fernández-Domínguez, and S. A. Gehrke, "A new procedure for processing extracted teeth for immediate grafting in post-extraction sockets. An experimental study in American Fox Hound dogs," *Annals of Anatomy*, vol. 217, pp. 14–23, 2018.

[17] T. Nampo, J. Watahiki, A. Enomoto et al., "A new method for alveolar bone repair using extracted teeth for the graft material," *Journal of Periodontology*, vol. 81, no. 9, pp. 1264–1272, 2010.

[18] S. T. Kao and D. D. Scott, "A review of bone substitutes," *Oral and Maxillofacial Surgery Clinics of North America*, vol. 19, no. 4, pp. 513–521, 2007.

[19] F. Graziani, S. Gennai, M. Petrini, L. Bettini, and M. Tonetti, "Enamel matrix derivative stabilizes blood clot and improves clinical healing in deep pockets after flapless periodontal therapy: a randomized clinical trial," *Journal of Clinical Periodontology*, vol. 46, no. 2, pp. 231–240, 2019.

[20] A. A. Krausz, E. E. Machtei, and M. Peled, "Effects of lower third molar extraction on attachment level and alveolar bone height of the adjacent second molar," *International Journal of Oral and Maxillofacial Surgery*, vol. 34, no. 7, pp. 756–760, 2005.

[21] D. Laurito, M. Lollobrigida, F. Graziani, F. Guerra, A. Vestri, and A. De Biase, "Periodontal effects of a transposed versus a conventional flap in mandibular third molar extractions," *The Journal of Craniofacial Surgery*, vol. 27, no. 3, pp. 708–711, 2016.

[22] D. Di Nardo, G. Mazzucchi, M. Lollobrigida et al., "Immediate or delayed retrieval of the displaced third molar: a review," *Journal of Clinical and Experimental Dentistry*, vol. 11, no. 1, pp. e55–e61, 2019.

[23] J. L. Calvo-Guirado, J. E. Maté-Sánchez de Val, M. L. Ramos-Oltra et al., "The use of tooth particles as a biomaterial in post-extraction Sockets. Experimental Study in Dogs," *Dentistry Journal*, vol. 6, no. 2, p. 12, 2018.

[24] R. S. Demetter, B. G. Calahan, and B. L. Mealey, "Histologic evaluation of wound healing after ridge preservation with cortical, cancellous, and combined cortico-cancellous freeze-dried bone allograft: a randomized controlled clinical trial," *Journal of Periodontology*, vol. 88, no. 9, pp. 860–868, 2017.

[25] A. J. Eskow and B. L. Mealey, "Evaluation of healing following tooth extraction with ridge preservation using cortical versus cancellous freeze-dried bone allograft," *Journal of Periodontology*, vol. 85, no. 4, pp. 514–524, 2014.

[26] R. A. Wood and B. L. Mealey, "Histologic comparison of healing after tooth extraction with ridge preservation using mineralized versus demineralized freeze-dried bone allograft," *Journal of Periodontology*, vol. 83, no. 3, pp. 329–336, 2012.

[27] S. Jambhekar, F. Kernen, and A. S. Bidra, "Clinical and histologic outcomes of socket grafting after flapless tooth extraction: a systematic review of randomized controlled clinical trials," *The Journal of Prosthetic Dentistry*, vol. 113, no. 5, pp. 371–382, 2015.

[28] K. Y. Peng, Y. C. Tseng, E. C. Shen, S. C. Chiu, E. Fu, and Y. W. Huang, "Mandibular second molar periodontal status after third molar extraction," *Journal of Periodontology*, vol. 72, no. 12, pp. 1647–1651, 2001.

[29] D. T. Richardson and T. B. Dodson, "Risk of periodontal defects after third molar surgery: an exercise in evidence-based clinical decision-making," *Oral Surgery, Oral Medicine, Oral Pathology, Oral Radiology, and Endodontics*, vol. 100, no. 2, pp. 133–137, 2005.

[30] R. Pippi, "Effectiveness of a personalized device in the evaluation of mandibular second molar periodontal healing after surgical extraction of adjacent third molar," *Annali Di Stomatologia (Roma)*, vol. 4, no. 3-4, pp. 218–229, 2013.

[31] G. H. Blakey, M. T. Jacks, S. Offenbacher et al., "Progression of periodontal disease in the second/third molar region in patients with asymptomatic third molars," *Journal of Oral and Maxillofacial Surgery*, vol. 64, no. 2, pp. 189–193, 2006.

[32] P. L. G. Coceancig, "Alveolar bone grafts distal to the lower second molar," *Journal of Maxillofacial and Oral Surgery*, vol. 8, no. 1, pp. 22–26, 2009.

[33] P. C. Passarelli, C. Lajolo, G. Pasquantonio et al., "Influence of mandibular third molar surgical extraction on the periodontal status of adjacent second molars," *Journal of Periodontology*, vol. 90, no. 8, pp. 847–855, 2019.

[34] H. Petsos, J. Korte, P. Eickholz, T. Hoffmann, and R. Borchard, "Surgical removal of third molars and periodontal tissues of adjacent second molars," *Journal of Clinical Periodontology*, vol. 43, no. 5, pp. 453–460, 2016.

[35] R. P. White Jr., E. L. Fisher, C. Phillips, M. Tucker, K. L. Moss, and S. Offenbacher, "Visible third molars as risk indicator for increased periodontal probing depth," *Journal of Oral and Maxillofacial Surgery*, vol. 69, no. 1, pp. 92–103, 2011.

[36] Y. K. Kim, S. G. Kim, P. Y. Yun et al., "Autogenous teeth used for bone grafting: a comparison with traditional grafting materials," *Oral Surgery, Oral Medicine, Oral Pathology, Oral Radiology*, vol. 117, no. 1, pp. e39–e45, 2014.

[37] F. Schwarz, V. Golubovic, K. Becker, and I. Mihatovic, "Extracted tooth roots used for lateral alveolar ridge augmentation: a proof-of-concept study," *Journal of Clinical Periodontology*, vol. 43, no. 4, pp. 345–353, 2016.

[38] J. L. Calvo-Guirado, A. Ballester-Montilla, P. N de Aza et al., "Particulated, extracted human teeth characterization by SEM˙EDX evaluation as a biomaterial for socket preservation: an in vitro study," *Materials (Basel)*, vol. 12, no. 3, p. 380, 2019.

[39] N. E. Saygin, Y. Tokiyasu, W. V. Giannobile, and M. J. Somerman, "Growth factors regulate expression of mineral associated genes in cementoblasts," *Journal of Periodontology*, vol. 71, no. 10, pp. 1591–1600, 2000.

[40] G. Serafini, M. Lopreiato, M. Lollobrigida et al., "Platelet Rich Fibrin (PRF) and Its Related Products: Biomolecular Characterization of the Liquid Fibrinogen," *Journal of Clinical Medicine*, vol. 9, no. 4, p. 1099, 2020.

[41] D. Laurito, M. Lollobrigida, F. Gianno, S. Bosco, L. Lamazza, and A. De Biase, "Alveolar ridge preservation with nc-HA and d-PTFE membrane: a clinical, histologic, and histomorphometric study," *The International Journal of Periodontics & Restorative Dentistry*, vol. 37, no. 2, pp. 283–290, 2017.

[42] Z. Mazor, R. A. Horowitz, H. Prasad, and G. A. Kotsakis, "Healing dynamics following alveolar ridge preservation with autologous tooth structure," *The International Journal of Periodontics & Restorative Dentistry*, vol. 39, no. 5, pp. 697–702, 2019.

[43] A. del Canto-Diaz, J. de Elio-Oliveros, M. del Canto-Diaz, M. A. Alobera-Gracia, M. del Canto-Pingarron, and J. M. Martinez-Gonzalez, "Use of autologous tooth-derived graft material in the post-extraction dental socket. Pilot study," *Medicina Oral, Patología Oral y Cirugía Bucal*, vol. 24, pp. e53–e60, 2018.

[44] A. Kuperschlag, G. Keršytė, G. M. Kurtzman, and R. A. Horowitz, "Autogenous dentin grafting of osseous defects distal to mandibular second molars after extraction of impacted third molars," *The Compendium of Continuing Education in Dentistry*, vol. 41, pp. 76–82, 2020.

5

Laterally Positioned Flap with Subepithelial Connective Tissue Graft Modified One-Stage Procedure for the Treatment of Deep Isolated Gingival Recessions in Mandibular Incisors

Alvaro Francisco Bosco,[1] **Juliano Milanezi de Almeida**,[1] **Belén Retamal-Valdes**,[2] **Renata Tavares**,[2] **Jessica M. Latimer**,[3] **Diego Messina**,[4] **Matheus Henke**,[4] **Laura Gantes Rodrigues Dias**,[4] **and Thiago Marchi Martins**[4]

[1]*Department of Surgery and Integrated Clinic, School of Dentistry, São Paulo State University, Araçatuba, São Paulo, Brazil*
[2]*Department of Periodontology, Dental Research Division, Guarulhos University, Guarulhos, São Paulo, Brazil*
[3]*Department of Oral Medicine, Infection, and Immunity, Harvard School of Dental Medicine, Boston, MA, USA*
[4]*Department of Semiology and Clinic, Periodontology Discipline, Federal University of Pelotas, Pelotas, Rio Grande do Sul, Brazil*

Correspondence should be addressed to Thiago Marchi Martins; thiagoperio@yahoo.com.br

Academic Editor: Giuseppe Colella

The laterally positioned flap (LPF) has been proposed as a promising treatment for isolated gingival recessions (GRs) in mandibular incisors. Several modifications have been proposed to reduce the risk of gingival recession (GR) at the donor tooth site. Therefore, the aim of this was to describe a modified one-stage procedure of performing the LPF associated with the subepithelial connective tissue graft (LPF + SCTG) with the modifications for the treatment of deep isolated GR in mandibular incisors. The modified one-stage technique (LPF + SCTG) is unique because it was presented being bilaminar with tunneled connective tissue graft (CTG) in the adjacent tooth and extended to the flap donor site, without a submarginal incision in the adjacent tooth, taking the entire band of the keratinized tissue (KT) into the flap. In addition, 3 clinical cases were described using this surgical technique. Three healthy patients with Cairo RT1 or RT2 GRs on teeth 31 or 41 were treated with the LPF + SCTG technique. Probing depth (PD), clinical attachment level (CAL), complete root coverage (CRC), mean root coverage (MRC), recession depth (RD), and keratinized tissue width (KTW) were assessed at baseline and in the follow-up periods of 18, 24, and 48 months, in the cases 1, 2, and 3, respectively. The LPF + SCTG with the modifications presented is a predictable approach for the treatment of deep isolated RT1 and RT2 GRs in mandibular incisors that are well positioned in the bone envelope with the presence of KTW adjacent to GR and adequate vestibule depth in the donor area of the flap.

1. Introduction

Gingival recession (GR) is the apical shift of the gingival margin with respect to the cementoenamel junction (CEJ), with exposure of the root surface to the oral environment [1]. This condition may promote the occurrence of dental hypersensitivity and root alterations in the cervical area. In addition, it may become one predisposing factor for plaque accumulation [2] or may be considered an esthetic problem by the patient [1]. The overall prevalence of GR in the adult population has been reported to be > 60% [3], while the central and lateral mandibular incisors were the most frequently affected teeth [4, 5].

Coronally advanced flap (CAF) with subepithelial connective tissue graft (SCTG) is now considered the gold standard procedure for the treatment of GR [6–8]. Due to unfavorable local anatomical conditions, the CAF has been contraindicated in some clinical situations [9]. Thus, the clinician should take into consideration the soft tissues located laterally to the recession defect into consideration to evaluate the possibility of performing the laterally positioned flap (LPF) [9, 10].

Numerous modifications to the original laterally sliding flap proposed by Grupe and Warren [11] have been published in order to reduce the risk of GR at the donor site [12, 13]. Bosco et al. [14] proposed an internal bevel performed in the graft recipient area. This modification in technique promotes better flap adaptation to the recipient area and favors the esthetic result by reducing visibility of the incision line perception after scarring. Zucchelli et al. [9] suggested the coronal advancement of the laterally moved flap and a different thickness during flap elevation with a submarginal incision in the adjacent tooth. Recently, other authors have proposed the association of an SCTG coverage by LPF without a submarginal incision in the adjacent tooth, taking the entire band of the keratinized tissue (KT) into the flap [15]. More predictable prognosis was associated with gingival thickness (GT) of 0.8–1.2 mm [16] and a thickness < 1 mm that could affect the percentage of complete root coverage (CRC) [17]. In this context, the modified one-stage technique (LPF + SCTG) is unique because it was presented being bilaminar [18], with tunneled CTG in the adjacent tooth and extended to flap donor site, without a submarginal incision in the adjacent tooth, taking the entire band of the keratinized tissue (KT) into the flap and the inversion of bevels in relation to Parkinson et al. [13]. Therefore, the aim of this manuscript was to describe a modified one-stage procedure of performing the laterally positioned flap with subepithelial connective tissue graft (LPF + SCTG) with the modifications for the treatment of deep isolated GR in mandibular incisors.

2. Case Description

2.1. Surgical Technique (LPF + SCTG Modified-Figure 1)

2.1.1. Clinical Indications and Contraindications. "This technique is a time-efficient, less invasive (one-stage procedure), and highly esthetic treatment option for managing isolated Cairo RT1 and RT2 GRs, in teeth well positioned in the bone envelope or slightly buccal where odontoplasty is possible, mainly in the mandible in the presence of a thin gingival phenotype and little or no band of KT, apical in the recession defect, with the presence of KT adjacent to GR (minimum of 2 mm), and adequate vestibule depth in the donor area of the flap. Instead, in the Cairo RT3 GRs, this technique would not be indicated due to the presence of extensive interproximal CAL and lack of predictability for root coverage".

After the full-mouth periodontal examination, all patients receive a dental prophylaxis including oral hygiene instruction (OHI), supragingival scaling, and professional tooth cleaning. For teeth with GR, a coronally directed roll tooth brushing technique is recommended to minimize toothbrushing trauma to the gingival margin. On the day of surgery, patients rinse with 15 ml of 0.12% chlorhexidine gluconate mouth rinse for 1 minute. In addition, anti-inflammatory medication (600 mg ibuprofen), 1 hour before the surgical procedure, is indicated.

Local anesthesia of the bilateral mental and lingual nerves is achieved with 2% mepivacaine (MEPIADRE 100, DFL). Only the portion of the exposed root with attachment loss should be instrumented with curettes. The roots are conditioned for two minutes with cotton pellets soaked with 100 mg/ml tetracycline hydrochloride solution, followed by abundant irrigation with saline solution [15].

The surgical technique begins at the level of CEJ with an internal bevel incision using a 15C blade (2 to 3 mm from root surface) extending in the direction of the alveolar mucosa, bypassing the apical portion of the GR defect continuing with an external bevel incision along the distal gingival margin (1 mm from root surface) ending at the dental surface at the level of the CEJ [14, 15] (modification that was made to the original one [13]) (Figure 1(a)). After an intrasulcular incision (Figure 1(b)), this area is deepithelialized with the use of a 15C blade kept parallel to the external gingival surface. Connective tissue area lateral and apical to the root exposure provides the LPF with an anchorage bed (Figure 1(c)).

In the tooth adjacent to the GR, an intrasulcular incision is performed in the horizontal direction in order to contour the mesial and distal papillae (modification that was made to the original one [9]), continuing with a vertical beveled incision that starts at the level of the base of the papilla on the mesiobuccal surface of the second or third tooth adjacent to GR, extending into the alveolar mucosa [15]. The flap of mixed thickness is elevated, with split thickness in the papillae (Figure 1(d)-purple color) and full thickness (Figure 1(d)-yellow color) in the center up to the limit of the mucogingival junction and long enough to cover the mesial-distal extension of the avascular root area of the GR defect (Figures 1(d) and 1(e)). Once the mucogingival line is reached, apical split-thickness flap elevation is continued, keeping the blade parallel to the bone surface. Flap elevation is terminated when it is possible to passively move the flap laterally above the exposed root and reach a level coronal to the CEJ (Figure 1(f)).The papillae of the recipient site (marginal area of prepared tunnel) is carefully deepithelialized with a 15c blade (Figure 1(d)-orange color). The CTG is harvested from the hard palate in the region between the maxillary first premolar and the second molar by de-epithelialized free gingival graft (D-FGG) [19] technique. The donor area of the palate received protection from the epithelialized portion of the graft stabilized by sutures [19]. Appropriately sized CTG is positioned mesially, inside the tunnel prepared, (Figure 1(d)-green color) (modification that were made to the original one [14]) with the remaining portion covering the defect area and the distally adjacent tooth (or teeth) at the level of CEJ. CTG must be stabilized with two simple interrupted sutures (absorbable thread 5.0), one on the tunnel prepared and one on the papilla opposite to the defect site (Figure 1(g)). Subsequently, the flap will then be laterally positioned and secured with suspensory sutures (monofilamentar thread 5.0) and simple interrupted sutures to approximate margins and secure the LPF margin in the recipient site (Figure 1(h)).

Patients receive strict postoperative instructions, including medication (600 mg ibuprofen, every 12 hours). They are also instructed not to brush their teeth in the treated area, but to rinse with 15 ml of 0.12% chlorhexidine gluconate solution, twice a day for 1 minute for 14 days. Sutures at the donor site are removed 7 days postoperatively, and sutures in the grafted site are removed 2 weeks postoperatively. The

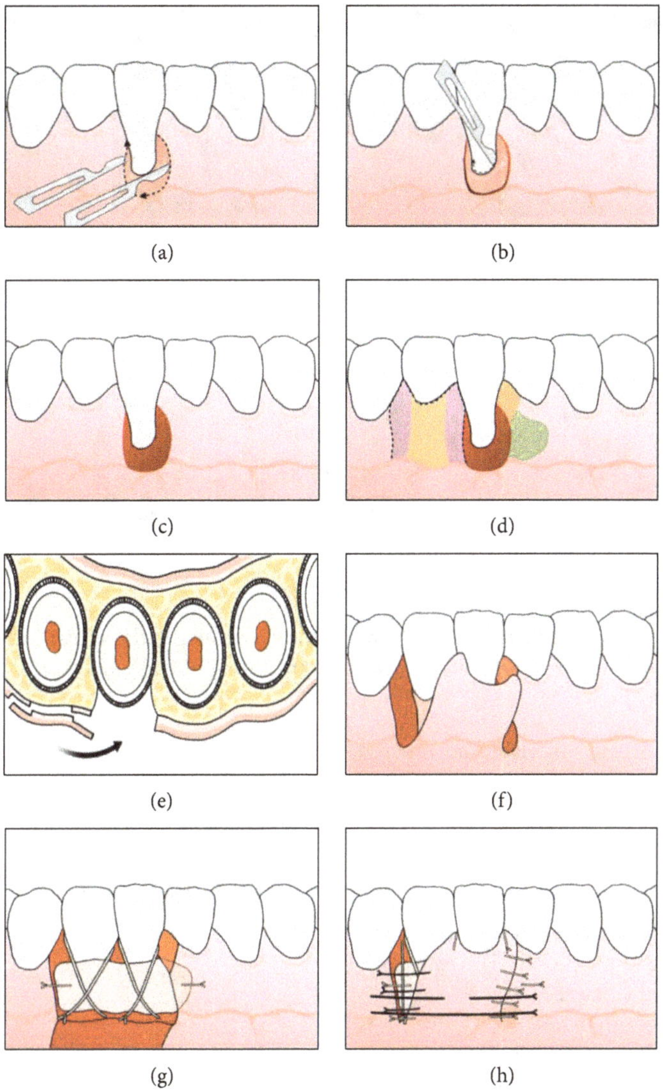

FIGURE 1: Schematic representation of the surgical technique. (a) Internal and external bevel incision, whereas flap will be positioned from tooth 42 to 41. (b) Intrasulcular incision in tooth 41. (c) Deepithelialization area providing laterally positioned flap (LPF) with an anchorage bed. (d) Delimitation of mixed thickness flap (purple color: split thickness; yellow color: full thickness) and preparation of surgical bed to receive connective tissue graft (CTG) (orange color: papilla deepithelialized; green color: tunnel). (e) Cross-section showing different thicknesses of flap that will be positioned laterally. (f) Flap prepared and positioned laterally. Papilla mesial of tooth 41 deepithelialized (orange color in (d)). (g) CTG positioned and stabilized in the created tunnel (green color in the (d)), over the gingival recession (GR) defect with extension to the flap donor area. (h) Flap positioned and stabilized with suture.

patients are again reinstructed with regard to mechanical plaque control of the treated area and must continue with the chlorhexidine rinse instructions for 14 additional days.

All patients were informed about the treatment plan, the surgical technique, postoperative recommendations, and possible complications, and informed consent was obtained from the patients.

2.2. Case 1. The patient, a 22-year-old Caucasian man, nonsmoker, systemically healthy, presented with the main complaint of difficulty with cleaning the region of tooth #41 and fear of losing the tooth, at the Department of Periodontology, Federal University of Pelotas (Pelotas, Rio Grande do Sul, Brazil), in April 2018. The patient had previously undergone orthodontic treatment. According to the clinical and radiographic examination, a RT2 RG was observed on the vestibular surface of the right mandibular central incisor (4 mm high and 3 mm wide at the height of the CEJ), with a probing depth (PD) of 3 mm in the proximal and 2 mm of 2 mm measured on the on free surfaces, clinical attachment level (CAL) of 6 mm on the buccal surface, radiographic interproximal bone loss mesial and distal sites, slight buccal prominence (dental linguoversion), slight dental extrusion, biofilm accumulation, protruding occlusal interference, and thin periodontal phenotype (Figure 2).

After supragingival periodontal therapy, the protrusive occlusal interference in #41 tooth was subsequently adjusted to balance the contacts and improve the distribution of forces. To adjust this, occlusal contact markings were made at maximum habitual intercuspation, protrusion, and right

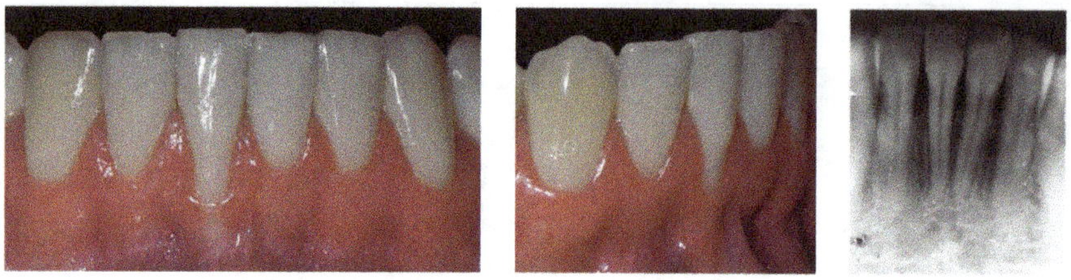

(a) (b) (c)

FIGURE 2: Case 1. (a) Frontal view, gingival recession of 4 mm high by 3 mm wide. (b) Right lateral view. (c) Periapical radiograph, 2 mm radiographic interproximal bone loss mesial and distal.

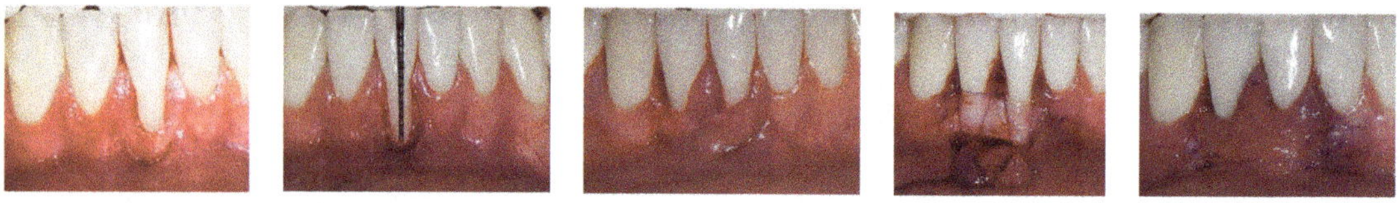

(a) (b) (c) (d) (e)

FIGURE 3: Case 1. (a) Vertical internal bevel incision extending into alveolar mucosa and external bevel incision along distal gingival margin of the recession defect and extending into alveolar mucosa. (b) Deepithelialized area after intrasulcular incision. (c) Flap of mix thickness. (d) Connective tissue graft positioned and stabilized. (e) Laterally positioned flap without tension and secured with sutures on recipient site.

and left laterality. For selective wear, spherical and tapered diamond (KG Sorensen, Cotia, São Paulo, SP, Brazil) tips were used, in addition to abrasive rubber, discs, and polishing paste (TDV Dental, Pomerode SC, Brazil), until the establishment of balanced contacts during mandibular movements were established, in order to maintain a mutually protected occlusion. Two weeks after the occlusal adjustment, periodontal surgical treatment was performed using the LPF + SCTG technique (T.M.M.), as previously described (Figure 3).

The CTG, with an average thickness of 1 mm, was removed from the palate, in the region between the first maxillary premolar and the first molar, using the D-FGG technique [19]. The CTG extended high enough into the mesiodistal direction, to cover teeth 41 and 42, high to cover the exposed root surface and remain within the tunnel created under the initial mesial incision of 41 tooth, in order to be covered by LPF later (Figure 3).

2.3. Case 2. The patient, a 21-year-old Caucasian woman, nonsmoker, systemically healthy, presented with main complaint of difficulty with cleaning the region of tooth #41 and esthetic change when smiling, at the Department of Periodontology, Federal University of Pelotas (Pelotas, Rio Grande do Sul, Brazil). According to the clinical and radiographic examination, a RT1 RG was observed on the buccal surface of the right mandibular central incisor (4 mm high and 3 mm wide at the height of the CEJ), with a PD of 2 mm in the proximal and 1 mm on free surfaces, CAL of 5 mm on the buccal surface, absence of interproximal bone loss, slight (dental linguoversion) on the buccal surface, biofilm accumulation, protruding occlusal interference, and thin periodontal phenotype (Figure 4).

Firstly, an adjustment of protrusive occlusal interference in tooth #41 was performed, as describe in case 1. Two weeks after the occlusal adjustment, periodontal surgical treatment

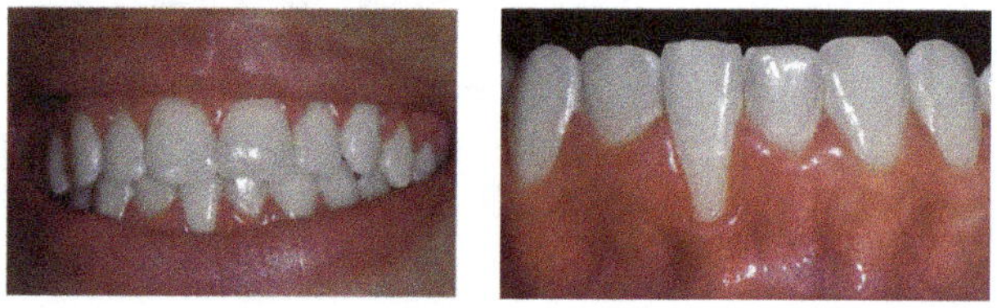

(a) (b)

FIGURE 4: Case 2. (a) Frontal aspect of smile. (b) Frontal view, gingival recession of 4 mm high by 3 mm wide.

was performed using the LPF + SCTG technique (T.M.M.; Figure 5).

2.4. Case 3. The patient, a 23-year-old, Caucasian woman, systemically healthy, presented with main complaint of fear of losing tooth #31 and dentin hipersensivity, at the Department of Surgery and Integrated Clinic, São Paulo State University (Araçatuba, São Paulo, Brazil), in April 2016. The patient was a nonsmoker and had previously undergone orthodontic treatment. According to the clinical and radiographic examination, an RT1 RG was observed in the buccal surface of the left mandibular central incisor (5 mm high and 3,5 mm wide at the height of the CEJ), with a PD of 2 mm in the proximal and 2 mm on free surfaces, CAL of 7 mm on the buccal surface, absence of interproximal bone loss, biofilm accumulation, and thin periodontal phenotype (Figure 6).

After 21 days of the supragingival periodontal therapy, the treatment using the LPF + SCTG technique was performed in a single surgical stage (J.M.A.). In this case, the flap was extended to two adjacent teeth distal tooth with GR, so that it remained of mixed thickness on the immediately adjacent tooth (tooth #32) and split thickness on the most distal tooth (tooth #33). The CTG was extended mesiodistal enough to cover tooth #31 to #33 (decision made due to the

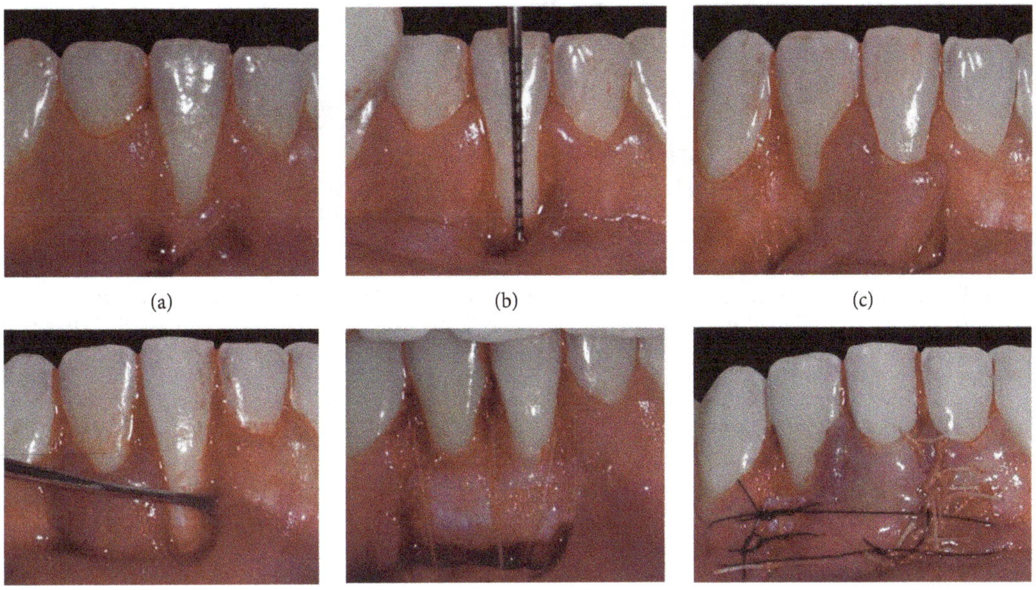

(a) (b) (c)

(d) (e) (f)

FIGURE 5: Case 2. (a) Vertical internal bevel incision extending into alveolar mucosa and external bevel incision along distal gingival margin of gingival recession (GR) defect. (b) Deepithelialized area after intrasulcular incision. (c) Flap of mix thickness. (d) Mesial papilla of tooth 41 deepithelialized and tunnel preparation. (e) Connective tissue graft (CTG) positioned and stabilized with sutures. (f) Laterally positioned flap without tension and secured with sutures on the recipient site.

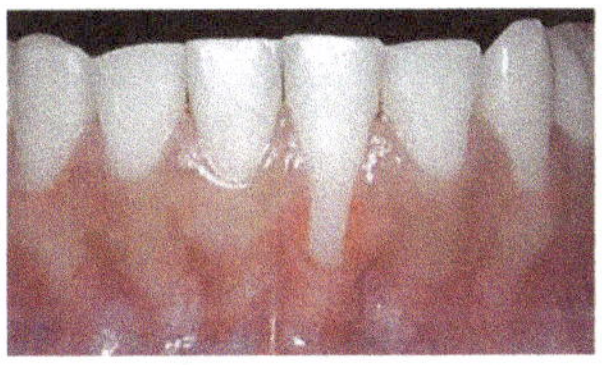

FIGURE 6: Case 3. Frontal view, gingival recession of 5 mm high by 3.5 mm wide.

width [3.5 mm] and height [5 mm] of the GR), to cover the exposed root surface and remain within the tunnel created under the initial mesial incision of tooth #31, to later be covered by LPF (Figure 7).

Three deep GRs were surgically treated with LPF + SCTG in three different patients. The periodontal characteristics of the three clinical cases are presented in Table 1. One hundred percent of the cases treated achieved CRC. An increase in the keratinized tissue width (KTW) was observed in all the cases. The follow-up time intervals were 18, 24, and 48 months, in cases 1, 2 and 3, respectively (Figures 8–10). No postsurgical complications were reported.

3. Discussion

This manuscript described a modified one-stage procedure to perform the LPF + SCTG as an effective therapeutic option for the treatment of deep isolated GRs in mandibular incisors. In time intervals of 18 (case 1), 24 (case 2), and 48 months (case 3) after surgeries, CRC was obtained in all defects treated. Mean RD and MRC changed from 4.33 ± 0.58 mm at baseline to 0.0 ± 0.0 mm ($p < 0.05$) in the last postoperative period of each case. The CRC was obtained not only in Cairo RT1 defects (cases 2 and 3) but also in the Cairo RT2 GR (case 1). Mean KTW changed from 0.0 ± 0.0 mm at baseline to 5.0 ± 2.0 mm ($p < 0.05$) in the follow-up period. The donor bed of the LPF showed no post-operative GR defect in follow-up time intervals. The patients reported absence of dentin hypersensitivity when cleaning the region of GR defects and an excellent esthetic result of periodontal tissues.

The treatment of deep buccal GRs in the mandibular anterior area represents a major clinical challenge owing to several anatomical conditions [20, 21]. In this case series, the decision-making to define the flap extension depended on the recession depth (GR ≥ 5 mm) and width (GR ≥ 3.5 mm) of the GR and on the presence or absence of compromising factors, such as buccal tooth position, root prominence, proximity of vital structures (e.g., mental nerve), and deep bone dehiscence [20].

The potential of the FGG (free gingival graft) for increasing the KTW has been documented and seems to explain the increase in KTW after the two-stage CAF procedures [21, 22]. Among the free graft procedures, the bilaminar techniques have been reported to be more predictable [23] and to provide more esthetic results [24] than the FGG. The surgical technique (LPF + SCTG) presented in this case reports has been shown to be effective in increasing KTW and root coverage in only one surgical procedure [8], thereby minimizing morbidity among surgical patients.

In a randomized controlled clinical study, [23] evaluated the treatment of isolated Miller Class I and II GR on mandibular incisors. Treatment was performed by means of CAF + SCTG with or without removal of labial submucosal tissue (LST). The results showed predictable recession coverage,

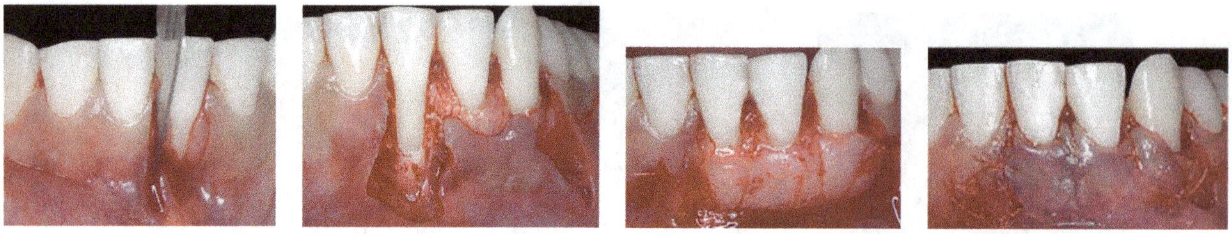

(a) (b) (c) (d)

Figure 7: Case 3. (a) Vertical internal bevel incision extending in alveolar mucosa and an external bevel incision along distal gingival margin of gingival recession (GR) defect. (b) Flap of mix thickness. (c) CTG positioned and stabilized with sutures. (d) Laterally positioned flap without tension and secured with sutures on the recipient site.

Table 1: Clinical characteristics of the three clinical cases, means (±SD), minimum (min), and maximum (max) of clinical parameters at baseline and follow-up.

Variable	Time point	Mean ± SD	Min	Max	p value Paired t-test
PD (mm)	Baseline	2.06 ± 0.42	1.67	2.50	>0.05
	Follow-up	1.83 ± 0.29	1.67	2.17	
PD-3b (mm)	Baseline	2.11 ± 0.51	1.67	2.67	>0.05
	Follow-up	1.89 ± 0.38	1.67	2.33	
PD-1b (mm)	Baseline	1.67 ± 0.58	1.00	2.00	≤0.001
	Follow-up	1.00 ± 0.00	1.00	1.00	
CAL (mm)	Baseline	1.56 ± 0.98	0.83	2.67	0.017
	Follow-up	0.44 ± 0.77	0.00	1.33	
CAL-3b (mm)	Baseline	2.44 ± 0.84	1.67	3.33	0.00
	Follow-up	0.44 ± 0.77	0.00	1.33	
CAL-1b (mm)	Baseline	6.00 ± 1.00	5.00	7.00	0.009
	Follow-up	0.00 ± 0.00	0.00	0.00	
KTW (mm)	Baseline	0.00 ± 0.00	0.00	0.00	0.049
	Follow-up	5.00 ± 2.00	3.00	7.00	
RD (mm)	Baseline	4.33 ± 0.58	4.00	5.00	0.005
	Follow-up	0.00 ± 0.00	0.00	0.00	
MRC (mm)	Follow-up	4.33 ± 0.58	4.00	5.00	—
CRC (100%)	Follow-up	Yes	Yes	Yes	—

Abreviations: CAL, Clinical Attachment Level (6 sites); CAL-3b, Clinical Attachment Level (3 buccal sites); CAL-1b, Clinical Attachment Level (1 buccal site); CRC, Complete Root Coverage; KTW, Keratinized Tissue Width; mm, millimeters; MRC: mean root coverage; PD: probing depth (6 sites); PD-3b: probing depth (3 buccal sites); PD-1b: probing depth (1 buccal site); RD: recession depth; SD: standard deviation. The significance of differences over time was assessed by paired t-test ($p < 0.05$).

while the additional removal of LST yielded a tension-free flap, resulting in less graft exposure and statistically significantly better CRC (48% vs 88%). These results were difficult to compare directly with those obtained in the present case series, which also included one case of RT2 GR, and the donor area of the flap was lateral to the GR defect. Nevertheless, both studies clearly pointed out the pivotal role of tension-free mobilization of the flap to obtain predictable CRC.

The results of the KTW gain obtained with LPF + SCTG (from 0.0 ± 0.0 mm at baseline to 5.0 ± 2.0 mm at follow up times) were similar to those found by César Neto et al. [20] who reported the results of root coverage in maxillary and mandible isolated Miller Class II or III deep GRs (≥ 5 mm), based on the decision-making algorithm. Similarly, Sculean and Allen [24] obtained KTW values of 1.41 ± 1.00 mm at baseline to 4.14 ± 1.67 mm at 12 months, generating a gain of 2.75 ± 1.52 mm, in a series of 24 patients treated by means of a novel surgical technique (the laterally closed tunnel, LCT) associated with CTG, specifically designed for Miller Class I, II, or III deep isolated mandibular GR (≥ 4 mm).

The use of the split thickness flap in the most distal portion of the flap as described in the surgical technique

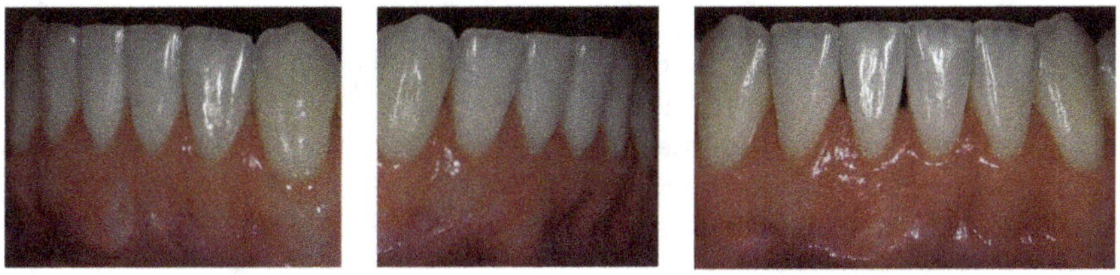

(a) (b) (c)

FIGURE 8: Case 1. Healing 18 months postoperatively. (a) Left side view showing complete root coverage. (b) Right side view showing maintenance of integrity of donor bed. (c) Front view showing keratinized tissue width gain and gingival tissue color very similar to that of the adjacent area.

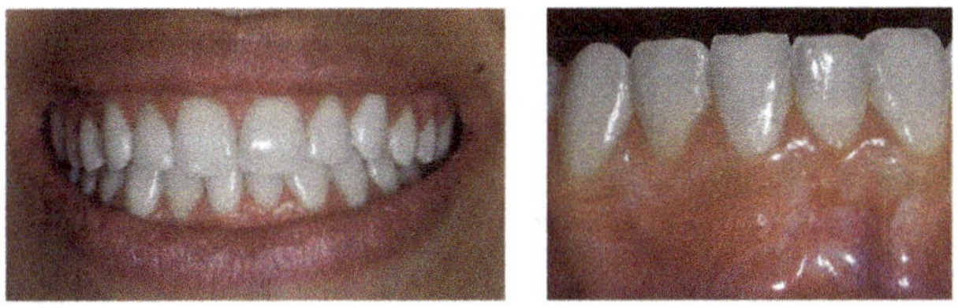

(a) (b)

FIGURE 9: Case 2. (a) Frontal aspect of smile with visualization after healing 24 months postoperatively. (b) Front view showing complete root coverage and keratinized tissue width gain.

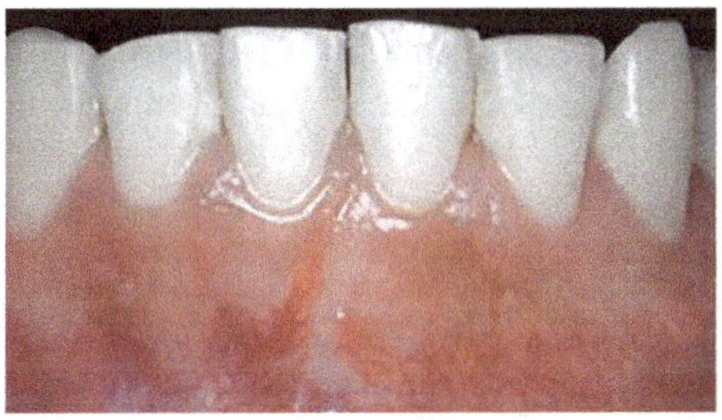

FIGURE 10: Case 3. Frontal view, healing 48 months postoperatively demonstrating complete root coverage; maintenance of integrity of the donor flap area, keratinized tissue width gain, and gingival tissue color very similar to that of the adjacent area.

prevented bone exposure and possible gingival recession in that area [26]. The performance of internal and external bevels characterizes the inversion of bevels concerning Parkinson et al. [13], which used an external bevel in the donor area and an internal bevel in the flap positioned laterally. In the present technique (LPF + SCTG), it is the opposite of this (Figure 1(a)). As the flap was positioned laterally, it is important to report that the flap bevel inversions [14, 15] were used to allow better adaptation at the time of suturing, in order to avoid overlapping the flap in the receiving area and thereby reducing visibility of the incision line perception after scarring.

Zucchelli et al. [9] evaluated the effectiveness concerning root coverage of a modified surgical approach of the laterally moved flap procedure with a submarginal incision and mix-thickness flap in the donor site, for the treatment of the isolated type of recession defects (Miller Class I or II). Specific features of the KT lateral to the defects were considered for indication: lateral keratinized tissue width (KTW donor) at least 6 mm greater than the width of the recession measured at the level of the CEJ and lateral keratinized tissue height (KTH donor) at least 2 mm greater than the buccal probing depth (PD) of the adjacent tooth/teeth (PD donor). Unlike the technique described by Zucchelli et al. [9], the present LPF + SCTG technique considers adding a tunneled CTG in the GR mesial and distally extended to protect and change the gingival phenotype to thicker areas adjacent to the GR defect. In the anterior mandible, a thin gingival phenotype is often found. It can be difficult to move the flap in the coronal direction due to muscle insertions and shallow vestibule [23]. In this context, the LPF + SCTG technique considers that the preservation of the entire band of KT adjacent to GR in the flap minimizes this need to move the flap also in the coronal direction to cover the GR defect.

A minimum amount of the attached keratinized tissue (KT) ($\geq$ 1 mm) is required to prevent significant apical displacement of the gingival margin in the long-term [27]. In addition, it was shown that gingival thickness > 1.2 mm at the level of the keratinized mucosa was a positive predictor of CRC [24]. In the presence of a thin gingival phenotype (< 1 mm GT), bilaminar procedures consisting of a LCT or a LPF in combination with an autogenous graft are recommended [15, 24, 26]. In the LPF + SCTG technique described, the graft is inserted into the created tunnel and extended distally to protect the donor area of the flap, even if a small portion of it is exposed in that area [27]. In this clinical setting, the gingival phenotype of the areas adjacent to the GR defect were modified by obtaining greater thickness and KTW gain, which may favor the stability of long-term root coverage results [15].

LPF + SCTG and CAF + SCTG are commonly used surgical approaches to treat deep localized GR in mandibular incisors. However, in the presence of a shallow vestibule, Cairo RT3 GRs or lack of the keratinized tissue (minimum of 2 mm) adjacent to GR results using these approaches has clear limitations [28]. These clinical situations may represent the main indications for the two-step surgical approach with flattening of the root surface and later LCT [28]. In this two-step approach, flattening of the root surface creates a new emergence in order to treat anterior mandibular localized GRs in the prominent teeth. This approach will provide more space for the graft, increase the thickness of the gingival margin, and provide extra soft tissue at the margins of the GR [28].

The mandibular incisors of the cases described were relatively well positioned in the bone envelope. Although we did not perform the cone-bean computed tomography to observe the buccal-lingual inclination of the roots and the occurrence of bone dehiscence in the teeth adjacent to the GR defect, this is considered an important complementary exam for making the treatment decision about whether to perform orthodontic treatment or concomitant odontoplasty to the surgical technique of root coverage [28].

Despite the excellent results obtained with the LPF + SCTG technique in the cases reported, these findings revealed the importance of well-designed randomized clinical studies that compare the effectiveness of different surgical techniques for the treatment of deep isolated GRs in the mandibular arch.

The present results indicated that the LPF-SCTG with the modifications presented is a predictable approach for the treatment of deep isolated RT1 and RT2 GRs in mandibular incisors that are well positioned in the bone envelope with the presence of KTW adjacent to GR and adequate vestibule depth in the donor area.

References

[1] P. Cortellini and N. F. Bissada, "Mucogingival conditions in the natural dentition: narrative review, case definitions, and diagnostic considerations," *Journal of Periodontology*, vol. 89, Supplement 1, pp. 204–213, 2018.

[2] P. Cortellini and G. Pini Prato, "Coronally advanced flap and combination therapy for root coverage. Clinical strategies based on scientific evidence and clinical experience," *Periodontology 2000*, vol. 59, no. 1, pp. 158–184, 2012.

[3] N. A. Chrysanthakopoulos, "Gingival recession: prevalence and risk indicators among young Greek adults," *Journal of Clinical and Experimental Dentistry*, vol. 6, no. 3, pp. e243–e249, 2014.

[4] S. R. Manchala, K. L. Vandana, N. B. Mandalapu, S. Mannem, and C. D. Dwarakanath, "Epidemiology of gingival recession and risk indicators in dental hospital population of Bhimavaram," *Journal of International Society of Preventive and Community Dentistry*, vol. 2, no. 2, pp. 69–74, 2012.

[5] M. Romandini, M. C. Soldini, E. Montero, and M. Sanz, "Epidemiology of mid-buccal gingival recessions in NHANES according to the 2018 world workshop classification system," *Journal of Clinical Periodontology*, vol. 47, no. 10, pp. 1180–1190, 2020.

[6] L. Chambrone and D. N. Tatakis, "Periodontal soft tissue root coverage procedures: a systematic review from the AAP regeneration workshop," *Journal of Periodontology*, vol. 86, Supplement 2, pp. S8–51, 2015.

[7] L. Chambrone, R. C. N. de Castro Pinto, and L. A. Chambrone, "The concepts of evidence-based periodontal plastic surgery: application of the principles of evidence-based dentistry for the treatment of recession-type defects," *Periodontology 2000*, vol. 79, no. 1, pp. 81–106, 2019.

[8] L. Chambrone, M. A. Salinas Ortega, F. Sukekava et al., "Root coverage procedures for treating localised and multiple recession-type defects," *Cochrane Database of Systematic Reviews*, vol. 10, no. 10, article CD007161, 2018.

[9] G. Zucchelli, C. Cesari, C. Amore, L. Montebugnoli, and M. De Sanctis, "Laterally moved, coronally advanced flap: a modified surgical approach for isolated recession-type defects," *Journal of Periodontology*, vol. 75, no. 12, pp. 1734–1741, 2004.

[10] R. B. Santana, F. E. de Mello, M. B. Furtado, C. M. M. de Santana, and S. Dibart, "Single-stage advanced versus rotated flaps in the treatment of gingival recessions: a 5-year longitudinal randomized clinical trial," *Journal of Periodontology*, vol. 90, no. 9, pp. 941–947, 2019.

[11] H. E. Grupe and R. F. Warren, "Repair of gingival defects by a sliding flap operation," *Journal of Periodontology*, vol. 27, no. 2, pp. 92–95, 1956.

[12] H. Staffileno, "Management of gingival recession and root exposure problems with periodontal disease," *Dental Clinics of North America*, vol. 3, pp. 111–120, 1964.

[13] W. M. Parkinson, M. A. Richards, and W. I. R. Davies, "A modified technique for the laterally repositioned flap," *Apex*, vol. 5, no. 2, pp. 51-52, 1971.

[14] A. F. Bosco, L. A. Milanezi, and E. Passanezi, "Contribution to the technique of covering the exposed roots," *Rev Reg Araçatuba Assoc Paul Cir Dent*, 1990, https://pesquisa.bvsalud.org/portal/resource/pt/biblio-858810.

[15] T. M. Martins, P. L. Faleiros, N. M. Pola, L. A. Fernandes, and A. F. Bosco, "Root coverage of adjacent gingival recessions with a combination of two surgical techniques," *RSBO Revista Sul-Brasileira de Odontologia*, vol. 12, no. 2, pp. 225–232, 2015.

[16] J. G. Woodyard, H. Greenwell, M. Hill, C. Drisko, J. M. Iasella, and J. Scheetz, "The clinical effect of acellular dermal matrix on gingival thickness and root coverage compared to coronally positioned flap alone," *Journal of Periodontology*, vol. 75, no. 1, pp. 44–56, 2004.

[17] C. Ahmedbeyli, S. D. Ipçi, G. Cakar, B. E. Kuru, and S. Yılmaz, "Clinical evaluation of coronally advanced flap with or without acellular dermal matrix graft on complete defect coverage for the treatment of multiple gingival recessions with thin tissue biotype," *Journal of Clinical Periodontology*, vol. 41, no. 3, pp. 303–310, 2014.

[18] S. W. Nelson, "The subpedicle connective tissue graft. A bilaminar reconstructive procedure for the coverage of denuded root surfaces," *Journal of Periodontology*, vol. 58, no. 2, pp. 95–102, 1987.

[19] A. F. Bosco and J. M. Bosco, "An alternative technique to the harvesting of a connective tissue graft from a thin palate: enhanced wound healing," *The International Journal of Periodontics & Restorative Dentistry*, vol. 27, no. 2, pp. 133–139, 2007.

[20] J. B. César Neto, M. C. Cavalcanti, R. T. Sekiguchi, C. M. Pannuti, G. A. Romito, and D. N. Tatakis, "Root coverage for single deep gingival recessions: outcomes based on a decision-making algorithm," *International Journal of Dentistry*, vol. 2019, Article ID 1830765, 9 pages, 2019.

[21] G. Zucchelli and M. De Sanctis, "Modified two-stage procedures for the treatment of gingival recession," *The European Journal of Esthetic Dentistry*, vol. 8, no. 1, pp. 24–42, 2013.

[22] L. Chambrone and G. Avila-Ortiz, "An evidence-based system for the classification and clinical management of non-proximal gingival recession defects," *Journal of Periodontology*, vol. 92, no. 3, pp. 327–335, 2021.

[23] G. Zucchelli, M. Marzadori, I. Mounssif, C. Mazzotti, and

M. Stefanini, "Coronally advanced flap + connective tissue graft techniques for the treatment of deep gingival recession in the lower incisors. A controlled randomized clinical trial," *Journal of Clinical Periodontology*, vol. 41, no. 8, pp. 806–813, 2014.

[24] A. Sculean and E. P. Allen, "The laterally closed tunnel for the treatment of deep isolated mandibular recessions: surgical technique and a report of 24 cases," *The International Journal of Periodontics & Restorative Dentistry*, vol. 38, no. 4, pp. 479–487, 2018.

[25] R. G. Caffesse and E. A. Guinard, "Treatment of localized gingival recessions. Part IV. Results after three years," *Journal of Periodontology*, vol. 51, no. 3, pp. 167–170, 1980.

[26] G. Agudio, L. Chambrone, and P. G. Pini, "Biologic remodeling of periodontal dimensions of areas treated with gingival augmentation procedure: a 25-year follow-up observation," *Journal of Periodontology*, vol. 88, no. 7, pp. 634–642, 2017.

[27] A. Dodge, J. Garcia, P. Luepke, Y. L. Lai, M. Kassab, and G. H. Lin, "The effect of partially exposed connective tissue graft on root-coverage outcomes: a systematic review and meta-analysis," *European Journal of Oral Sciences*, vol. 126, no. 2, pp. 84–92, 2018.

[28] J. Núñez, J. Sanz-Esporrin, R. Caffesse, and M. Sanz, "A two-step surgical approach with flattening of the root surface to treat localized gingival recessions affecting mandibular incisors: a case series report," *The International Journal of Periodontics & Restorative Dentistry*, vol. 38, no. 5, pp. 683–690, 2018.

6

Multidisciplinary Oral Rehabilitation of a Severely Compromised Dentition

Carlo Maiorana,[1] Dario Andreoni,[2] Paola Polacco,[1] and Pier Paolo Poli[1]

[1]*Implant Centre for Edentulism and Jawbone Atrophies, Maxillofacial Surgery and Odontostomatology Unit, Fondazione IRCCS Cà Granda Ospedale Maggiore Policlinico, University of Milan, Milan, Italy*
[2]*Private Practice, Via Milano 19, 20871 Vimercate, Monza Brianza, Italy*

Correspondence should be addressed to Pier Paolo Poli; pierpaolo_poli@fastwebnet.it

Academic Editor: Samir Nammour

The decision-making process of complex clinical cases should involve multiple specialists to obtain a predictable result on a long-term basis. In view of the above, the present report is aimed at describing the multidisciplinary management of a partially edentulous female patient presenting with a severely compromised residual dentition. To improve function and aesthetics, the treatment combined multiple extractions, temporary rehabilitation with a complete removable denture, guided bone regeneration and implant insertion, soft tissue management, tooth alignment, and restorative dentistry. Thus, several dental branches were embraced during the treatment phases, including oral surgery and implantology, periodontology, orthodontics, and prosthodontics. The involvement of different specialists ensured the achievement of a good result from biological, functional, and aesthetic aspects. The patient was satisfied with the final outcome. In conclusion, to meet the patient's expectations particularly in complex clinical situations, the interdisciplinary approach becomes essential from the early phases in order to identify the ideal treatment plan with the correct time sequence.

1. Introduction

The long-lasting failing dentition is a frequent and insidious day-to-day clinical challenge. Common features include heavily restored teeth, incongruous prostheses, residual roots, periapical lesions, abundant deposits of dental calculus, and periodontal disease. The progression of periodontitis is strictly combined with alveolar bone loss, which is mediated by the host immune and inflammatory response to the microbial challenge. For such reason, it is not unusual to observe at the radiographic examination an extensive horizontal bone resorption eventually associated with vertical bony defects at the expense of the alveolar process. Bone remodelling is exacerbated by the use of conventional removable dentures that leads to a pronounced reduction of the mandibular ridge and consequent forward-upward rotation of the mandible. In the lower jaw, this results in the reduction of ridge height and consequent prosthetic retention problems. The lack of fit and stability negatively influence patients' comfort during chewing and speaking.

All these factors are responsible for the low oral health-related quality of life perceived by the patients wearing removable dentures [1]. This explains why a better quality of life can be achieved with implant-retained prosthesis compared to conventional dentures in terms of physical pain and disability, psychological discomfort and disability, and functional limitations [2]. It must be noted that edentulism can lead to a significant functional impairment together with unfavourable aesthetic and psychological changes in patients. Problems include restrictions in diet and limited ability to eat certain foods, speech impairment, loss of support for facial musculature, and decreased vertical dimension. All these drawbacks taken together have made the edentulism to be recognized by the World Health Organization as a physical handicap [3].

All these findings taken together suggest the importance of saving teeth with modest tooth-associated ailments at least during the early stages and usage of dental implants to replace hopeless and/or missing teeth. Therefore, a comprehensive evaluation that implies a multidisciplinary approach

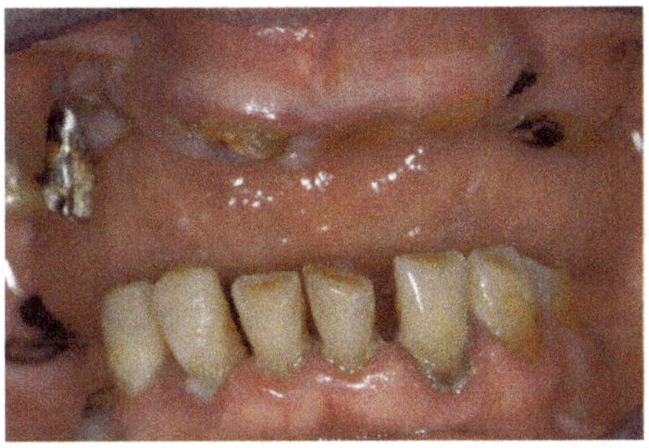

(a)

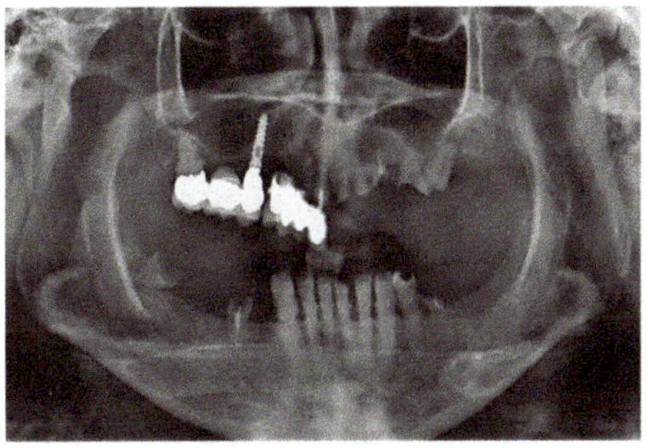

(b)

Figure 1: (a) Baseline clinical view of the severely compromised residual dentition; (b) baseline orthopantomograph.

is crucial to establish the correct treatment plan based on individual characteristics worked out to meet the patient's expectations on a long-term basis.

In view of the aforesaid, the aim of the present report was to describe the full-mouth rehabilitation of a partially edentulous patient seeking for a fixed rehabilitation adopting a multidisciplinary approach involving the oral surgeon, the orthodontist, and the prosthodontist.

2. Case Presentation

The present case was conducted according to the 1964 Helsinki declaration and its later amendments or comparable ethical standards and was reported in compliance with the CARE guidelines (http://www.care-statement.org).

A 67-year-old female patient presented with the chief complaint of tooth mobility, pain while chewing, masticatory limitations, and unsatisfying aesthetic appearance. The patient was healthy, nonsmoking, and with a noncontributory medical history except for a well-controlled hypertension (ASA II according to the American Society of Anesthesiologists physical status classification system).

At the clinical intraoral examination, in the maxilla, it was possible to observe a metal-ceramic dental bridge in the frontal right maxilla and an implant-tooth-supported metal-ceramic bridge in the posterior right maxilla. In the mandible, periodontally compromised malpositioned natural elements with calculus deposits were present from the right canine to the first left premolar. In both the jaws, few residual roots were identified. Oedematous and inflamed soft tissues with generalized bleeding on probing and loss of clinical attachment were evident (Figure 1(a)).

The baseline orthopantomograph showed an extensive pneumatization of the maxillary sinuses, with a generalized horizontal bone resorption in both the maxilla and the mandible (Figure 1(b)).

From clinical and radiological findings, both maxillary right metal-ceramic bridges were judged hopeless due to extensive crown structure loss and periodontal disease. Conversely, the maxillary implant was affected by a mild peri-implant mucositis with no loss of supporting bone at the threaded portion, and the residual mandibular teeth could be maintained. Therefore, the preliminary treatment plan consisted of full-mouth extractions of all compromised teeth and residual root stumps and nonsurgical periodontal therapy with manual instruments and piezoelectric ultrasonic unit to eliminate plaque and calculus deposits in the remaining natural elements. Nonsurgical therapy of the implant affected by peri-implant mucositis has been performed with Teflon curettes, ultrasonic scaling with polyether ether ketone- (PEEK-) coated scaler tips, and 0.2% chlorhexidine irrigation. Detailed domiciliary oral health instructions and motivation were given to the patient. A temporary complete removable denture was delivered immediately after the extractions.

After a healing period of 3 months, new clinical and radiological examinations by means of orthopantomograph and cone-beam computed tomography scan were conducted to define possible treatment objectives aimed at restoring function and aesthetic. At this point, two different treatment options were discussed with the patient, namely, a removable or a fixed solution. Following explanation of advantages and disadvantages, the patient refused to wear removable prostheses and preferred fixed implant-supported prosthetic rehabilitations with orthodontic alignment of the mandibular teeth followed by additive composite reconstructions. At the acceptance of the treatment plan, signed informed consent was obtained before starting with the multidisciplinary rehabilitation.

The first step consisted in the insertion of 5 implants (AnyOne®, MegaGen Implant Co. Ltd., Daegu, South Korea) in the maxilla. Both clinical and radiographic evaluations showed a narrow edentulous ridge with significant bone resorption in the buccopalatal dimension. After the elevation of a full-thickness flap, implants were placed according to the manufacturer's instructions with an insertion torque of roughly 30 Ncm. The ideal position of the implants was achieved with the aid of a surgical stent based on the preliminary prosthetic wax-up equipped with a 2 mm diameter guiding hole. Implants were located in correspondence with right and left canines, right and left central incisors, and left second premolar. The prosthetically guided insertion resulted in bone dehiscences and fenestrations of the buccal plate around the implants (Figures 2(a) and 2(b)). Hence, guided bone regeneration (GBR) was performed by grafting autogenous bone chips retrieved from the drilling sequence in direct contact with the exposed implant threads (Figure 2(c)) and deproteinized bovine bone mineral particles (Bio-Oss®, Geistlich Biomaterials, Wolhusen, Switzerland) to overcorrect the bone defect (Figures 2(d) and 2(e)). The graft was then covered with double-layer resorbable collagen membranes

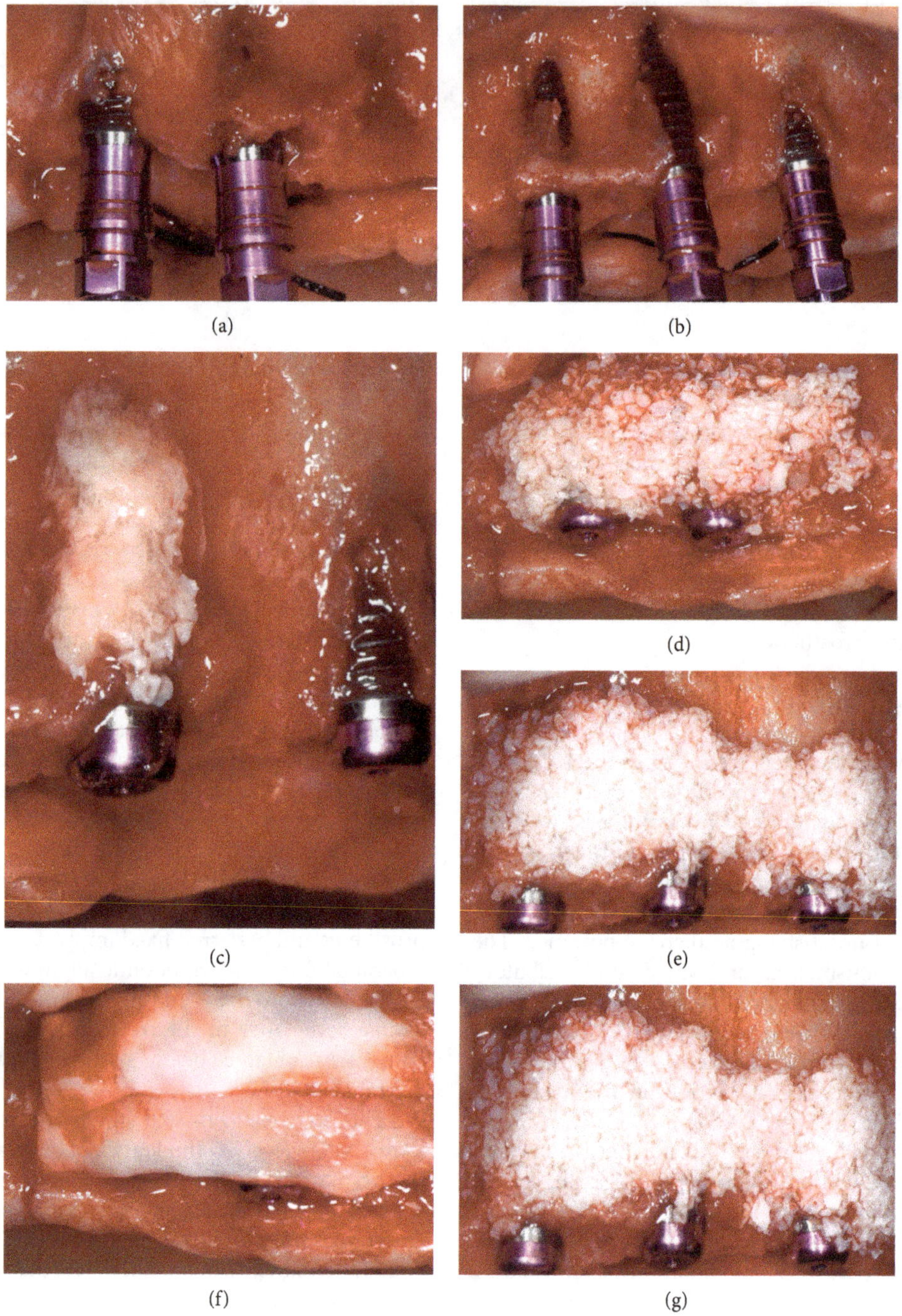

Figure 2: (a, b) Prosthetically guided implant insertion resulting in dehiscences and fenestrations of the buccal bone; (c) autogenous bone particles retrieved from the implant bed preparation in direct contact with the exposed implant threads; (d, e) deproteinized bovine bone particles grafted to overcorrect the bone defect; (f, g) resorbable collagen membranes used with a double-layer technique to cover the graft.

(Bio-Gide®, Geistlich Biomaterials, Wolhusen, Switzerland) to create a secluded space and promote undisturbed healing (Figures 2(f) and 2(g)). In the same surgical session, a lateral antrostomy was performed to access the left maxillary sinus. After careful elevation of the Schneiderian membrane, deproteinized bovine bone mineral particles (Bio-Oss®, Geistlich Biomaterials, Wolhusen, Switzerland) were grafted to complete the maxillary sinus floor elevation. This procedure was performed as a preventive measure allowing placement of an additional implant in case the most distal right fixture would have been lost during the subsequent phases. Following horizontal periosteal releasing incisions of the buccal flap, a tension-free first-intention healing was achieved with 5-0 monofilament nylon suture (Ethilon™, Ethicon Inc., Somerville, NJ, USA).

Almost the same surgical procedure was performed after one month in the mandible. A total of 3 implants (AnyOne®, MegaGen Implant Co. Ltd., Daegu, South Korea) were inserted with a torque of approximately 35 Ncm to replace one premolar and one molar in the right side and one molar

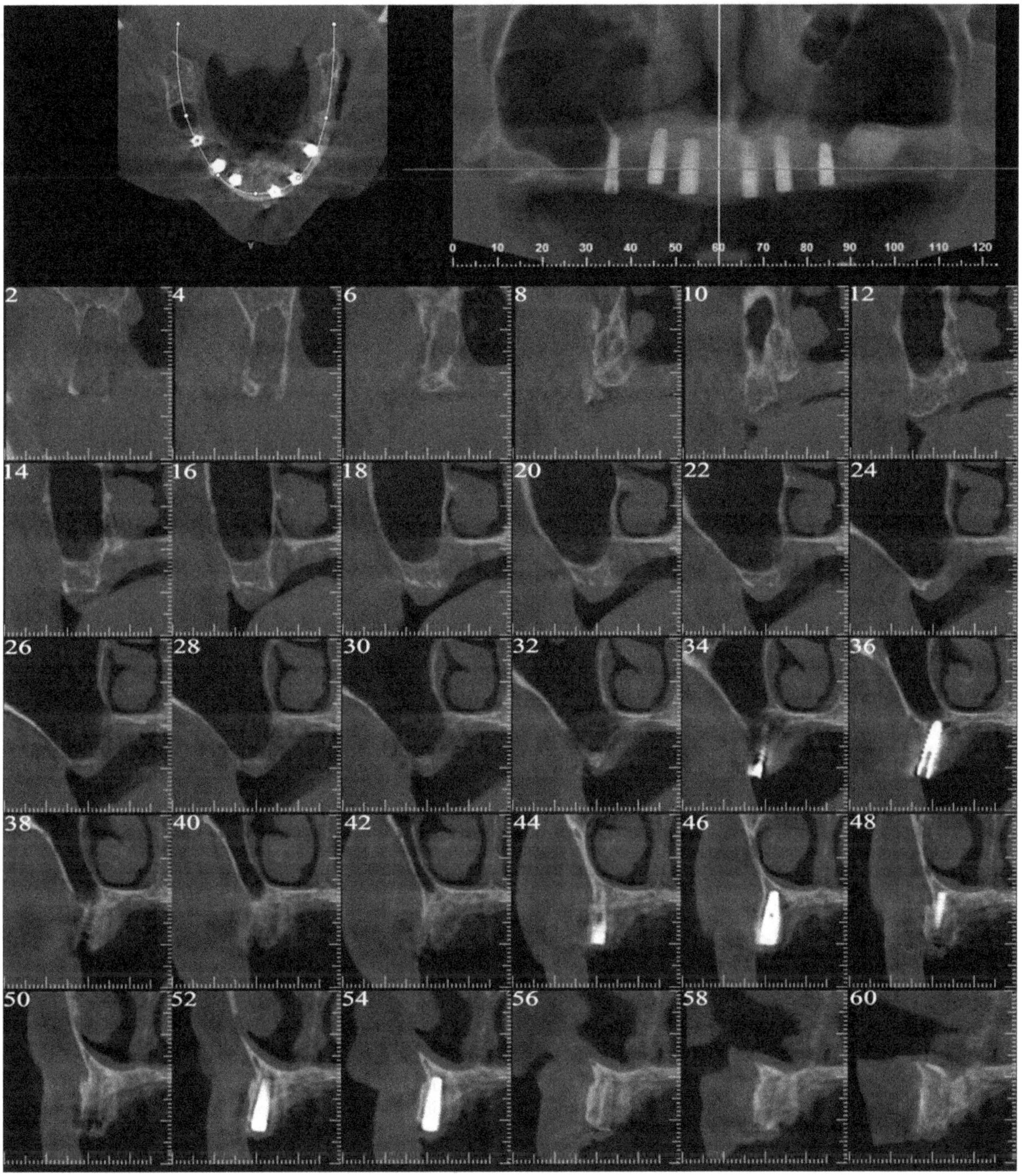

FIGURE 3: Postoperative tomographic scan showing radiopaque regenerated newly formed bone at the buccal aspect of the implants.

in the left side. Bone augmentation procedures were unnecessary in this region due to an adequate amount of bone in both horizontal and vertical dimensions.

The healing proceeded uneventfully, and the reentry surgery was performed to connect the healing abutments after 6 months in the maxilla and 4 months in the mandible. Before the second stage surgery, a tomographic scan of the maxilla was obtained to evaluate the amount of bone regeneration (Figure 3). In the upper jaw, an apically repositioned flap with the crestal incision slightly displaced toward the palatal aspect was carried out to gain keratinized mucosa at the buccal aspect of the implants. The soft tissues around the implant already present in correspondence with the right second premolar were enhanced by means of an epithelialized free-gingival graft harvested from the homolateral hemipalate. With respect to the mandible, a simple crestal incision was performed to split the keratinized mucosa and uncover the implants.

With regard to the pharmacological management of the surgical interventions, the patient was prescribed antibiotics

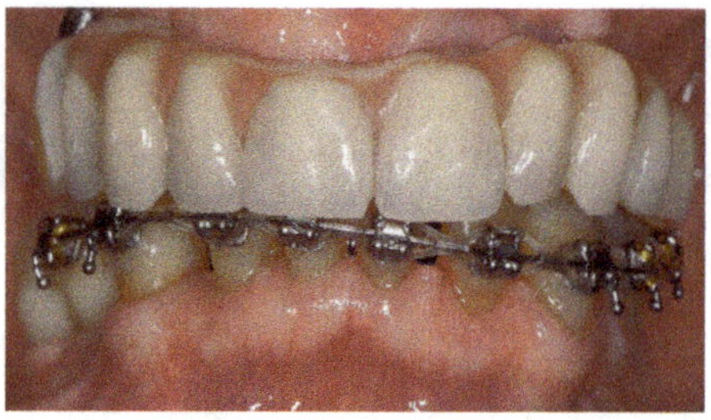

FIGURE 4: Intraoral clinical view of the interim prostheses in situ during the soft tissue conditioning of peri-implant tissues and orthodontic alignment of the lower teeth.

(amoxicillin clavulanate 875/125 mg tablets) to prevent postoperative surgical site infections, nonsteroidal anti-inflammatory drugs (ibuprofen 600 mg effervescent granules) for pain relief, and 0.2% chlorhexidine gluconate oral rinse to reduce the bacterial load. The patient was also instructed to apply ice packs topically for 3 hours postoperatively.

Following the initial adaptation of the soft tissues, impressions were taken to begin with the prosthetic phases. An implant-supported screw-retained fixed temporary prosthesis was delivered in the maxilla, while implant-supported provisional resin crowns were screwed to the mandibular implants for soft tissue conditioning.

The interim prostheses were left in situ for approximately 7 to 8 months to allow proper maturation of the peri-implant soft tissues. During this timeframe, the orthodontist proceeded with the alignment of the lower teeth (Figure 4). The final rehabilitation consisted of definitive implant-supported screw-retained fixed dental prostheses associated with additive composite reconstructions of the mandibular teeth performed by the prosthodontist (Figure 5(a)). The main goals of the treatment were achieved restoring stable and functional occlusion and chewing and speech abilities, together with a pleasant aesthetic.

The patient was enrolled in a regular supportive peri-implant/periodontal therapy consisting of supra- and submucosal biofilm removal at the treated implants using titanium or carbon fibre curettes and ultrasonic devices and professional prophylaxis at residual teeth in association with oral hygiene reinforcement. Recall visits were scheduled every 3 months for the first year and twice a year thereafter.

The follow-up orthopantomograph performed after 2 years showed a radiologically healthy situation characterized by stable peri-implant bone levels and no further bone loss around natural teeth compared to the baseline (Figure 5(b)).

3. Discussion

Loss of teeth affects the function of the stomatognathic system, particularly if left untreated over an extended period of time. Edentulism not only affects the adjacent teeth that may move undesirably or the opposing teeth that tend to extrude. It has been demonstrated that dimensional ridge resorption inevitably occurs following tooth loss [4, 5]. Advanced resorption of the alveolar bone associated with the physiological pneumatization of the maxillary sinus may preclude proper insertion of dental implants to replace missing teeth. Bone atrophy associated with long-standing malocclusion leads to a decline in masticatory and speech function, compromises the aesthetic appearance, renders the management of oral hygiene more difficult, and becomes a risk factor in the development of periodontal disease.

Such a progressive decay has been well represented by the case reported herein. A partially edentulous patient with atrophic edentulous ridges presented with an extremely compromised residual dentition, generalized chronic periodontitis, impaired function, and unpleasant aesthetic appearance.

The initial aim was to extract the hopeless teeth, bearing in mind that teeth even compromised because of periodontal disease or endodontic problems may have a longevity that surpasses by far that of the average implant [6]. Thus, any nonextractive treatment that is aimed primarily at dental element preservation has been considered before tooth extractions.

At the same time, periodontal disease had to be controlled on the remaining dentition before implant insertion. This is of paramount importance, since patients diagnosed or with a history of periodontitis have a higher risk of developing peri-implantitis than healthy subjects [7]. In patients with a history of periodontitis, putative periodontal pathogens appear to predominate in the microbiome of diseased peri-implant tissues, which confirms previous observations of periodontitis-associated species in deepened pockets around implants [8]. To strengthen the association between periodontitis and peri-implantitis, culture techniques have suggested that the microflora present in the oral cavity before implantation determines the composition of the newly establishing microflora on implants [9]. Given that natural teeth may act as a reservoir for pathogens colonizing implants, and patients with a history of periodontitis are at higher risk to develop peri-implantitis, an initial nonsurgical periodontal therapy has been performed before implant insertion. In the present case, active nonsurgical periodontal therapy consisted of meticulous supra- and subgingival scaling and root planing of all teeth involved by means of ultrasonic and hand instruments. According to the present case, in patients with adult periodontitis, active nonsurgical periodontal therapy yielded effective results, particularly in the case of single-rooted front teeth and premolars [10]. As a result, the patient treated herein showed no residual bleeding on probing and probing pocket depths < 5 mm around the remaining teeth before implantation. The combination of amoxicillin-metronidazole has demonstrated synergic effects, and it has been recommended as an adjuvant to nonsurgical periodontal treatment in the management of periodontitis. However, adjunctive systemic antibiotics shall only be considered according to the severity and extent of the disease. In compliance with recent recommendations, in the present case, antibiotics were not prescribed because the patient is aged >56 years and showed probing depths > 4 mm in less than 35% of sites [11].

At this point, implant insertion was needed to replace the missing teeth according to the patient's wishes. It is needless to say that an adequate amount of bone volume is mandatory at the recipient site to obtain predictable functional and aesthetic results. In reconstructed atrophic ridges,

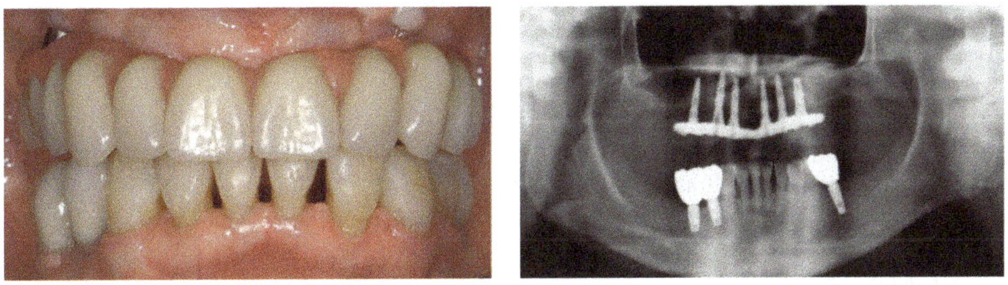

(a) (b)

Figure 5: (a) Maxillary and mandibular definitive implant-supported screw-retained fixed dental prostheses associated with additive composite reconstructions of the mandibular teeth; (b) follow-up orthopantomograph performed 2 years after the conclusion of the multidisciplinary treatment.

dental implant rehabilitations provided encouraging survival rates on the long term [12, 13]. Amongst the techniques used to augment resorbed edentulous sites, implants placed in association with GBR procedures presented safe and predictable long-term clinical results [14]. In brief, as performed in the present clinical case, bone regeneration is achieved by promoting the repopulation of solely slower-growing osteoprogenitor cells into the bone defect. Barrier membranes are therefore used to prevent the migration of rapidly proliferating epithelium and connective tissue cells and other non-osteogenic tissues into the site to be augmented. By exploiting the barrier function of the membrane, undisturbed new bone formation can occur inside a secluded compartment starting from the surface of the pristine bone [15, 16]. According to modern concepts, implants should be inserted in the ideal position in bone augmented so as to closely match and fully support the rehabilitation plan. In this way, the original concept of restoration-driven implant placement is combined with modern prosthetically guided bone regeneration aimed at following the prosthetic needs in order to achieve the anticipated treatment outcome. In the present case, due to the centripetal and apical resorption pattern of the maxillary alveolar bone, the maxillary osseous base was internal to the tooth position. For such reason, in the present case, GBR procedures were performed in conjunction with prosthetically driven implant insertion to augment horizontally the supporting bone on the buccal aspect of the implants. The outcome of the horizontal augmentation was clearly visible in the 6-month computed tomography scan showing mineralized newly formed bone buccal to the implants.

The management of the soft tissues is a key issue that should not be underestimated. Although there is no consensus available that identifies the absence of keratinized mucosa as a risk factor for peri-implantitis [17], emerging evidence suggests that a reduced width of keratinized tissue around dental implants might be considered a risk indicator for severity of peri-implant mucositis [18]. The fact that peri-implant mucositis is considered to be the precursor of peri-implantitis supports the finding that the absence of keratinized tissue is strongly associated with peri-implant lesions [19]. For such reasons, in the present case, soft tissue augmentation procedures have been performed to improve the quality of peri-implant soft tissues and to increase the width of keratinized mucosa around the implants. It is worth mentioning that both apically positioned flap and autogenous soft tissue grafts result in more favourable peri-implant health in terms of gingival index values and marginal bone level stability [20].

The present report emphasizes the importance of a multidisciplinary approach required for comprehensive care and optimal posttreatment functional and aesthetic outcomes. A thorough knowledge of the relationship between the bone morphology, the periodontal and peri-implant soft tissues, and the three-dimensional position of teeth and implants, with the aid of restorative and prosthetic dentistry, is essential to obtain a good result based on an individualized patient-centred treatment plan.

References

[1] S. Shaghaghian, M. Taghva, J. Abduo, and R. Bagheri, "Oral health-related quality of life of removable partial denture wearers and related factors," *Journal of Oral Rehabilitation*, vol. 42, no. 1, pp. 40–48, 2015.

[2] M. Sanchez-Siles, J. F. Ballester-Ferrandis, N. Salazar-Sanchez, F. J. Gomez-Garcia, R. Moraleja-Ruiz, and F. Camacho-Alonso, "Long-term evaluation of quality of life and satisfaction between implant bar overdentures and conventional complete dentures: a 23 years retrospective study," *Clinical Implant Dentistry and Related Research*, vol. 20, no. 2, pp. 208–214, 2018.

[3] World Health Organization, *International Classification of Functioning, Disability and Health (ICF)*, World Health Organization, Geneva, Switzerland, 2001.

[4] C. Maiorana, P. P. Poli, M. Deflorian et al., "Alveolar socket preservation with demineralised bovine bone mineral and a collagen matrix," *Journal of Periodontal & Implant Science*, vol. 47, no. 4, pp. 194–210, 2017.

[5] V. Natale Junior, F. A. Souza, E. Vedovatto, R. S. Nishioka, P. P. Poli, and P. S. P. de Carvalho, "Preservation of dental sockets filled with composite bovine bone. A single-blind randomized clinical trial," *Brazilian Dental Journal*, vol. 29, no. 6, pp. 583–591, 2018.

[6] W. V. Giannobile and N. P. Lang, "Are dental implants a panacea or should we better strive to save teeth?," *Journal of Dental Research*, vol. 95, no. 1, pp. 5-6, 2016.

[7] S. D. Ferreira, C. C. Martins, S. A. Amaral et al., "Periodontitis as a risk factor for peri-implantitis: systematic review and meta-analysis of observational studies," *Journal of Dentistry*, vol. 79, pp. 1–10, 2018.

[8] D. Apatzidou, D. F. Lappin, G. Hamilton, C. A. Papadopoulos, A. Konstantinidis, and M. P. Riggio, "Microbiome of peri-implantitis affected and healthy dental sites in patients with a history of chronic periodontitis," *Archives of Oral Biology*, vol. 83, pp. 145–152, 2017.

[9] A. Mombelli, M. Marxer, T. Gaberthüel, U. Grander, and N. P. Lang, "The microbiota of osseointegrated implants in patients with a history of periodontal disease," *Journal of Clinical Periodontology*, vol. 22, no. 2, pp. 124–130, 1995.

[10] G. A. Van der Weijden (Fridus), G. J. Dekkers, and D. E. Slot, "Success of non-surgical periodontal therapy in adult periodontitis patients-a retrospective analysis," *International Journal of Dental Hygiene*, vol. 17, no. 4, pp. 309–317, 2019.

[11] B. Pretzl, S. Sälzer, B. Ehmke et al., "Administration of systemic antibiotics during non-surgical periodontal therapy-a consensus report," *Clinical Oral Investigations*, vol. 23, no. 7, pp. 3073–3085, 2018.

[12] C. Maiorana, P. P. Poli, A. E. Borgonovo et al., "Long-term retrospective evaluation of dental implants placed in resorbed jaws reconstructed with appositional fresh-frozen bone allografts," *Implant Dentistry*, vol. 25, no. 3, pp. 400–408, 2016.

[13] C. Maiorana, P. P. Poli, A. Mascellaro, S. Ferrario, and M. Beretta, "Dental implants placed in resorbed alveolar ridges reconstructed with iliac crest autogenous onlay grafts: a 26-year median follow-up retrospective study," *Journal of Cranio-Maxillo-Facial Surgery*, vol. 47, no. 5, pp. 805–814, 2019.

[14] M. Beretta, M. Cicciù, P. P. Poli et al., "A retrospective evaluation of 192 implants placed in augmented bone: long-term follow-up study," *The Journal of Oral Implantology*, vol. 41, no. 6, pp. 669–674, 2015.

[15] C. Dahlin, A. Linde, J. Gottlow, and S. Nyman, "Healing of bone defects by guided tissue regeneration," *Plastic and Reconstructive Surgery*, vol. 81, no. 5, pp. 672–676, 1988.

[16] C. Dahlin, L. Sennerby, U. Lekholm, A. Linde, and S. Nyman, "Generation of new bone around titanium implants using a membrane technique: an experimental study in rabbits," *The International Journal of Oral & Maxillofacial Implants*, vol. 4, no. 1, pp. 19–25, 1989.

[17] H. Dreyer, J. Grischke, C. Tiede et al., "Epidemiology and risk factors of peri-implantitis: a systematic review," *Journal of Periodontal Research*, vol. 53, no. 5, pp. 657–681, 2018.

[18] J. Grischke, A. Karch, A. Wenzlaff, M. M. Foitzik, M. Stiesch, and J. Eberhard, "Keratinized mucosa width is associated with severity of peri-implant mucositis. A cross-sectional study," *Clinical Oral Implants Research*, vol. 30, no. 5, pp. 457–465, 2019.

[19] P. P. Poli, M. Beretta, G. B. Grossi, and C. Maiorana, "Risk indicators related to peri-implant disease: an observational retrospective cohort study," *Journal of Periodontal & Implant Science*, vol. 46, no. 4, pp. 266–276, 2016.

[20] D. S. Thoma, N. Naenni, E. Figuero et al., "Effects of soft tissue augmentation procedures on peri-implant health or disease: a systematic review and meta-analysis," *Clinical Oral Implants Research*, vol. 29, pp. 32–49, 2018.

7

Metastatic Carcinoma of the Breast Presenting as Gingival Swelling in the Maxilla: A Case Report

Arun Sadasivan,[1] K. Rakul Nambiar,[2] Deepu George Mathew,[3] Elizabeth Koshi,[1] Roshni Ramesh,[4] and Ashna Mariya Benny[1]

[1]*Department of Periodontics, Sree Mookambika Institute of Dental Sciences, Kulashekaram, Tamil Nadu, India*
[2]*Sree Mookambika Cancer Centre, Kulasekharam, Tamil Nadu 629161, India*
[3]*Department of Oral and Maxillofacial Pathology, Annoor Dental College, Muvatupuzha, Kerala, India*
[4]*Department of Periodontics, Government Dental College, Trivandrum, Kerala, India*

Correspondence should be addressed to Arun Sadasivan; sadasivan_arun@hotmail.com

Academic Editor: Pia L. Jornet

Background. Metastatic cancers in the oral cavity are usually very rare and are usually an indication of widespread malignancy. In some cases, oral metastasis was found to be the first presentation of distant site tumours. Even though oral metastatic lesions may be found anywhere in the oral cavity, they commonly present in the posterior areas of the jaw bones. Among the soft tissues, the gingiva is the most common site. The presence of inflammation in the gingiva and the role of periodontal microbiota are suggested to play a role in the attraction of metastatic cells. The purpose of this case report is to present a rare case of metastatic breast carcinoma presenting as a gingival enlargement in the maxillary anterior region. *Case Presentation.* A 37-year-old female patient who underwent modified radical mastectomy for invasive ductal breast carcinoma reported to the dental clinic with a gingival enlargement in the anterior maxillary region. Clinical and radiographic examination showed a rapidly enlarging gingival lesion with destruction of the underlying bone. A wide excision of the entire lesion was done. Histopathological and immunohistochemical (IHC) evaluations were suggestive of infiltrating poorly differentiated adenocarcinoma. *Conclusion.* This case report presents a metastatic oral lesion in the maxillary anterior region of the primary breast cancer site. The young age of patient and an uncommon site of metastatic lesion are the striking features of this case. We would like to highlight the importance of a thorough clinical, radiological, and histological evaluation of any gingival swelling as it could be a metastatic lesion. IHC staining helps in the diagnosis of the primary site of metastatic carcinomas. An early diagnosis and intervention could reduce the morbidity of the lesion and improve the survival rate.

1. Introduction

Metastatic cancers in the oral cavity are a rare occurrence and represent less than 1% of all malignancies reported in the oral cavity [1]. The most common metastatic malignancies in women are from primary tumours in the thyroid glands, breast, colorectal region, kidneys, and genital organs [2]. Breast cancer is one of the most common malignancies affecting females. It does have a wide metastatic pattern, the most commonly reported includes those in the lungs, lymph nodes, bone, pleura, and liver [3].

Oral metastatic lesions have been more frequently reported in the mandible rather than the maxilla, with a site predilection for the posterior areas of the mandible. The presence of hematopoietic bone marrow, multiple blood vessel branching, and slow flow of blood have been speculated as reasons for the site predilection [4]. Clinically, oral metastases often present as areas of inflammation, pain, paraesthesia, or swelling. They may often be misdiagnosed as giant cell granulomas, pyogenic granulomas, bone cysts, osteomyelitis, Paget's disease, and fibrous epulis among the differential diagnoses [5]. Only about 33% of oral metastatic lesions are found in the soft tissues, with the lung being reported as the most common source [4]. In soft tissues, the attached gingiva, alveolar mucosa, and the tongue are said to be the most common sites for metastasis [6]. In a study by Allon et al. in 2014 demonstrated a significant association between the presence of teeth and gingival metastatic lesions. In the presence of teeth, 80% of the patients had gingival metastases compared to one-third of the edentulous patients [7]. Hirshberg et al. in 1993 have suggested an important role for inflammation in attracting metastatic tumour cells to the gingiva [4]. Gingival metastatic lesions typically present as highly vascular exophytic lesions, which strongly resemble reactive or hyperplastic lesions such as fibroma, pyogenic granulomas, peripheral giant cell granulomas or fibrous epulis [7, 8]. Akheel et al. in 2013 have reported that in about 25% of cases, oral lesions are found to be the first sign of metastatic spread and in 23% of cases; oral metastatic lesions could be an indication of an unidentified primary tumour at a distant site [9].

Most often, metastases to the oral cavity occur in the end stages of cancer lesions and cause severe morbidity to the patients. This is often considered as a sign of widespread cancer and is an indicator of poor prognosis, with a 5-year survival rate below 5% [6]. Due to these reasons, it is important to detect oral metastases early. They need to be considered in the differential diagnosis of inflammatory and reactive lesions of the gingiva [4]. In this case report, we describe a case of gingival metastasis from invasive ductal carcinoma of the breast, which occurred 9 months after detection of breast cancer.

2. Case Presentation

A 37-year-old female patient reported to the Department of Periodontics, Sree Mookambika Institute of Dental Sciences, Kulashekaram, Tamil Nadu, India, with a chief complaint of swelling of gums in the upper front tooth region. The medical history revealed that the patient reported to the hospital 9 months back as she felt a lump on her left breast. An incision biopsy was done and was pathologically diagnosed as invasive ductal carcinoma of histological grade II. Modified radical mastectomy (lumpectomy with axillary clearance) was done to remove the lump and involved axillary lymph nodes (levels I and II). Following the surgical removal, the patient was advised to start a course of radiotherapy and chemotherapy. The patient delayed the treatment by one month and later reported to the hospital with a complaint of memory loss, following which a positron emission tomography (PET) scan was done which showed the presence of brain metastasis. Palliative whole brain radiotherapy of 3000 cGy was administered, divided into 10 fractions. While on radiation treatment, the patient presented with multiple flaccid blisters, erythematous erosions spread throughout the body and was diagnosed as Steven Johnson syndrome (probably anti-epileptic drug induced) and this was managed conservatively. The patient was then started on chemotherapy 14 days later with paclitaxel. During chemotherapy, the patient developed a swelling of the gums which was symptomatic and hence was referred to the Periodontics department for further management. The swelling occurred 9 months after the initial breast swelling was noticed.

On intra-oral clinical examination, a dumbbell-shaped swelling of the gums was seen extending from the buccal aspect through the interdental space to the palatal aspect in the upper maxillary teeth (between 11 and 21). The swelling on the buccal aspect appeared smooth and shiny, while the palatal swelling had a more irregular surface. The swelling was reddish pink in color. The dimension of the buccal swelling was 16 mm × 11 mm and the palatal swelling was 13 × 12 mm approximately (Figures 1(a) and 1(b)). The patient reported that the swelling was initially small and grew at a rapid rate to the current size within a span of 2 weeks, causing an increase in space between the central incisors. The patient also had a history of occasional pain and bleeding from the palatal side of the swelling. Plaque and calculus deposits were present with generalized gingival inflammation. On general examination, the patient presented with cancer cell deposits, presenting as a painless nodular swelling with a central necrotic crust on the tip of the middle finger of the right hand involving the fingernail, chin, scalp, and the upper arm (Figure 2).

Radiographic analysis was done to check for bony involvement and periapical radiographs showed bone loss extending beyond the middle third of the root in relation to 11 and 21. Cone beam computed tomography (CBCT) evaluation revealed that the height of maximum bone loss in the mid-alveolus region of 11 and 21 measured about 10.80 mm (Figures 1(c) and 1(d)). A panoramic radiograph was also taken to rule out the presence of other lytic bony lesions involving the jaw bones. Prior to surgery, routine hematological investigations were done and the reports showed that the blood parameters were just above the normal range.

A wide excision of the lesion was planned to remove the entire swelling with a 2 mm margin of healthy tissue using a 15c blade. On the removal of the lesion, the exposed underlying bone showed a moth-eaten appearance, which is characteristic of lytic lesions of the bone (Figure 3). The large defect was sealed with a gelatin sponge, sutures were given, and a periodontal dressing was placed to shield the surgical site. The patient was prescribed antibiotics and analgesics. Post-operative review after 3 months revealed satisfactory healing of the wound.

Histopathology of the hematoxylin and eosin-stained soft tissue section showed an atrophic ulcerated stratified squamous epithelium in association with a fibrovascular connective tissue. The connective tissue showed infiltrating solid islands of malignant epithelial tumour cells arranged in groups and clusters. The tumour cells were polygonal with eosinophilic cytoplasm and open-faced nuclei. Cells have pleomorphic hyperchromatic nuclei. The tumour cells showed numerous mitotic figures. Some of the dysplastic islands showed central necrosis resembling comedonecrosis. Focal areas of the tumour cells showed cytoplasmic clearing. The associated connective tissue was fibrovascular and scanty. The histopathological features were suggestive of infiltrating poorly differentiated adenocarcinoma (Figure 4). The tissue specimens were sent for immunohistochemistry (IHC) for confirmatory diagnosis. IHC evaluation showed that tumour cells were positive for cytokeratin (Pan CK)

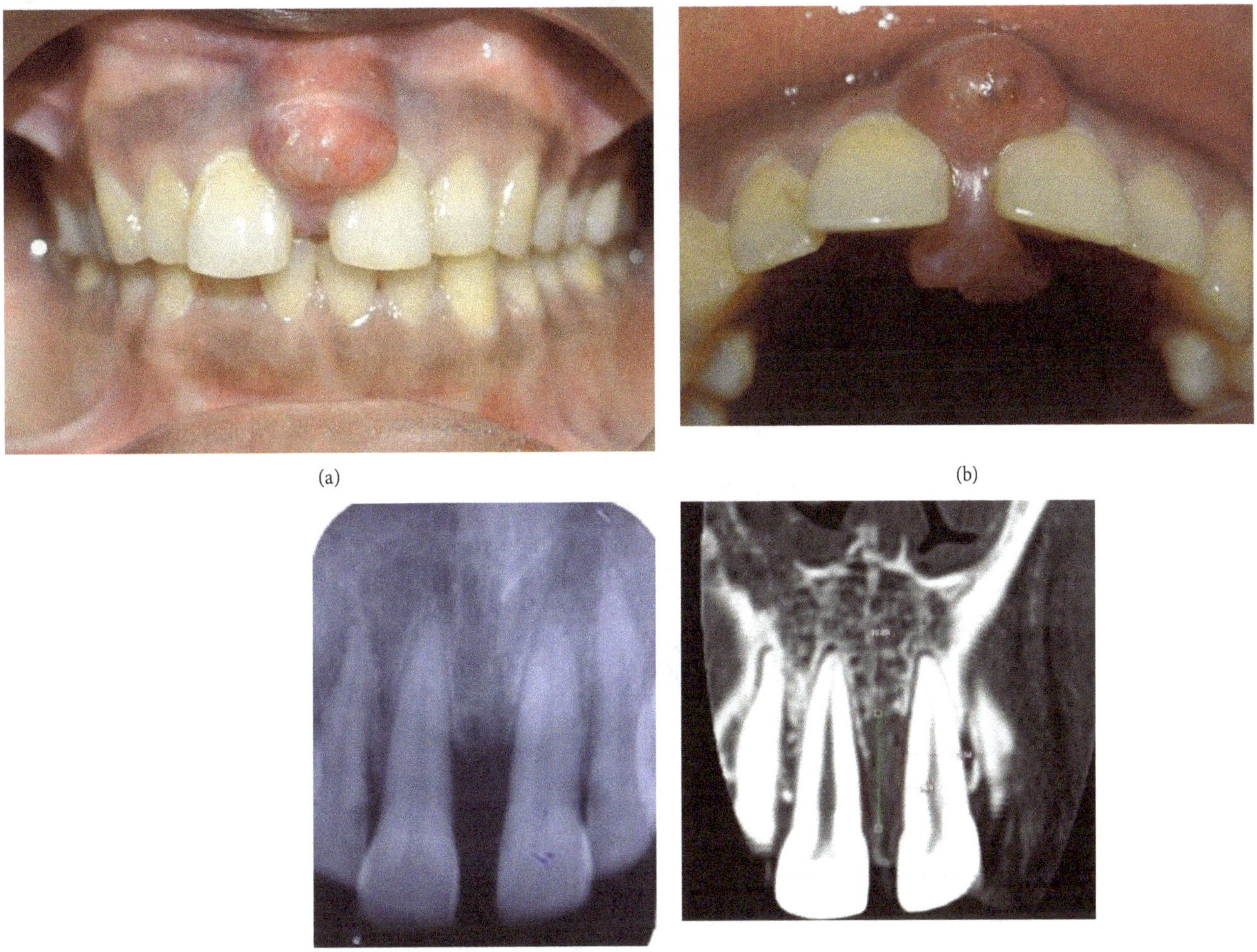

(a) (b) (c) (d)

FIGURE 1: (a) and (b) Dumbbell-shaped swelling involving the buccal and palatal aspect. (c) Intra-oral peri-apical radiograph showing interdental bone loss between maxillary central incisors; (d) CBCT showing bone loss in the mid-alveolus region.

and specifically for CK7 while showing negative results for oestrogen receptor (ER), human epidermal growth factor receptor (HER)-2, GATA binding protein (GATA) 3, and thyroid transcription factor (TTF)1.

After excision of the gingival enlargement, a PET scan was done which revealed extensive Fluorodeoxyglucose (FDG) avid metastases in the brain, lung, liver, pancreas, nodes, subcutaneous and intramuscular soft tissue nodules, and sacrum (Figure 5). FDG avid lesions in both breasts were also seen. Compared with the previous PET-CT, the reports suggested progression of the disease. The patient was started on chemotherapy—Eribulin in view of disease progression. Unfortunately, fourteen months after the detection of the primary breast cancer tumour the patient passed away.

3. Discussion

Metastasis is said to represent the end stage of the invasion cascade, it includes the dissemination of tumour cells to distant organ sites and their adaptation to foreign tissue microenvironment [7]. Kwon et al. in 2006 described three criteria for the diagnosis of a metastatic tumour as (1) histological verification of the primary tumour, (2) the metastatic tumour and primary tumour must possess histological similarity, (3) exclusion of the possibility of direct spread from the primary tumour [10]. Hirshberg et al. in 2014 have described that a metastatic colony is due to a process known as the 'invasion-metastasis cascade'. This involves a series of sequential steps including invasion through the surrounding extracellular matrix of the primary site, intravasation into the blood vessels, and the survival of circulating tumour cells (CTC) in circulation. The CTCs settle in the microvasculature of the target tissues and extravasate through the vessel wall. The cancer cells then reinitiate their proliferative properties at the target site leading to the formation of clinically detectable neoplastic lesions [11]. Metastasis to distant organs depends on the site and tissue-specific activities. It is now speculated that for a successful metastasis to occur, it needs a pre-metastatic niche, which allows the invading tumour cells to colonize, survive, and expand to form a macro-metastasis [12]. For men, the most common primary sites are the prostate, lung, liver, and kidney. For women, the most common primary sites

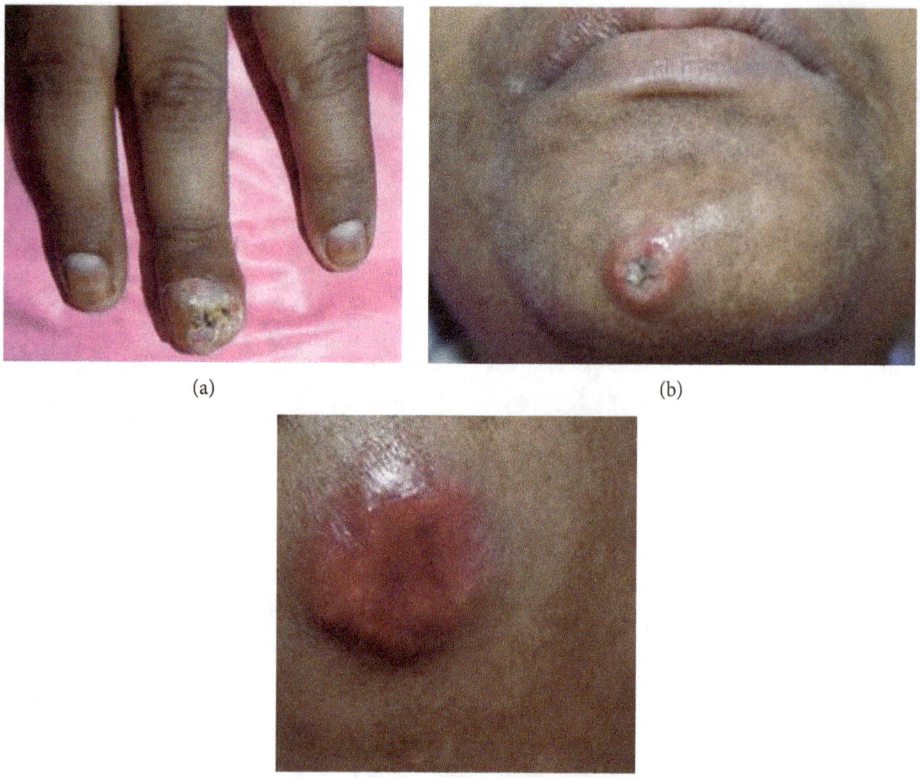

(a) (b) (c)

FIGURE 2: (a) Distal phalanx lesion on the third digit of the right hand. (b) and (c) Lesion with central necrotic crust involving the chin and forearm.

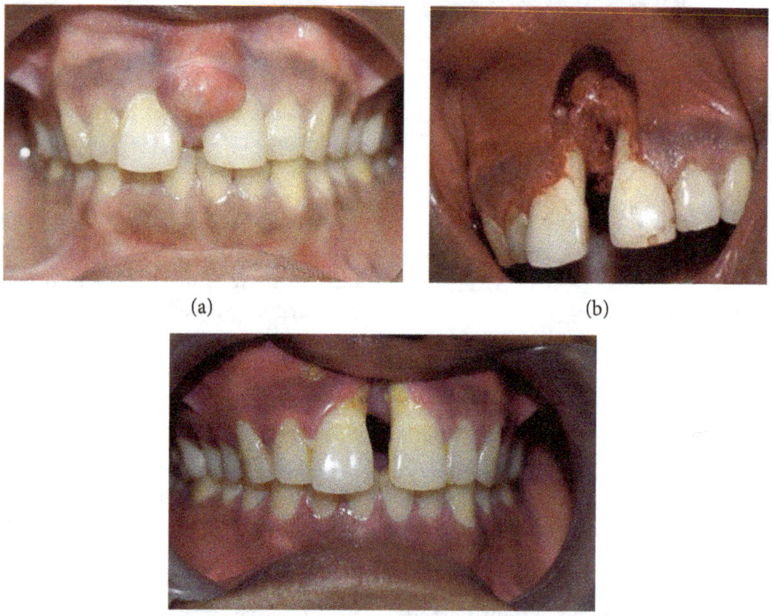

(a) (b) (c)

FIGURE 3: (a) Pre-operative view of growth. (b) Immediate post-operative view after excision of the lesion. (c) 3 months post-operative view.

are the breast, kidney, female genital organs, and colorectum [13]. Reports suggest that prostate and breast cancers usually metastasize to the jaw bones, while oral soft tissue metastases are frequently seen in lung carcinomas. Retrospective studies have reported a male predilection over females in metastases in the oral region [14]. Most of the patients presenting with oral cavity metastases are in the age group between 50 and 70 years, although variations in

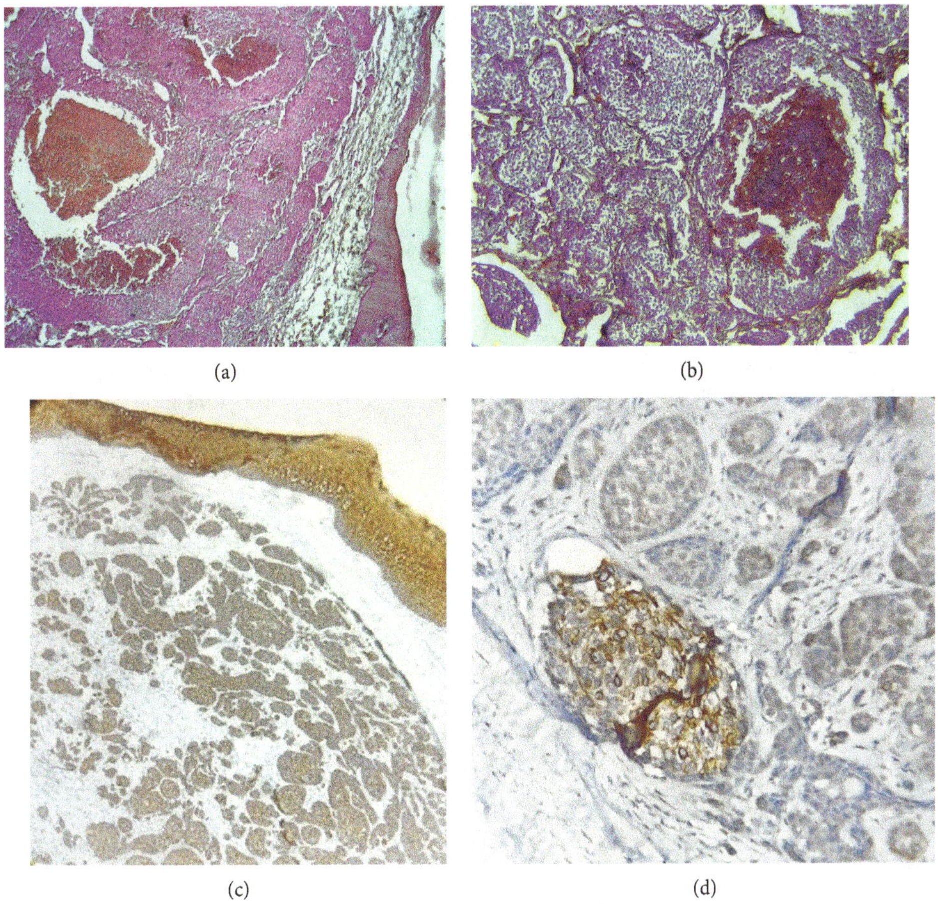

FIGURE 4: (a) Scanner view showing cohesive islands of tumour epithelial islands separated from the overlying surface epithelium by a grenz zone. Some tumour islands show central necrosis (4×); (b) Low power view shows cohesive islands of tumour epithelial islands and some tumour islands show central necrosis. (10×). (c) The surface epithelium and infiltrating epithelial tumour islands in the connective tissue were positive for Pan CK (4×). (d) IHC showing positive CK7 staining.

age have been reported [6]. However, in our case, the patient was only 37 years old.

Invasive ductal carcinoma is the most common form of breast cancer and accounts for 50–70% of invasive breast cancers [15]. Irani in 2016, in a review of 412 metastatic lesions that occurred in oral soft tissues, showed that gingiva was the most common site for metastases. The possible routes of oral metastasis include arterial, lymphatic, circulation, venous, and Batson's plexus. The majority of gingival metastases were reported in posterior areas. Anterior gingival metastases were seen only in 3.9% of cases [16]. In our case, the metastatic lesion was seen in the maxillary anterior region; a site that has not been commonly reported in the literature.

Allon et al. in 2014 have reported that in the soft tissues of the oral cavity, about 60% of the metastatic lesions are found in the attached gingiva followed by the tongue (18%). They also reported that in the presence of teeth, 80% of patients had metastasis in the gingiva when compared with one-third of edentulous patients [7]. The presence of inflammation in conditions such as gingivitis and periodontitis is speculated to be the critical factor regulating metastasis. Inflammation in the gingiva leads to vascular network proliferation as well as destruction of the basement membrane, which could attract metastatic cells [17]. There is growing evidence of the role of gingival inflammation acting as a cofactor in attracting metastatic tumour cells and resulting in gingival metastatic lesions. Spano and Zollo in 2012 have suggested a metastatic niche model, which suggests that it is necessary for the presence of a suitably conducive microenvironment referred to as the pre-metastatic niche for tumour cells to invade and proliferate at secondary sites [18]. There has been speculation on the role of gingival inflammation in the dissemination of gingival metastasis. Chronically inflamed gingiva may provide a suitable niche for metastatic tumour cells to colonize and proliferate [7]. The inflamed gingiva provides a permissive niche for metastatic tumour cells, which favours angiogenesis, immune evasion, and formation of a supporting stroma [19]. Periodontal disease results in the release of proinflammatory cytokines such as interleukin 1 (IL-1) and tumour necrosis factor α (TNF-α) which stimulate angiogenesis and formation of extracellular matrix, which facilitates metastatic progression. The cytokines may also induce or attract tumour-associated macrophages [20].

The involvement of the gingiva and underlying bone in metastatic lesions is an area of controversy. It remains

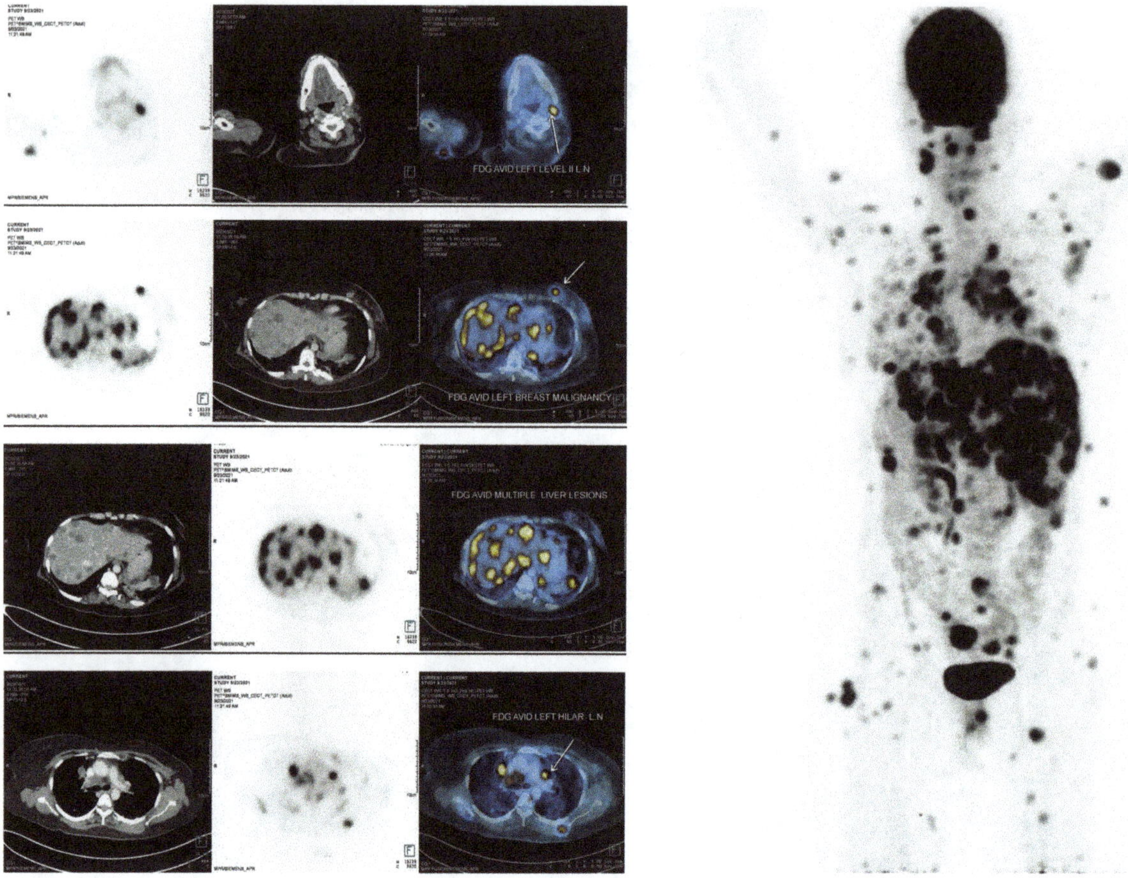

FIGURE 5: PET scan images showing extensive FDG avid metastases all over the body.

unclear whether cancer cells initially metastasize to the gingiva or whether it is a bone metastasis, which subsequently involves the gingiva or whether the patient develops both metastases simultaneously [21]. In our case, the clinical presentation was that of a gingival swelling which on surgical excision revealed underlying bone destruction.

It is clinically difficult to distinguish between gingival metastatic lesions and benign lesions. Some of the benign inflammatory lesions include gingival hyperplasia, fibrous epulis, and pyogenic granuloma. However, malignancy needs to be suspected if there is a definitive diagnosis of a primary tumour elsewhere in the body. Other clinical presentations for suspecting a malignant lesion could be a rapid rate of gingival overgrowth, abnormal bleeding tendency, and unexplained rapid changes in occlusion. Gingival metastatic lesions may cause progressive pain, discomfort, bleeding, superinfection, interference with mastication, dysphagia, and disfigurement [13]. It is therefore mandatory to perform a biopsy of any suspicious overgrowth. The histopathological features in our case were suggestive of infiltrating poorly differentiated adenocarcinoma.

To recognize a lesion as a metastasis, it is important to differentiate between primary intra-oral malignancies from a metastatic tumour. Soft tissue malignant tumours rarely originate intra-orally and therefore should be worked up as a metastatic lesion rather than a primary tumour. Immunohistochemical (IHC) phenotyping of metastatic tumour cells is now considered helpful in determining the site of the primary tumour [22]. If the patient presents with a history of cancer, it is important that the histopathological features of the metastatic lesion should be compared with those of the primary tumour. Special staining techniques like IHC can be helpful in identifying the nature of the lesion. Lesimple et al. in 2003 have given clinical practical guidelines for the diagnosis of carcinomas of an unknown primary site in which they mentioned an initial IHC panel, which includes antibodies against epithelial antigens (broad spectrum anti-pan-cytokeratin antibody cocktail), lymphoid antigen (CD 45/CD20/CD3) and melanocyte-differentiation antigens (S100, SOX 10) [23]. IHC is used to distinguish three histopathological subtypes among carcinoma metastases: (1) adenocarcinoma (in about 50% of cases), (2) poorly differentiated carcinoma (in about 30% of cases), and (3) squamous cell carcinoma (in about 15% of cases). Based on the expression profiles of CK7 and CK20, different subsets of carcinomas have been defined [24]. Studies have shown that the different expression patterns of CK (7 and 20) are among the most discriminant markers in the differential diagnosis of breast adenocarcinoma. The additional markers include ER/PR, GCDFP-15, and mammaglobin [25]. A detailed mapping of cytokeratin 20 (CK20) and cytokeratin 7 (CK7) profiles will help in directing the clinical investigations in most of the common types of adenocarcinomas [26]. The majority of oral metastatic tumours are of epithelial origin with adenocarcinoma being the most common type [4]. Among the breast cancers, adenocarcinoma is said to be one of the most common sources of distant metastases.

Several studies have shown that the $CK20^-/CK7^+$ immunophenotype are typical for breast carcinomas. Malzahn et al. in 1998 have evaluated the cytokine profiles in a series of 101 Ductal breast carcinomas. They have reported only three $CK20^+$ cases, all of which were poorly differentiated, whereas the majority of the tumours were $CK7^+$ [27]. Tibor Tot in 1999, in a study of 123 invasive breast carcinomas, 92% metastases showed to be CK 20 negative while 98% of the tumours were CK7 positive [28]. The diagnostic workflow suggests that once the CK7/CK20 expression profile is detected, complementary organ-specific antibody studies will allow precise guidance towards the primary origin of the tumour. Mhawech-Fauceglia et al. in 2012 have mentioned that the most classical IHC markers that can be used to identify the adenocarcinoma of unknown origin along with $CK7^+/CK20^-$ profile are thyroid transcription factor (TTF) 1, GATA binding protein (GATA) 3, paired box gene (PAX) 8, and Wilms Tumour (WT) 1 [29].

If the primary site of origin of tumour is the breast and with expression of $CK7^+/CK20^-$ profiles, IHC tumour staining patterns include oestrogen receptor (ER)+/Progesterone receptor $(PgR)^+$, GATA binding protein (GATA) 3^+, gross cystic disease fluid protein (GCDFP) $15^{-/+}$, mammaglobin $(MGB)^{+/-}$, thyroid transcription factor (TFF) 1^- [30]. In our case, IHC evaluation showed that tumour cells are positive for CK7 and negative for CK20. The cells were also negative for ER, Her-2, GATA 3 and TTF1. Janick Selves has reported in his article that around 5% of metastatic tumours especially poorly differentiated ones will not provide the clues to its origin during IHC investigations. They have also reported that some tumour-specific antibodies may show a less intense signal or no signal at metastatic sites [31]. In our case we had an identifiable primary site with metastatic deposits showing histologic features resembling ductal carcinoma and correlating with the IHC findings, a diagnosis of metastasizing poorly differentiated adenocarcinoma of the breast was made.

Metastatic tumours in the oral cavity do not usually present typical pathognomonic radiographic appearances. Most often, osteolytic changes with ill-defined and irregular margins may be seen. In the present case, there was a solitary gingival enlargement in the maxillary anterior region, radiographic evidence of bone loss was seen, which was clinically confirmed after excision of the lesion. In the majority of the oral metastatic tumours reported in the literature, there is a known primary tumour, which has been diagnosed. In our patient, breast cancer was the primary tumour and multiple metastatic lesions were present throughout the body. However, in some patients the oral lesions may be the first presentation with the primary tumour being unknown. This presents a clinical challenge. The prognosis and treatment are said to depend on the site of the primary tumour and the degree of spread of metastasis [32]. The time between the diagnosis of oral metastatic lesions and the patient's death varies from month to years, with a median survival ranging between a few months to 5 years. A mean survival of 6 to 9 months has been reported in studies by Hirshberg et al., van der Waals et al., and Oliver-Puigdomènech et al. [13, 33, 34].

In the present case, a 37-year-old patient presented with invasive ductal carcinoma of the breast as the primary tumour. Within a period of 9 months, PET scan revealed extensive metastases in the brain, lung, liver, pancreas, nodes, subcutaneous and intramuscular soft tissue nodules, and sacrum. She presented with a solitary gingival enlargement in the maxillary anterior attached gingiva region. The time interval from the detection of primary tumour and detection of oral metastasis was 9 months. The lesion was excised and was histopathologically diagnosed as infiltrating poorly differentiated adenocarcinoma. She was on chemotherapy, but the extensive spread of cancer all over the body and as oral metastasis is usually seen late in disease progression meant that her disease prognosis was poor. The time interval between the diagnosis of the primary tumour and death in our case was 14 months.

4. Conclusion

This paper presents the clinicopathological features of gingival metastasis from breast cancer in a 37-year-old woman. The rarity of this case was that it occurred in a young patient involving the maxillary anterior gingiva, which has not been commonly reported in the literature. Early diagnosis and treatment of oral cavity metastases presents a therapeutic challenge for the clinician, which can play an important role in improving the patient's quality of life and prolonging survival. It is mandatory to differentiate malignancies from inflammatory and reactive lesions of the gingiva. Therefore, it is of utmost importance to take a detailed patient history, a thorough clinical and radiographic examination in case of gingival swelling. We therefore recommend a biopsy for any gingival swelling in the context of previous malignancy and an IHC evaluation to determine the site of primary tumour.

Abbreviations

IHC: Immunohistochemistry
PET: Positron emission tomography
cGY: Centigray
CBCT: Cone beam computed tomography
CK: Cytokeratin
ER: Oestrogen receptor
HER-2: Human epidermal growth factor receptor 2
GATA 3: GATA binding protein 3
TTF 1: Thyroid transcription factor 1
FDG: Fluorodeoxyglucose
CTC: Circulating tumour cells
IL-1: Interleukin 1
TNF-α: Tumour necrosis factor α
CD 45/CD20/CD3: Cluster of Differentiation 45/20/3
S100 protein: These proteins are soluble in 100%, i.e. saturated, ammonium sulfate at neutral pH
SOX 10: Sry-related HMg-Box gene 10.

Consent

As the patient described in the case report passed away, consent for publication was sought from her next of kin, her husband. Written informed consent was obtained for publication of this case report and associated clinical photographs.

References

[1] J. P. Servato, L. F. de Paulo, P. R. de Faria, S. V. Cardoso, and A. M. Loyola, "Metastatic tumours to the head and neck: retrospective analysis from a Brazilian tertiary referral centre," *International Journal of Oral and Maxillofacial Surgery*, vol. 42, no. 11, pp. 1391–1396, 2013.

[2] R. E. Friedrich and M. Abadi, "Distant metastases and malignant cellular neoplasms encountered in the oral and maxillofacial region: analysis of 92 patients treated at a single institution," *Anticancer Research*, vol. 30, no. 5, pp. 1843–1848, 2010.

[3] Y. T. Lee, "Breast carcinoma: pattern of metastasis at autopsy," *Journal of Surgical Oncology*, vol. 23, no. 3, pp. 175–180, 1983.

[4] A. Hirshberg, P. Leibovich, and A. Buchner, "Metastases to the oral mucosa: analysis of 157 cases," *Journal of Oral Pathology & Medicine*, vol. 22, no. 9, pp. 385–390, 1993.

[5] N. J. D'Silva, D. J. Summerlin, K. G. Cordell et al., "Metastatic tumors in the jaws," *Journal of the American Dental Association*, vol. 137, no. 12, pp. 1667–1672, 2006.

[6] I. Kaplan, V. Raiser, A. Shuster et al., "Metastatic tumors in oral mucosa and jawbones: unusual primary origins and unusual oral locations," *Acta Histochemica*, vol. 121, no. 8, article 151448, 2019.

[7] I. Allon, A. Pessing, I. Kaplan, D. M. Allon, and A. Hirshberg, "Metastatic tumors to the gingiva and the presence of teeth as a contributing factor: a literature analysis," *Journal of Periodontology*, vol. 85, no. 1, pp. 132–139, 2014.

[8] A. Hirshberg, P. Leibovich, I. Horowitz, and A. Buchner, "Metastatic tumors to postextraction sites," *Journal of Oral and Maxillofacial Surgery*, vol. 51, no. 12, pp. 1334–1337, 1993.

[9] M. Akheel, S. S. Tomar, and S. M. Hussain, "Metastatic oral soft-tissue lesions: an incidental finding in four cases," *South Asian Journal of Cancer*, vol. 2, no. 3, p. 146, 2013.

[10] M. S. Kwon, S. O. Ko, N. P. Cho et al., "Gastric signet-ring cell adenocarcinoma metastatic to the gingiva: a case report," *Oral Surgery, Oral Medicine, Oral Pathology, Oral Radiology, and Endodontics*, vol. 102, no. 1, pp. 62–66, 2006.

[11] A. Hirshberg, R. Berger, I. Allon, and I. Kaplan, "Metastatic tumors to the jaws and mouth," *Head and Neck Pathology*, vol. 8, no. 4, pp. 463–474, 2014.

[12] B. Psaila and D. Lyden, "The metastatic niche: adapting the foreign soil," *Nature Reviews. Cancer*, vol. 9, no. 4, pp. 285–293, 2009.

[13] A. Hirshberg, A. Shnaiderman-Shapiro, I. Kaplan, and R. Berger, "Metastatic tumours to the oral cavity - pathogenesis and analysis of 673 cases," *Oral Oncology*, vol. 44, no. 8, pp. 743–752, 2008.

[14] A. Hirshberg, P. Leibovich, and A. Buchner, "Metastatic tumors to the jawbones: analysis of 390 cases," *Journal of Oral Pathology & Medicine*, vol. 23, no. 8, pp. 337–341, 1994.

[15] H. P. Erickson and A. Hamao-Sakamoto, "Breast cancer metastasis to a mandibular extraction socket: a case report and discussion on clinical detection of metastasis to the oral cavity," *Journal of Oral and Maxillofacial Surgery, Medicine, and Pathology*, vol. 26, no. 2, pp. 262–267, 2014.

[16] S. Irani, "Metastasis to the oral soft tissues: a review of 412 cases," *Journal of International Society of Preventive and Community Dentistry*, vol. 6, no. 5, pp. 393–401, 2016.

[17] A. F. Chambers, A. C. Groom, and I. C. MacDonald, "Dissemination and growth of cancer cells in metastatic sites," *Nature Reviews Cancer*, vol. 2, no. 8, pp. 563–572, 2002.

[18] D. Spano and M. Zollo, "Tumor microenvironment: a main actor in the metastasis process," *Clinical & Experimental Metastasis*, vol. 29, no. 4, pp. 381–395, 2012.

[19] D. Nelson and R. Ganss, "Tumor growth or regression: powered by inflammation," *Journal of Leukocyte Biology*, vol. 80, no. 4, pp. 685–690, 2006.

[20] M. Bickel, B. Axtelius, C. Solioz, and R. Attström, "Cytokine gene expression in chronic periodontitis," *Journal of Clinical Periodontology*, vol. 28, no. 9, pp. 840–847, 2001.

[21] A. Tiwari, N. Kumar, R. Bajpai, and P. Lal, "Bone metastasis from ovarian cancer," *Journal of Cancer Research and Therapeutics*, vol. 3, no. 1, pp. 34–36, 2007.

[22] R. W. Brown, L. B. Campagna, J. K. Dunn, and P. T. Cagle, "Immunohistochemical identification of tumor markers in metastatic adenocarcinoma. A diagnostic adjunct in the determination of primary site," *American Journal of Clinical Pathology*, vol. 107, no. 1, pp. 12–19, 1997.

[23] T. Lesimple, J. J. Voigt, A. Bataillard et al., "Clinical practice guidelines: standards, options and recommendations for the diagnosis of carcinomas of unknown primary site," *Bulletin du Cancer*, vol. 90, no. 12, pp. 1071–1096, 2003, French.

[24] A. Bahrami, L. D. Truong, and J. Y. Ro, "Undifferentiated tumor: true identity by immunohistochemistry," *Archives of Pathology & Laboratory Medicine*, vol. 132, no. 3, pp. 326–348, 2008.

[25] C. Pepper, I. Pai, A. Hay et al., "Investigation strategy in the management of metastatic adenocarcinoma of unknown primary presenting as cervical lymphadenopathy," *Acta Oto-Laryngologica*, vol. 134, no. 8, pp. 838–842, 2014.

[26] M. J. Sack and S. A. Roberts, "Cytokeratins 20 and 7 in the differential diagnosis of metastatic carcinoma in cytologic specimens," *Diagnostic Cytopathology*, vol. 16, no. 2, pp. 132–136, 1997.

[27] K. Malzahn, M. Mitze, M. Thoenes, and R. Moll, "Biological and prognostic significance of stratified epithelial cytokeratins in infiltrating ductal breast carcinomas," *Virchows Archiv*, vol. 433, no. 2, pp. 119–129, 1998.

[28] T. Tot, "Patterns of distribution of cytokeratins 20 and 7 in special types of invasive breast carcinoma: a study of 123 cases," *Annals of Diagnostic Pathology*, vol. 3, no. 6, pp. 350–356, 1999.

[29] P. Mhawech-Fauceglia, D. Wang, T. Menesses et al., "Pax-8 is a reliable marker in making the diagnosis in advanced stage epithelial ovarian carcinoma and primary peritoneal carcinoma for neoadjuvant chemotherapy on cell block and biopsy specimens," *Histopathology*, vol. 60, no. 6, pp. 1019–1020, 2012.

[30] P. G. Chu and L. M. Weiss, "Keratin expression in human tissues and neoplasms," *Histopathology*, vol. 40, no. 5, pp. 403–439, 2002.

[31] J. Selves, E. Long-Mira, M. C. Mathieu, P. Rochaix, and M. Ilié, "Immunohistochemistry for diagnosis of metastatic carcinomas of unknown primary site," *Cancers*, vol. 10, no. 4, p. 108, 2018.

[32] G. Sánchez Aniceto, A. García Peñín, P. R. de la Mata, and J. J. Montalvo Moreno, "Tumors metastatic to the mandible: analysis of nine cases and review of the literature," *Journal of Oral and Maxillofacial Surgery*, vol. 48, no. 3, pp. 246–251, 1990.

[33] R. I. van der Waal, J. Buter, and I. van der Waal, "Oral metastases: report of 24 cases," *The British Journal of Oral & Maxillofacial Surgery*, vol. 41, no. 1, pp. 3–6, 2003.

[34] C. Oliver-Puigdomènech, B. González-Navarro, C. Polis-Yanes, A. Estrugo-Devesa, E. Jané-Salas, and J. López-López, "Incidence rate of metastases in the oral cavity: a review of all metastatic lesions in the oral cavity," *Medicina Oral, Patología Oral y Cirugía Bucal*, vol. 26, no. 5, pp. e619–e625, 2021.

8

Combined Surgical and Restorative Procedures to Treat Maxillary Canine with Gingival Recession and Cervical Wear

Dler Ali Khursheed and Faraedon Mostafa Zardawi

Department of Periodontics, University of Sulaimani, Sulaymaniyah, Kurdistan Region, Iraq

Correspondence should be addressed to Faraedon Mostafa Zardawi; faraedon.mostafa@univsul.edu.iq

Academic Editor: Andrea Scribante

Introduction. Gingival recession (GR) with cervical tooth wear is a major concern for patients on the prominent maxillary canines, from both esthetic and dentine hypersensitivity points of view. Hypersensitivity could be treated nonsurgically; however, esthetics remain the major patients' concern that mostly requires surgical intervention for covering the denuded root surface. Several surgical procedures are applied successfully for covering single and multiple gingival recession; however, these procedures are sensitive procedures and not always predictable. Semilunar coronally repositioned flap (SCRF) is a very simple procedure that found to be very predictable for covering a single recession in presence of sufficient keratinized gingiva apical to the recession. The procedure provides better clinical outcome by involving less adjacent papillary tissue that maintains greater blood supply and achieves maximum flap stability with mattress sutures with minimal postoperative complications. Therefore, this case report is aimed at explaining the simplicity of this surgical procedure in the presence of wide keratinized tissue around the recession and starting the restorative procedure after a sufficient soft tissue healing period. *Case Presentation.* 42-year-old systemically healthy female patient referred with a single wide gingival type 1 (RT1) and cervical wear around tooth #43. A semilunar coronally repositioned flap was released and advanced coronally to cover the denuded root totally; then, the flap stabilized by three mattress sutures, and complete root coverage was achieved. Six months later, the cervical lesion was restored with composite filling material. Sixteen-month and 32-month postoperative follow-up revealed full coverage of the denuded root surface with firm stable gingiva; later, the gingiva in the area looked stable and healthy. *Conclusion.* Using SCRF in treating RT1 recession in the presence of wide keratinized gingiva is very promising surgical intervention for receded root coverage that requires less technical skill.

1. Background

Gingival recession is defined as the shift of the free gingival margin apical to the cementoenamel junction [1]. Localized attachment loss with GR is very common on the facial surfaces of teeth in patients with high standards of oral hygiene care [2]. Treatment approaches for cervical tooth wear with GR can be nonsurgical, surgical, or combined surgical-restorative [3]. Gingival recession is treated and based on esthetic and functional consideration either nonsurgically by using topical desensitizing agents to reduce dentine hypersensitivity, or in cases of esthetic demands, gingival recession is managed by advanced coronal or lateral pedicle flaps combined with free connective tissue graft. In the current case, the recession was treated by advanced partial flap with semilunar incision with slight variation in clinical outcome [4, 5].

Probiotics were used to prevent cervical tooth decay and further recession due to gingivitis or periodontitis, which are considered as the primary cause of gingival recession [5].

The major goal of periodontal plastic surgery is to achieve complete root coverage with an esthetic outcome, rendering a thicker gingival biotype to maintain long-term stability [6, 7]. Subepithelial connective tissue graft (SCTG)

is regarded as the most predictable root coverage procedure in single and multiple GRs [8]. However, SCRF may have advantages over SCTG in terms of simplicity and avoidance of two surgical procedures and tissue morbidity. Moreover, its predictability and esthetic results are considered promising. The following benefits are considered for SCRE, such as lack of tension on the flap or changes in the vestibular depth; further, the papillae mesial and distal to the tooth being treated remain intact from an esthetic point of view provides greater blood supply to the flap [9]. This case report attempts to show the potential of SCRF in respect to esthetic outcome, healing time, and patient comfort during the healing period.

2. Clinical Presentation

A 42-year-old nonsmoker female patient attended the dental clinic complaining of tooth sensitivity and elongation of tooth number #43 (Figure 1). RT1 of 4 mm with cervical wear was detected on clinical examination of # (Figures 2(a) and 2(b)). Probing depth at the mesial, midlabial, and distal thirds facially measured 1 mm, respectively. A wide band of keratinized tissue was existed adjacent to the recession, and about 3 mm of attached keratinized gingiva was found apical to the recession (Figure 2(c)). Periodontally and systemically, the patient was fit for surgery.

Before performing the surgical procedures, the patient was provided with an information sheet including the benefits, risks, alternative treatments, and consequences of non-treatment which were discussed in detail with the patient and a signed consent was achieved from the patient. Further, the study was registered at the Scientific Committee of College of Dentistry (N 24 at 3rd Sept. 2019), and ethical approval was obtained from the ethical committee of University of Sulaimani.

The patient then signed a consent form.

3. Case Management

The patient was instructed to rinse with 0.2% chlorhexidine gluconate mouthwash before the operation. Local anesthesia was given to the area, and the semilunar flap was designed based on the amount of keratinized gingiva at either sides and apical to the recession.

The exposed root was properly instrumented with a Gracey 3/4 curette and frequently irrigated with normal saline (Figure 3(a)). The root was then conditioned with EDTA gel for 2 minutes, followed by profound irrigation (Figure 3(b)). Using a 15C blade, sulcular incision of about 3 mm was performed laterally and apically to raise a partial thickness flap. The apical margin of the partial thickness flap was excised to make a semicircular flap (Figure 3(c)). The adjacent interdental gingival papillae were maintained with lesser undermining to provide the flap with maximum blood supply. The flap was further advanced coronally and fixed with 3 superficial horizontal mattress sutures, and the wound was covered with periodontal dressing to provide further support and protection from the external environment. The sutures were held by flowable composite on dry, etched, and bonded enamel (Figure 3(d)). Antibiotics and analgesics were not prescribed. She was also instructed to not brush the surgical area for at least two months.

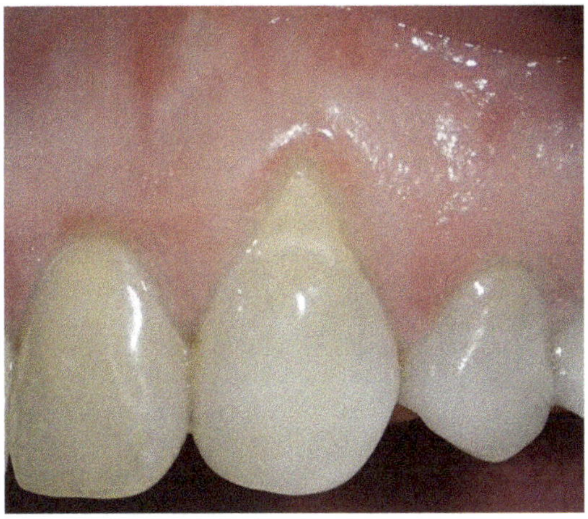

FIGURE 1: Tooth #43 class I Miller recession with root exposure and abrasion.

4. Clinical Outcomes

After 10 days, the periodontal dress and sutures were removed, and the recession was fully covered (Figure 4(a)). No surgical recession was observed after 10-day, 20-day, one-month, and two-month follow-ups (Figure 4(b)). The donor area was red and covered with granulation tissue after 10 days and more scar-like at 20 days. The tissue was firmly attached to the root surface with 1 mm sulcular depth at two-month and 6-month follow-up time (Figure 4(c)). The complete tissue remodeling was seen, and the cervical wear was restored with adhesive filling material. Sixteen months later, the gingiva and the restoration looked very stable (Figure 4(d)).

5. Discussion

Semilunar advanced coronal flap is a simple and predictable procedure for treatment of RT1 when a wide band of keratinized gingival is present apical to a recession [9]. The major differences between SCTG and SCRF are that the SCTG blood supply comes from the inner surface of stretched alveolar mucosal tissue and underlined periosteum, while the SCRF is a bilateral pedicle graft. It has profound collateral blood supply from interdental gingival tissues because the interdental papillae remain intact [10]. Additionally, a larger area of lateral papillary connective tissue remains undissected with SCRF.

Further, the procedure is simple and requires less time to be performed with less postoperative swelling and bleeding compared to other root coverage procedures.

EDTA was applied to render a clean root surgical interface free of any bacterial products and residual smear layer to enhance interaction between root surface collagen fibrils and connective tissue cells [11, 12], and therefore, higher

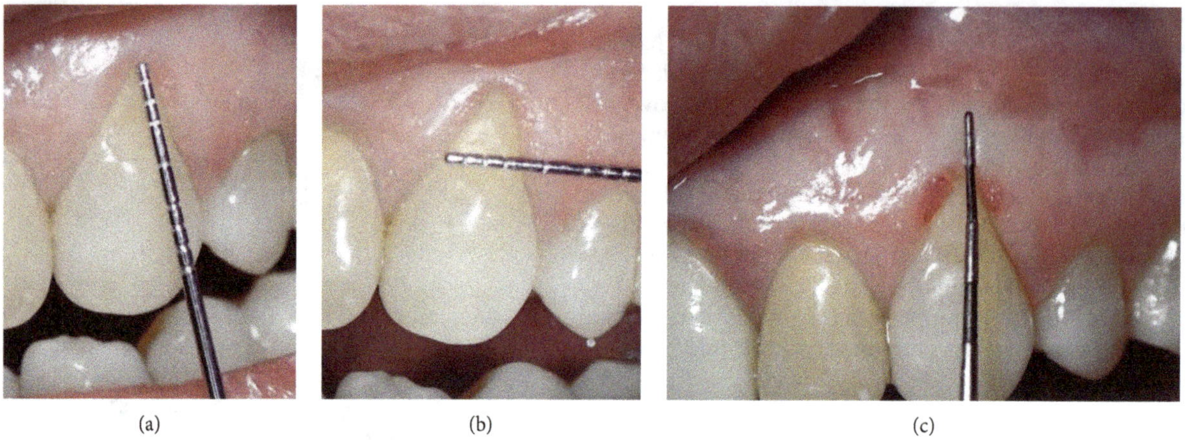

FIGURE 2: (a, b) Vertical and horizontal dimensions of the recession using Michigan probe. (c) Measuring the amount of attached keratinized gingiva around the recession by using Marquis periodontal probe.

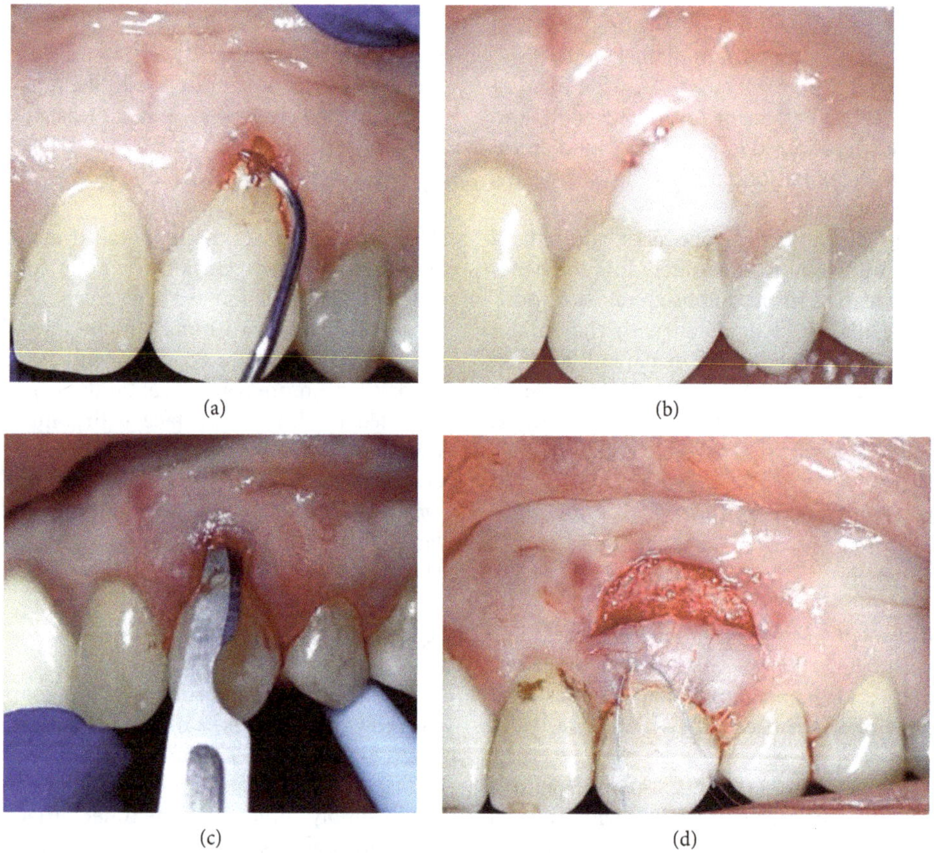

FIGURE 3: (a) Root planing using sharp Gracey curette. (b) Root detoxification using EDTA gel for 2 minutes. (c) Using 15C blade to make partial thickness flap. (d) The coronally repositioned semilunar flap was secured by three horizontal mattress sutures and fixed with flowable composite to the crown of the tooth.

penetration resistance was shown to probing the recession site after two months, which could be attributed to proper integration of connective tissue with root dentine. At this stage, the cervical lesion was restored to achieve an integrated soft and hard tissue between the restored cervical lesion and color and position and consistency of the gingiva at the area of the recession 6 months postoperatively.

The procedure first published by Tarnow in Journal of Clinical Periodontology 1986. It was found to be a successful method for covering a single recession without suturing the flap, when sufficient zone of keratinized gingiva is present apical to the recession [10].

There is no fundamental modification or novelty performed in this study; however, the procedure was simplified

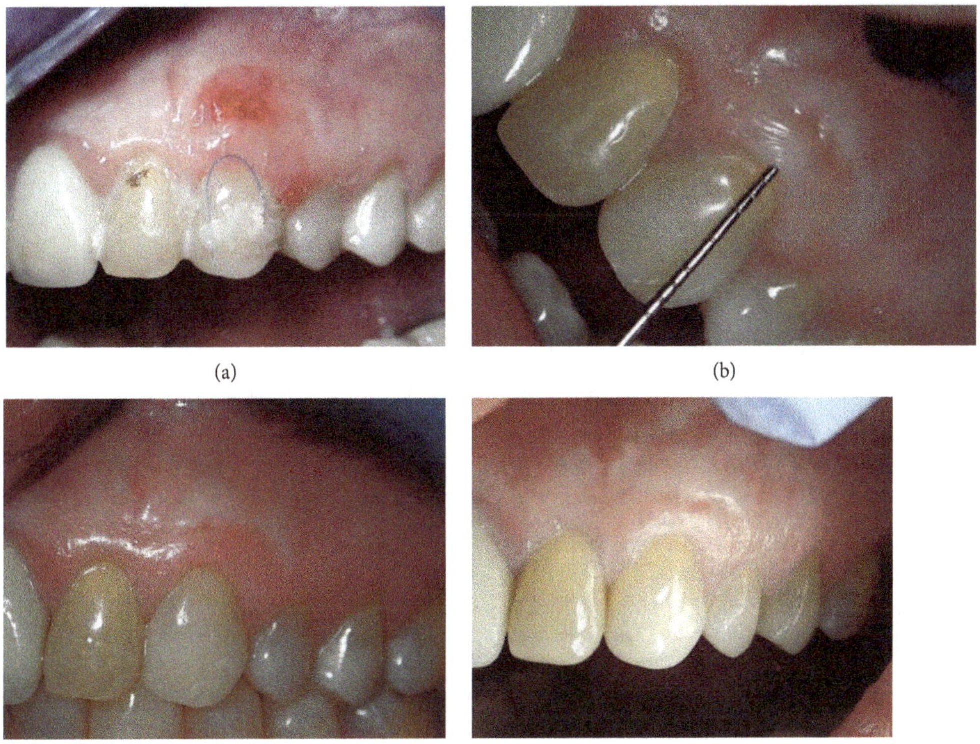

(a) (b) (c) (d)

FIGURE 4: (a) Ten days after removing the periodontal dressing and sutures. (b) Two months later, the gingiva was very stable and showed resistance to the periodontal probe. (c) At six months, the gingiva remained very stable with small amount of scar tissue on the donor area and was filled with composite filling. (d) 32 months postoperatively, the gingiva looked very stable and healthy.

by a small partial thickness flap without lateral extension with semilunar incision at the apical area, and the keratinized tissue was retracted and fixed coronally with composite by three superficial horizontal mattress sutures (Figures 3(a)–3(d)).

Keratinized gingiva was retracted coronally to cover the recession and remain stable, immobilized during the healing period. The procedure is now minimally invasive with less postoperative patient complaints and better clinical outcome for a single root coverage surgical procedure with similar color and texture of gingival tissue specially the area is an esthetic zone such as maxillary canine.

After complete heeling, the survival tooth wear was treated by composite restoration to avoid further tooth wear of cervical dentine and future recession at the area. After thirty-two months postoperatively, still full coverage of the denuded root is achieved and maintained (Figure 2(d)).

Additional Points

Key Finding. Semilunar coronally positioned flap is an appropriate choice to treat gingival recession in the presence of wide keratinized gingiva. *Why is this case new information?* Semilunar flap is aneffective and simple procedure choice to restore the defect in the presence of thick gingival biotype around the recession. Suturing techniques provide maximum stability to the graft. *What are the keys to successful management of these cases?* Maintaining maximum blood supply to semilunar flap from collateral blood supply by involving less of the adjacent interdental tissues. Presence of thick and wide gingiva apically and interdentally. *What are the primary limitations to success in these cases?* Amount of keratinized tissue around the recession and presence of receded adjacent interdental papillae. Apical and lateral extensions of the recession. Healing may show scare tissue at the site of the incision.

References

[1] American Academy of Periodontology, *Glossary of Periodontal Terms*, The American Academy of Periodontology, Chicago, 3rd edition, 1992.

[2] G. Serino, J. Lindhe, and L. Eneroth, "The prevalence and distribution of gingival recession in subjects with a high standard of oral hygiene," *Journal of Clinical Periodontology*, vol. 21, no. 1, pp. 57–63, 1994.

[3] S. Bittencourt, É. D. P. Ribeiro, E. A. Sallum, A. W. Sallum, F. H. Nociti Jr., and M. Z. Casati, "Semilunar coronally positioned flap or subepithelial connective tissue graft for the

treatment of gingival recession: a 30-month follow-up study," *Journal of Periodontology*, vol. 80, no. 7, pp. 1076–1082, 2009.

[4] R. B. Antana, C. M. Mattos, and S. Dibart, "A clinical comparison of two flap designs for coronal advancement of the gingival margin: semilunar versus coronally advanced flap," *Journal of Clinical Periodontology*, vol. 37, no. 7, pp. 651–658, 2010.

[5] A. Butera, S. Gallo, C. Maiorani et al., "Probiotic alternative to chlorhexidine in periodontal therapy: evaluation of clinical and microbiological parameters," *Microorganisms*, vol. 9, no. 1, p. 69, 2021.

[6] I. Bignozzi, C. Littarru, A. Crea, G. Vittorini Orgeas, and L. Landi, "Surgical treatment options for grafting areas of gingival recession association with cervical lesions: a review," *Journal of Esthetic and Restorative Dentistry*, vol. 25, no. 6, pp. 371–382, 2013.

[7] U. Pagliaro and G. Pini-Prato, "Evidenced-based mucogingival therapy. Part 2: ordinary and individual patient data meta-analyses of surgical treatment of recession using complete root coverage as the outcome variable," *Journal of Periodontology*, vol. 74, no. 5, pp. 741–756, 2003.

[8] M. Roccuzzo, M. Bunino, I. Needleman, and M. Sanz, "Periodontal plastic surgery for treatment of localized gingival recessions: a systematic review," *Journal of Clinical Periodontology*, vol. 29, pp. 178–194, 2002.

[9] L. Chambrone, F. Sukekava, M. G. Araújo, F. E. Pustiglioni, L. A. Chambrone, and L. A. Lima, "Root-coverage procedures for the treatment of localized recession-type defects: a Cochrane systematic review," *Journal of Periodontology*, vol. 81, no. 4, pp. 452–478, 2010.

[10] D. P. Tarnow, "Semilunar coronally repositioned flap," *Journal of Clinical Periodontology*, vol. 13, no. 3, pp. 182–185, 1986.

[11] S. Bittencourt, É. D. Ribeiro, E. A. Sallum, A. W. Sallum, F. H. Nociti, and M. Z. Casati, "Root surface biomodification with EDTA for the treatment of gingival recession with a semilunar coronally repositioned flap," *Journal of Periodontology*, vol. 78, no. 9, pp. 1695–1701, 2007.

[12] A. Ruggeri Jr., C. Prati, A. Mazzoni et al., "Effects of citric acid and EDTA conditioning on exposed root dentin: an immunohistochemical analysis of collagen and proteoglycans," *Archives of Oral Biology*, vol. 52, no. 1, pp. 1–8, 2007.

9

A Rare Case of Plasma Cell Gingivitis with Cheilitis

Yashodeep Chauhan, Shaleen Khetarpal, Madhu Singh Ratre, and Manish Varma

Department of Periodontology, Govt. College of Dentistry, Indore, M.P., India

Correspondence should be addressed to Yashodeep Chauhan; yashodeep.chauhan@rediffmail.com

Academic Editor: Kevin Seymour

Background. Plasma cell gingivitis (PCG) is a rare condition of the gingiva, characterized histopathologically by infiltration of plasma cells in connective tissue. Hypersensitivity reaction due to antigen is considered as primary etiological factor. *Case Presentation.* The present case is of an 18-year-old male patient suffering from gingival enlargement along with cheilitis. Histopathological and immunohistochemistry of tissue revealed lesion as plasma cell gingivitis. After gingivectomy, the follow up of the patient was done for 8 months. Gradual reduction of lip swelling was observed after gingivectomy during subsequent visits. *Conclusion.* Early diagnosis is essential as plasma cell gingivitis has similar pathologic changes seen clinically as in leukemia, multiple myeloma, discoid lupus erythematosus, atrophic lichen planus, desquamative gingivitis, or cicatricial pemphigoid which must be differentiated through hematologic examination.

1. Introduction

Plasma cell gingivitis (PCG) is a rare benign inflammatory condition of the gingiva. Various synonyms of plasma cell gingivitis are atypical gingivostomatitis, idiopathic gingivostomatitis, allergic gingivostomatitis, and plasma cell gingivostomatitis [1]. The lesion was first described in the year 1952 when Zoon referred to the term as "plasma-cell infiltrate." These conditions have also been reported on the lips, tongue, vulva, conjunctiva, nasal aperture, larynx, and epiglottis [2]. PCG is caused by allergen which induces hypersensitivity reaction. Various allergens documented are chewing gums, certain components of toothpastes, cinnamon, mint, red pepper, and khat leaves [3]. However, PCG has been classified into three categories, based on the etiology as follows: PCG due to allergens, PCG due to neoplastic origin, and PCG due to unknown cause [4]. Clinically, PCG is characterized by sharply demarcated erythematous and edematous gingiva often extending to the mucogingival junction. Moreover, the gingiva appears red, friable, and bleeds easily on provocation [1]. PCG mimics lesions associated with discoid lupus, lichen planus, cicatricial pemphigoid, leukemia, and myeloma; thus, an early diagnosis in such cases is vital to the patient's interest [1]. The case presented here is a PCG associated with cheilitis in an 18-year-old male patient.

2. Case Presentation

Patient, aged 18 years old, male, reported to the Department of Periodontics with the chief complaint of unaesthetic swelling of the gums in the maxillary and mandibular regions of the teeth since 4 to 5 years. Extraoral examination revealed cheilitis (Figure 1). Intraoral examination revealed generalized severe gingival enlargement covering up to the middle third of the clinical crowns. Gingiva was red, oedematous, and friable, with the absence of stippling, and easily bleeds on provocation. Gingival enlargement extends from teeth 14 to 27 in the maxilla and 37 to 43 in the mandible (Figure 2). Minimal local deposits were found in the mouth. There was no loss of attachment; however, generalized pseudo pockets ranged from 6 mm to 8 mm were recorded. The medical, dental, and personal history of the patient was noncontributory. Investigative hematologic examination did not reveal any significant findings. There was a negative Nikolsky's sign with no cutaneous lesion. Excisional biopsy was done to rule out PCG.

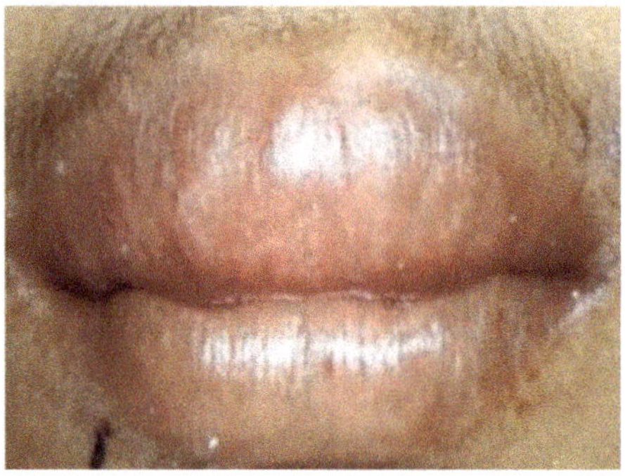

FIGURE 1: Cheilitis in the lips.

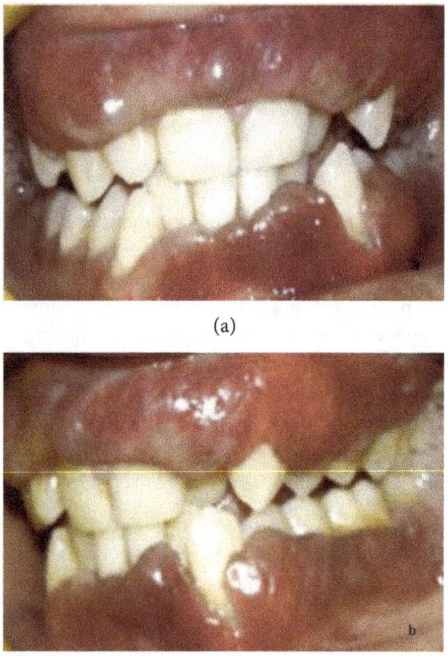

(a)

(b)

FIGURE 2: Gingival enlargement.

Histopathological examination revealed parakeratinized stratified squamous epithelium of varying thickness with regions of thinned-out epithelium and sharp rete ridges (Figure 3). Connective tissue was composed of dense diffuse chronic inflammatory cell infiltrate predominantly of plasma cells, lymphocytes, collagen fibers, and endothelium lined blood vessels. Above features were indicative of plasma cell gingivitis. The immunohistochemistry study further confirmed the lesion with the aid of kappa and lambda light chain reactivity (Figure 4). No relevant radio graphical finding was present.

After diagnosis, treatment was planned as phase I therapy followed by external bevel gingivectomy procedure under local anesthesia. The procedure was explained to the patient, and consent was taken. Postsurgical healing was satisfactory, and no recurrence was observed at consecutive follow-up visits. Follow-up of the patient was done at 1 week, 2 weeks, 3 weeks, 1 month, 3 months, 6 months, and 8 months

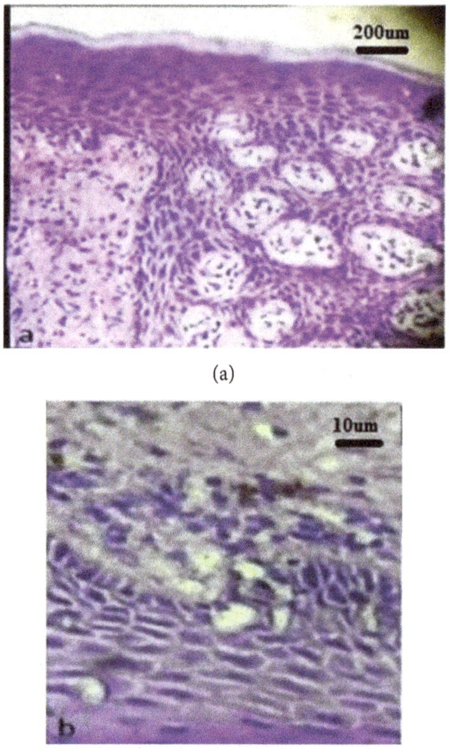

(a)

(b)

FIGURE 3: Histopathology: (a) 20x magnification and (b) 100x magnification.

(Figures 5–8). Gradual decrease in lip swelling was observed (Figure 9).

3. Discussion

PCG is a rare inflammatory condition, characterized by diffuse and massive infiltration of the plasma cells into the connective tissue [5]. Kerr and Kenneth in 1981 reported gingival enlargement in gum chewers, which disappeared following the discontinuation of the chewing habit [6]. Gargiulo et al. classified PCG as an immunological reaction to allergens, neoplasia, or of unknown origin [4]. Antigenic identification is necessary for proper diagnosis of the condition along with clinical, histopathological, and hematological screening [5]. However, in the present case, identification of antigen was unattainable; therefore, it was classified as the third variant of PCG. PCG resembles histologically as multiple myeloma and plasmacytoma, clinically as acute leukemia. Clinically, PCG is characterized as oedematous swelling with diffuse erythema clearly demarcated from mucogingival junction [1]. In the present cases, gingival enlargement was confined to both maxillary and mandibular teeth which was fiery red in color and obstinate to oral prophylaxis. These findings are consistent with earlier cases as documented by Joshi and Sukla [1]. Although in contrast to the present case, Arduino et al. found a decrease in gingival enlargement after phase I therapy [7]. In contrast to the case reported by Kumar et al., in present case, loss of attachment and severe bone loss were not appreciated [8]. In

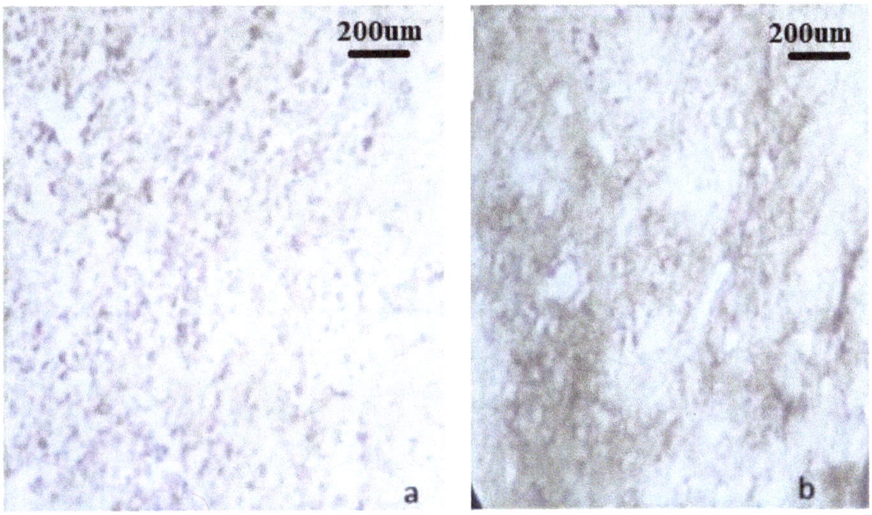

(a) (b)

Figure 4: Immunohistochemistry showing positive reactivity for (a) kappa chain and (b) lambda chain.

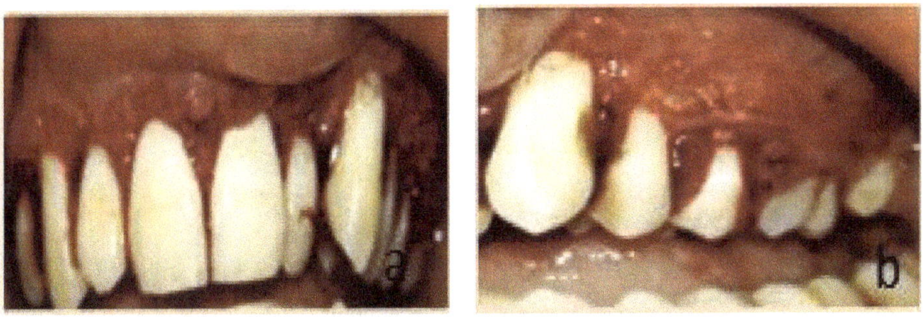

(a) (b)

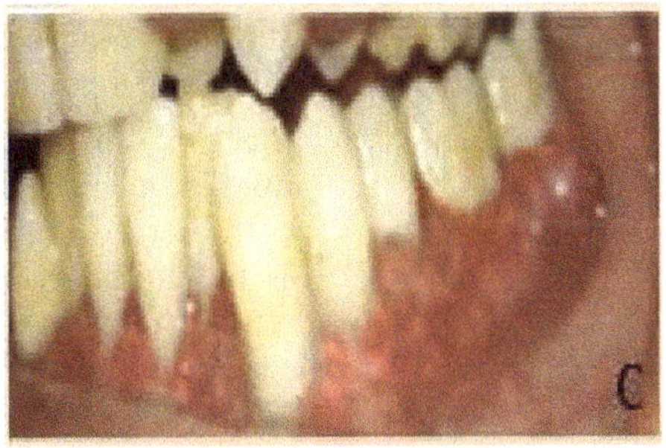

(c)

Figure 5: Immediate postoperative view: (a, b) maxilla and (c) mandible.

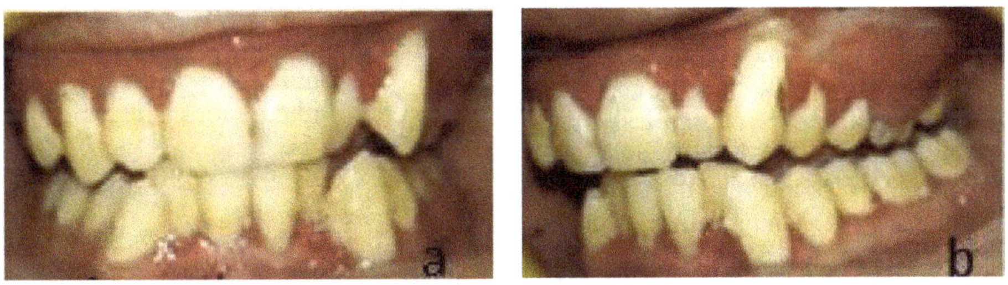

(a) (b)

Figure 6: Follow-up at 1 month.

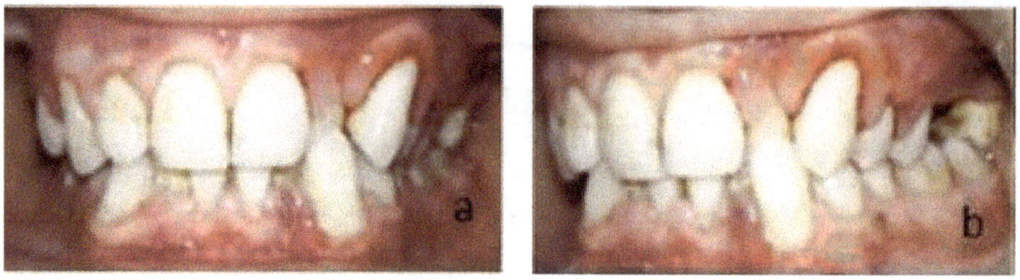

(a) (b)

FIGURE 7: Follow-up at 3 months.

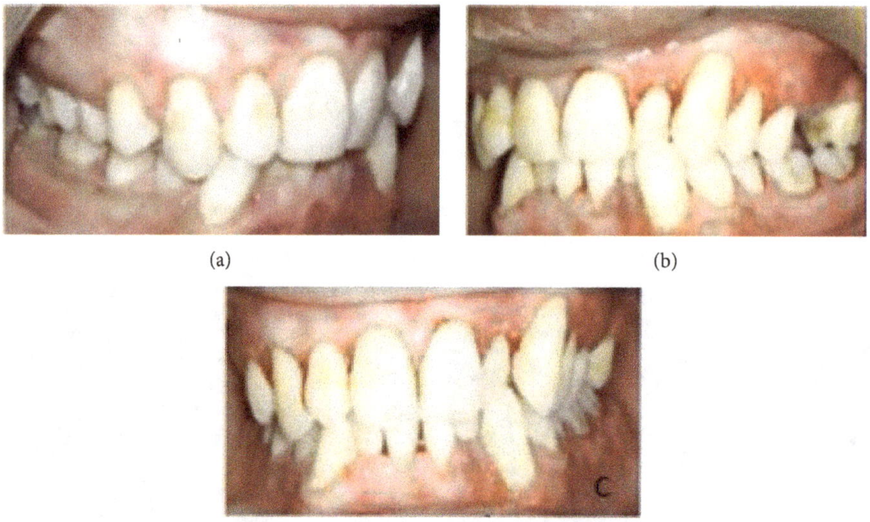

(a) (b)

(c)

FIGURE 8: Follow-up at 8 months.

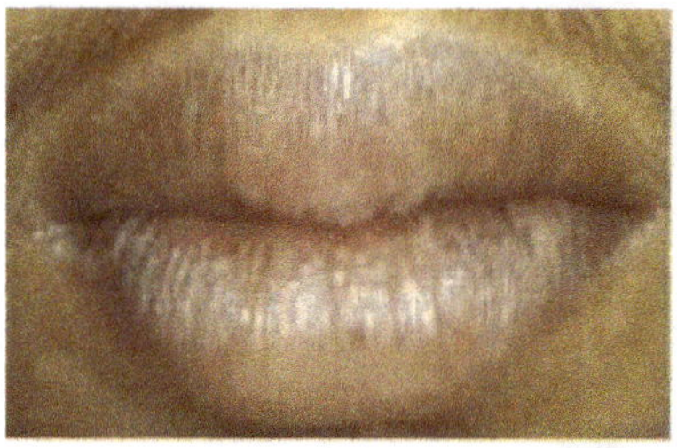

FIGURE 9: Reduction in lip swelling.

contrast to the present case, Makkar et al. reported a case of PCG in a 17-year-old female with generalized aggressive periodontitis [9]. As presented in a most recent case series by Prasanna et al., a similar case of PCG associated with cheilitis, they also reported subsiding of cheilitis after treatment as in our case [5]. Gingivitis, cheilitis, and glossitis have been described as a triad for plasma cell gingivostomatitis [6]. In the present case, removal of the gingival lesion by gingivectomy resulted in the reduction of lip swelling suggesting that the combined lesion of the lip and gingiva could be due to contact dermatitis as labial mucosa was in close contact of the gingiva as reported by Abhishek and Rashmi [10]. Histopathologically, it is crucial to differentiate PCG from various plasma cell tumors. The gingival contour and texture were stable after 8 months of gingivectomy. Gradual decrease in lip swelling was observed during consecutive follow-up visits. Diagnosis by clinical exclusion, haematological, histopathological examination, and immunohistochemistry helps to arrive at a diagnosis of PCG and inflammatory cheilitis.

4. Conclusion

As PCG mimics various other fatal conditions such as leukemia and multiple myeloma, early diagnosis and prompt treatment of the lesion are necessary. Therefore, a careful case history taken along with hematological, histopathological, and immunohistochemical examination is necessary so as to exclude other lesions and come to a proper diagnosis.

Consent

Patient was explained about the lesion, and informed consent was taken.

References

[1] C. Joshi and P. Shukla, "Plasma cell gingivitis," *Journal of Indian Society of Periodontology*, vol. 19, no. 2, pp. 221–223, 2015.

[2] C. C. Román, C. M. Yuste, M. A. González, A. P. González, and G. López, "Plasma cell gingivitis," *Cutis*, vol. 69, no. 1, pp. 41–45, 2002.

[3] P. Marker and A. Krogdahl, "Plasma cell gingivitis apparently related to the use of khat: report of a case," *British Dental Journal*, vol. 192, no. 6, pp. 311–313, 2002.

[4] A. V. Gargiulo, J. A. Ladone, and P. A. Ladone, "Case report: plasma cell gingivitis A," *CDS Review*, vol. 88, no. 3, pp. 22-23, 1995.

[5] J. S. Prasanna, D. A. Mutyap, V. R. Pantula, S. Akula, and B. Chinthapalli, "Plasma cell Gingivits-A conflict of diagnosis," *Journal of Clinical and Diagnostic Research*, vol. 10, pp. ZD01–ZZD0, 2016.

[6] D. A. Kerr, K. D. McClatchey, and J. A. Regezi, "Allergic gingivostomatitis (due to gum chewing)," *Journal of Periodontology*, vol. 42, no. 11, pp. 709–712, 1971.

[7] P. G. Arduino, F. D'Aiuto, C. Cavallito et al., "Professional oral hygiene as a therapeutic option for pediatric patients with plasma cell gingivitis: preliminary results of a prospective case series," *Journal of Periodontology*, vol. 82, no. 12, pp. 1670–1675, 2011.

[8] V. Kumar, A. K. Tripathi, C. S. Saimbi, and J. Sinha, "Plasma cell gingivitis with severe alveolar bone loss," *BMJ Case Reports*, vol. 2015, article bcr2014207013, 2015.

[9] A. Makkar, S. Tewari, K. Kishor, and S. Kataria, "An unusual clinical presentation of plasma cell gingivitis related to "Acacia" containing herbal toothpaste," *Journal of Indian Society of Periodontology*, vol. 17, no. 4, pp. 527–530, 2013.

[10] K. Abhishek and J. Rashmi, "Plasma cell gingivitis associated with inflammatory cheilitis: a report on a rare case," *Ethiopian Journal of Health Sciences*, vol. 23, no. 2, pp. 183–187, 2013.

10

A Journey toward Immediate Denture: Overcoming Bitter Reality with Psychotherapy

R. Varsha,[1] P. S. Manoharan,[1] Vigneshvar Chandrasekaran,[2] and K. Savitha[3]

[1]*Department of Prosthodontics, Indira Gandhi Institute of Dental Sciences, Sri Balaji Vidyapeeth Deemed-to-Be University, Pillaiyarkuppam, Puducherry 607 402, India*
[2]*Department of Psychiatry, Mahatma Gandhi Medical College and Research Institute, Sri Balaji Vidyapeeth, Deemed-to-Be University, Pillaiyarkuppam, Puducherry 607 402, India*
[3]*Department of Prosthodontics, Mahatma Gandhi Postgraduate Institute of Dental Sciences, Kalaivaanar Nagar, Puducherry 605006, India*

Correspondence should be addressed to P. S. Manoharan; manodent_2000@yahoo.com

Academic Editor: Márta Radnai

The loss of teeth affects the aesthetics, function (mastication and speech), confidence, mental state, and the overall quality of life of an individual. Aggressive periodontitis is a destructive condition leading to loss of teeth at early stages of the disease. Individuals facing this inevitable condition of losing the teeth and replacement at a younger age experience formidable psychological distress. The prosthodontic procedure when supported with psychotherapeutic interventions can support the patient in accepting the prognosis and treatment. We report the scenario where psychological intervention was provided in a systematic manner adopting the SPIKES protocol for a 42-year-old man presenting with aggressive periodontitis.

1. Introduction

The loss of teeth, apart from affecting the structural integrity, nutrition, mastication, and taste perception associated with the functions of teeth, also affects the emotional stability, self-image, confidence leading to disturbances in physical and overall well-being of an individual [1].

Aggressive periodontitis is a condition leading to early tooth loss. It is characterized by rapid loss of periodontal ligament and the alveolar and the interproximal attachment loss that affects more than three teeth during or even before the onset of puberty. Furthermore, the symptoms of mobility are noticed quite late when the destruction of teeth have progressed to a higher severity. In severe presentations of the disease, individuals present with mobile teeth and an inability to eat. In such individuals, the prognosis of the condition is considered very poor, leaving the dentist with fewer options apart from the definitive solution of removing all the teeth with prosthetic rehabilitation [2]. Aggressive periodontitis can be managed by mechanical debridement accompanied by antimicrobial agents, scaling, and root planing effectively; however, it may not ensure long term stability [3, 4].

Due to the unawareness of the aggressive nature of the disease, the patients' acceptance of the prognosis and the rehabilitation measures are limited. The provision of a systematic psychological intervention for "breaking the bad news" can lead to improved acceptance and outcomes in such individuals [5]. It is expected of a dentist to understand, diagnose, and carefully plan the treatment considering the benefits of psychological interventions [6]. The literature opines that training of undergraduate and postgraduate should encompass a well-structured training module for providing the appropriate knowledge, attitude, and communication skills, which are needed to counsel patients [7]. In this report, we discuss about a middle aged male with aggressive periodontitis who was provided psychological intervention as a part of management and rehabilitation.

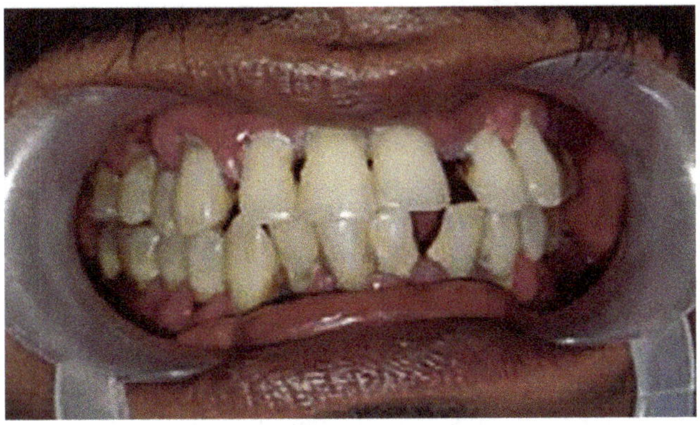

Figure 1: Clinical oral examination.

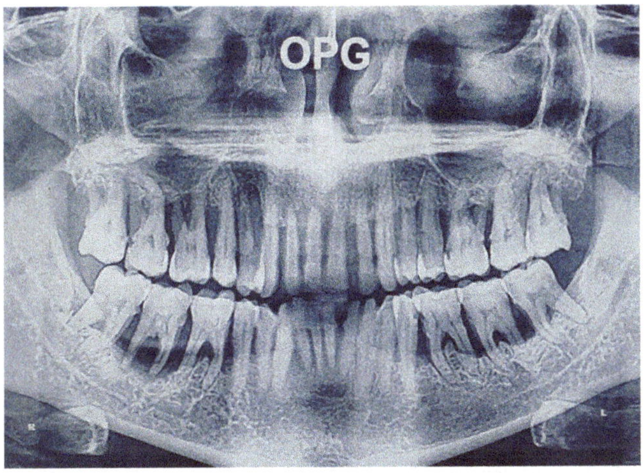

Figure 2: Orthopantomograph examination.

1.1. Case Presentation. A 42-year-old male patient reported to the Department of Prosthodontics, complaining of severely mobile maxillary and mandibular teeth and the inability to chew with the existing dentition. The patient had been diagnosed of diabetes and was on regular medications for past 5 years. On examination the patient presented with Grade II mobility in the anterior and Grade III mobility and Grade II to III gingival recession and furcation involvement (Figure 1). The examination findings were explained to the patient and was emphasized the need for further investigations. Orthopantomograph revealed generalized severe vertical bone loss around all the teeth (Figure 2). The prognosis of all the remaining natural teeth was hopeless as per the opinion of the periodontist.

A diagnosis of aggressive periodontitis was made according to the guidelines presented by AAP [1999] classification by the periodontists and reported that all the teeth had hopeless prognosis, with the advanced bone loss and clinical attachment loss in all the teeth. Total extraction and replacement of teeth was considered as the only option. The patient owns a business where he would have to face customers on a daily basis due to which the impending loss of teeth would be quite distressful and unacceptable for the patient.

The bad news was communicated using the SPIKES protocol [8] as follows (Table 1).

Table 1: The SPIKES protocol.

Setting ambience and privacy	A private counseling set up was planned for the patient along with his spouse without any external interruptions.
Perception (how much the patient knows)	He was totally unaware of the condition and may never accept the aforementioned treatment.
Invitation or information	The patient was explained about the situation with all the supporting radiographs and diagnostic casts on the severity of the condition.
Knowledge sharing	Simple words were used and practical issues related to understanding of the disease was conveyed gradually in a piece meal approach.
Empathy	The anxiety of the patient and the bystander was very evident from their body language as the severity of the problem was revealed to its fullest. We felt a stoic silence and they were trying to conceal disappointment and emotional distress. We asked them to express what they felt at that moment. We did not get any response or reply but a silent pause and an anticipation of some hope.
Summarize	At that point we decided to disclose to the patient that, it was very unfortunate that his remaining teeth had a very hopeless prognosis. The patient was also explained that retaining his remaining teeth will in no manner alleviate the present situation.
Strategise	Although the patient and the relatives came to terms with the reality, they wanted to know possible options for an alternative. The plan of sequential extraction and immediate denture was explained to the patient. The patient was given four different treatment options based on the diagnostic work up.

All the possible pros and cons for each treatment option was explained in simple words. Educational models and videos were used to explain all the treatment options. The patient was given ample opportunity to ask questions and express his limitations in terms of affordability and time. The patient opted for immediate denture based on the factor that he could not be without teeth owing to his profession and affordability. After the patient chose the option, photographs of other patients with a similar condition were shown for better appreciation of the course of treatment. The need for relining within the first year was also explained to the patient [9].

The treatment plan for a conventional immediate denture was adopted [10]. The patient was reviewed after 3 months (Figure 3). The patient had performed well with

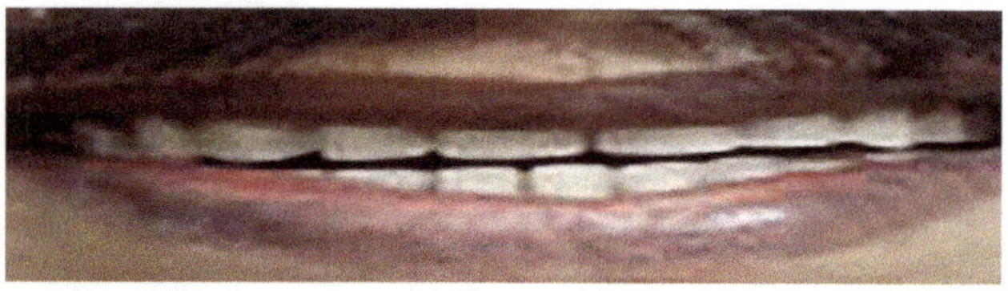

Figure 3: Oral examination after Immediate denture replacement (after 3 months).

Table 2: Models of breaking bad news.

Model	Characteristics
ABCDE model	A—Advance preparation B—Build a therapeutic environment/relationship C—Communicate well D—Deal with patient and family reactions E—Encourage and validate emotions (reflect back emotions) [15]
PACIENTE protocol	P—Prepare A—Assess how much the patient knows and how much they want to know C—(*Convite à verdade*, in Portuguese) Invite the patient to the truth I—Inform E—Emotions N—(*Não abandone o paciente*, in Portuguese) Do not abandon the patient TE—(*trace uma estratégia*, in Portuguese) Outline a strategy P-A-C-I-E-N-T-E stands for ("patient," in Portuguese) [16]
BREAKS protocol	B—Background R—Rapport E—Explore A—Announce K—Kindling S—Summarize [17]

the dentures with respect to day-to-day functions of mastication and speech. The patient also mentioned that he would consider replacement with implants as an option at a later date [11]. The OHIP EDENT questionnaire was used to assess the patient before and after the usage of dentures, and it was found that the oral health quality of life had improved for the patient after the usage of dentures.

2. Discussion

The level of emotional distress, loss of confidence, and self-image is often overlooked during the treatment of aggressive periodontitis [12]. The wholesome management including psychotherapy of such patients would help the patient to go through a smooth transition from a dentate to an edentate individual with the prosthesis [13].

In the literature pertaining to dentistry, breaking the bad news involves informing about a suspicious lesion, information on loss of teeth, information of a surgical procedure or a procedure with poor prognosis, or the information of a lesion that reflects a likely systemic condition. Other models of breaking bad news such as ABCDE model, PACIENTE protocol, and BREAKS protocol have been mentioned to be used as guidelines for breaking the bad news [14] (Table 2).

In this case report, we have adopted the SPIKES protocol in systematically educating and motivating the patient toward accepting his disability, the poor prognosis, and possible treatment options [8]. The patient gained confidence and assurance from the operator and was quite ready when the last day of extraction of anterior teeth were planned. The patient understood the need for future procedures such as reline and accepted to undergo other further definitive options at a later date.

Tooth loss has a significant impact on the emotional well-being of the patient and should be handled in a systematic and scientific manner. Adequate use of guidelines for breaking bad news by trained personnel would alleviate the apprehension and the associated anxiety and distress ultimately leading to acceptance of prosthodontic rehabilitation.

References

[1] R. J. Shah, F. J. Diwan, M. J. Diwan, V. J. Chauhan, H. S. Agrawal, and G. C. Patel, "A study of the emotional effects of tooth loss in an edentulous Gujarati population and its association with depression," *Journal of Indian Prosthodontic Society*, vol. 15, no. 3, pp. 237–243, 2015.

[2] D. Priyadarshini, P. Nadig, N. Deshpande, and A. Deshpande, "Role of psychotherapy in managing a case of generalised aggressive periodontitis," *BML Case Reports*, vol. 2014, article bcr2013200851, 2014.

[3] W. Teughels, R. Dhondt, C. Dekeyser, and M. Quirynen, "Treatment of aggressive periodontitis," *Periodontology 2000*, vol. 65, no. 1, pp. 107–133, 2014.

[4] F. Sgolastra, A. Petrucci, R. Gatto, and A. Monaco, "Effectiveness of systemic amoxicillin/metronidazole as an adjunctive therapy to full-mouth scaling and root planing in the treatment of aggressive periodontitis: a systematic review and meta-analysis," *Journal of Periodontology*, vol. 83, no. 6, pp. 731–743, 2012.

[5] A. V. Naik and R. C. Pai, "Study of emotional effects of tooth loss in an aging north Indian community," *ISRN Dentistry*, vol. 2011, no. 2011, 4 pages, 2011.

[6] B. J. Scott, K. C. Leung, A. S. McMillan, D. M. Davis, and J. Fiske, "A transcultural perspective on the emotional effect of tooth loss in complete denture wearers," *The International Journal of Prosthodontics*, vol. 14, no. 5, pp. 461–465, 2001.

[7] J. T. Newton and J. Fiske, "Breaking bad news: a guide for dental healthcare professionals," *British Dental Journal*, vol. 186, no. 6, pp. 278–281, 1999.

[8] S. Curtin and M. McConnell, "Teaching dental students how to deliver bad news: S-P-I-K-E-S model," *Journal of Dental Education*, vol. 76, no. 3, pp. 360–365, 2012.

[9] V. Bhat and S. S. Balaji, "Immediate partial denture prosthesis-a case report," *Journal of Health and Allied Sciences NU*, vol. 3, no. 4, pp. 120–124, 2013.

[10] M. Handa and P. Marya, "Rehabilitation of a patient with an immediate complete denture: a case report," *Indian Journal of Dental Advancements*, vol. 10, no. 1, pp. 56–59, 2018.

[11] S. Kraljević, J. Pandurić, T. Badel, and R. Ćelić, "Immediate complete denture," *Acta Stomatologica Croatica*, vol. 35, no. 2, pp. 281–285, 2001.

[12] P. F. Allen and A. S. McMillan, "A review of the functional and psychosocial outcomes of edentulousness treated with complete replacement dentures," *Journal of the Canadian Dental Association*, vol. 69, no. 10, p. 662, 2003.

[13] A. R. Mysore and M. A. Aras, "Understanding the psychology of geriatric edentulous patients," *Gerodontology*, vol. 29, no. 2, pp. e23–e27, 2012.

[14] P. Güneri, J. Epstein, and R. W. Botto, "Breaking bad medical news in a dental care setting," *Journal of the American Dental Association (1939)*, vol. 144, no. 4, pp. 381–386, 2013.

[15] M. W. Rabow and S. J. McPhee, "Beyond breaking bad news: how to help patients who suffer," *The Western Journal of Medicine*, vol. 171, no. 4, pp. 260–263, 1999.

[16] C. R. Pereira, M. A. M. Calônego, L. Lemonica et al., "The P-A-C-I-E-N-T-E protocol: an instrument for breaking bad news adapted to the Brazilian medical reality," *Revista da Associação Médica Brasileira*, vol. 63, no. 1, pp. 43–49, 2017.

[17] V. Narayanan, B. Bista, and C. Koshy, "BREAKS. Protocol for breaking bad news," *Indian Journal of Palliative Care*, vol. 16, no. 2, pp. 61–65.

11

Morphological and Molecular Characterization of Human Gingival Tissue Overlying Multiple Oral Exostoses

Luca Francetti,[1,2] **Claudia Dellavia**,[1] **Stefano Corbella**,[1,2] **Nicolò Cavalli**,[1,2] **Claudia Moscheni**,[3] **Elena Canciani**,[1] **and Nicoletta Gagliano**[4]

[1]*Department of Biomedical, Surgical and Dental Sciences, Università degli Studi di Milano, via L. Mangiagalli 31, 20133 Milan, Italy*
[2]*IRCCS Istituto Ortopedico Galeazzi, Via R. Galeazzi, 4, 20161 Milan, Italy*
[3]*Department of Biomedical and Clinical Sciences "L. Sacco", Università degli Studi di Milano, via G.B. Grassi 74, 20157 Milan, Italy*
[4]*Department of Biomedical Sciences for Health, Università degli Studi di Milano, via L. Mangiagalli 31, 20133 Milan, Italy*

Correspondence should be addressed to Nicoletta Gagliano; nicoletta.gagliano@unimi.it

Academic Editor: Jamil Awad Shibli

Gingival and osseous augmentations are reported as hypertrophic or hyperplastic reactions to different factors including chronic traumatisms and surgeries such as free gingival graft (FGG) that induce an abnormal growth of both hard and soft tissues in genetically predisposed subjects. Since an imbalance in collagen turnover plays a key role in the development of gingival overgrowth leading to an accumulation of collagen in gingival connective tissue, in this study we described the histological and molecular features of three oral overgrowths obtained from a 34-year-old woman previously operated for FGG in order to evaluate a possible relationship between exostoses and overgrown tissue. Healthy and overgrown gingiva were analyzed by histological methods, and the expression of genes and proteins involved in collagen synthesis, maturation, and degradation was assessed in cultured fibroblasts obtained from gingival fragments at the molecular level. Our results show that general morphology and collagen content were similar in healthy and overgrown gingivae. However, fibroblasts obtained from the overgrown gingiva revealed an anabolic phenotype characterized by an increased collagen turnover and maturation. These findings indicate that an exostosis could act as a mechanical stimulus stretching the overlying connective tissue and triggering an anabolic phenotype of gingival fibroblasts and suggest to use minimally invasive surgical techniques to avoid traumatizing the periosteal tissues for the eradication of the exostosis with minimal relapses.

1. Introduction

Exostoses are described in literature as benign localized overgrowths of the bone of unknown etiology [1]. They may appear as nodular, flat, or pedunculate protuberances and may be found in different anatomical areas; the most frequent are palatal and mandibular *tori*, but vestibular exostoses can also be present. Vestibular exostoses are most common in the maxilla and are less frequently found on the mandibular surface. Multiple exostoses are present less regularly [1, 2]. Exostoses may appear as a rare side effect of free gingival graft (FGG) resulting from periosteal traumatism during site preparation that induces the activation of osteoprogenitor cells and of fibroblasts contained in the connective tissue of the graft, leading to bone and soft tissue overgrowth [1, 3].

Several studies have tried to explain the etiology, and different hypotheses have been proposed. Chambrone and Chambrone evaluated nine exostoses where FGG surgery was performed to augment the amount of keratinized gingiva. The authors have observed that in each of the examined cases, intentional or accidental periosteal fenestration during the surgical approach has occurred [1]. Considering the hypotheses of periosteal trauma acting as the main etiologic agent, frenectomies can also be involved in exostosis formation. In fact, the linear micro-fenestrations that occur during the preparation of a receiving site can evoke bone stimulation leading to the development of exostoses [2]. In three cases described in literature, the exostoses appeared in grafted areas associated with teeth that had supported removable or fixed prostheses. It is possible that the combination of periosteal fenestration and occlusal function as a continuous irritation factor is responsible for this osseous proliferation [4–6]. Pechenkina and coworkers in 2002 studied bone exostosis development in 66 well-preserved crania from Neolithic China to establish a possible etiopathological association [7]. The role of ethnic and genetic predispositions seemed to be important in the occurrence of such exostoses. In the same study, authors considered other factors as potentially related to exostosis formation such as masticatory hyperfunction (clenching or bruxism), occlusal stress, a compensatory response of periodontal disease, and chemical agents and concluded that every periodontal microdamage or inflammation can evolve in exostoses in genetically predisposed subjects. Severe occlusal stress, associated with temporomandibular joint disorders, was hypothesized to be a major environmental factor predisposing to exostosis development [7]. Echeverria and colleagues in 2001 presented a report about the formation of exostoses following FGG surgical procedure [8]. The authors postulated that surgical trauma combined with occlusal stress and genetic factors could cause the occurrence of exostoses. They also noticed that most of the post-FGG exostoses appeared in the premolar area, probably due to excessive chewing forces. The histological examination of hard and soft tissues of exostoses showed dense and mature lamellar bone surrounded by fibrous tissue with the presence of acanthosis, pseudoepitheliomatous hyperplasia, parakeratosis, and reactive fibrosis [8]. Likewise, other authors proposed the same potential etiological explanation, suggesting that the periodontal trauma and surgical damage of soft tissue (plastic surgery of the vestibule, gingival graft, and, notably, fenestration occurred in the periosteum) can evolve in buccal bony exostoses in genetically predisposed patients [3, 9–14].

Since the mechanisms leading to the overgrowth of gingival connective tissue overlying the exostosis are not completely known, the aim of this study was to characterize the gingival connective tissue in the case of multiple exostoses following FGG by histological and molecular analysis.

2. Case Presentation

2.1. Patient. A female patient, 34 years old at the time of the first visit, was referred to us to correct her gingival esthetic problem caused by the formation of gingival/mucosal overgrowths. Gingival outgrowths localized in the second, third, and fourth quadrants, corresponding to the position of premolars and canine roots, were identified during an oral examination. Their consistency appeared hard and unmovable, and they presented a normal gingival color. The lesions were asymptomatic, and the morphology did not change over time (Figure 1).

The anamnestic investigation revealed a history of FGG surgery in 2004 (8 years before our first examination) in each site that was treated for gingival recessions; allergic reactions to nonsteroidal anti-inflammatory drugs, paracetamol, cephalosporin, penicillin and its derivatives, and macrolide antibiotics; absence of any systemic conditions affecting metabolism; and altered wound healing (cutaneous keloids and hypertrophic scars).

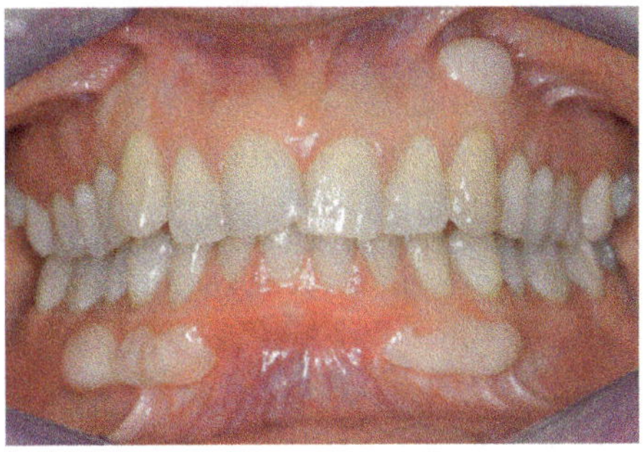

Figure 1: Clinical aspect at baseline.

The hypothesis of exostosis formation was suggested by the following clinical observations: benign aspect, nodular and hyperplastic tissue, hard and stable on palpation, not symptomatic, and localized in canine and premolar areas involved in a surgical procedure that could have acted as a promoter event.

We decided to perform an excisional surgery, followed by a histologic and molecular evaluation. The Review Board of the Research Center in Oral Implantology of the Università degli Studi di Milano in Milan, Italy, approved the treatment and research protocol before the first surgery.

All procedures were in accordance with the ethical standards of the institutional and/or national research committee and with the 1964 Helsinki declaration and its later amendments or comparable ethical standards. The patient was informed about the formulated medical hypothesis and the need for surgical intervention to remove the lesions and analyze the specimen. The patient agreed to the surgery and signed a written informed consent form. The surgery was planned after a complete evaluation of the patient's systemic conditions that confirmed an absence of clinical contraindications.

2.2. Surgical Procedures. All surgeries were performed in three different sessions by the same operator, with more than ten years of experience in the field of oral surgery (LF), and following the same protocol. The first surgical event involved a lesion localized in the second quadrant. Local anesthesia was performed with articaine 4% + epinephrine 1 : 100.000, voiding injection in the lesion area. The lesion was first isolated by incisions with a microblade following its external border; after that, the incision was continued above the periosteum, removing the tissue covering the exostosis. Then, with a 15C blade, a full-thickness incision was performed coronally to the lesion and the exostosis surface was exposed using a periosteal elevator. The full-thickness incision was extended in the mesiodistal direction in order to have a better view of the surgical site. Gingival fragments obtained from the overgrown gingiva were collected for histological and molecular characterization. A carbide bur, mounted on a rotary instrument and under sterile saline solution irrigation, was used to remove the bone structure in order to recreate a plane surface. To obtain a primary closure of the flap after the removal of the lesion, a partial thickness incision was performed in the free alveolar mucosa. The flap was then sutured with a 6/0 nonresorbable suture (ETHILON™ Nylon Suture, Ethicon ®, Cincinnati, OH, United States). After flap closure, an infiltration of 4 mg corticosteroid (BENTELAN 4 mg/2 mL, Defiante Farmaceutica S.A., Madeira, Portugal) was performed, to prevent the recurrence of overgrowths in the short term. The last surgical procedure was performed within 4 months of the first visit.

The follow-up visits revealed small relapses after 18 months from the surgical intervention that were asymptomatic and did not affect aesthetics and function. The recurrences observed in the second and fourth quadrants were linearly arranged along the incision of the periosteum that occurred during the surgery, while the lesion treated in the third quadrant showed a more evident relapse.

2.3. Histological Analysis. One gingival fragment was processed for histological analysis while another fragment was cultured for in vitro evaluations. Moreover, to characterize the pathological gingiva, a fragment from the healthy papilla was obtained from the same patient for comparison.

Immediately after surgery, each tissue fragment was fixed in 4% formalin in 0.1 M phosphate-buffered saline (PBS), pH 7.4, routinely dehydrated and paraffin-embedded. Serial sections of 5 μm were obtained. Sections were stained with freshly made hematoxylin-eosin (Sigma-Aldrich, St Louis, MO, United States) to evaluate cell and tissue morphology.

To evaluate fibrillary collagen, slides were deparaffinized and immersed for 30 minutes in saturated aqueous picric acid containing 0.1% Sirius Red F3BA (Sigma-Aldrich, St. Louis, MO, United States), a staining method that specifically marks collagen [15]. The sections were observed under a light and polarized microscope (Nikon Eclipse E600, Nikon, Tokyo, Japan) and photographed with a calibrated digital camera (DXM1200, Nikon, Tokyo, Japan) at a 20x magnification.

2.4. Cell Cultures. Human gingival fibroblasts were obtained from a gingival fragment covering the exostosis and from a gingival fragment obtained from the patient's healthy gingiva. Tissue fragments were washed with sterile PBS, plated in T25 flasks, and incubated in DMEM containing 10% heat-inactivated fetal bovine serum (FBS) and antibiotics (100 U/mL penicillin, 0.1 mg/mL streptomycin) at 37°C in a humidified atmosphere with 5% CO_2. Fibroblasts that grew out from the explant were trypsinized (0.025% trypsin-0.01% EDTA) for secondary cultures and plated in T75 flasks, as previously described [16, 17]. Human gingival fibroblasts were used between the fourth and fifth passages. Molecular evaluations were performed in samples cultured for 24, 48, and 72 h. All evaluations were performed on duplicate cultures for each sample.

2.5. Cell Morphology and Viability. Cell morphology of cultured gingival fibroblasts was analyzed by phase-contrast microscopy using a Leica DM IL microscope. Cell viability was determined by Trypan blue exclusion. Growth curves were obtained after plating cells in 6-well plates (150,000 cells/well). After the attachment, the cells were counted after 24, 48, and 72 h.

2.6. Real-Time RT-PCR. Total RNA was isolated from cultured fibroblasts as previously described [17]. Briefly, 1 μg of total RNA was reverse-transcribed in a 20 μL final volume of reaction mix (Bio-Rad, Segrate, Milan, Italy). Gene expression for the tissue inhibitor of matrix metalloproteinase 1 (TIMP-1), lysyl oxidase (LOX), and focal adhesion kinase (FAK) was assessed. GAPDH was used as internal control for normalization of the differences in the amount of total RNA in each sample. The following primers were used: GAPDH: sense CCCTTCATTGACCTCAACTACATG, antisense TGGGATTTCCATTGATGACAAGC, antisense GGAACCAGGATGACCAGATGTACC; TIMP-1: sense GGCTTCTGGCATCCTGTTGTTG, antisense AAGGTG GTCTGGTTGACTTCTGG; LOX: sense GGATACGGCAC TGGCTACTT, antisense GACGCCTGGATGTAGTAGGG; and FAK: sense GTCTGCCTTCGCTTCACG, antisense GAATTTGTAACTGGAAGATGCAAG.

Amplification was performed in a 96-well plate in a final volume of 20 μL per well containing 10 μL of 1x SYBR Green Supermix (Bio-Rad, Italy), 2 μL of template, and 300 pmol of each primer, and each sample was analyzed in triplicate in an iQ5 thermal cycler (Bio-Rad, Italy) after 40 cycles. After determining the cycle threshold (Ct), gene expression levels relative to that of GAPDH were calculated by the $2^{\Delta Ct}$ method.

2.7. Slot Blot. Slot blot analysis was used to assess type I collagen (COL-I), type III collagen (COL-III), and matrix metalloproteinase-1 (MMP-1) protein levels secreted by gingival fibroblasts in cell culture supernatants, as previously described [17]. Briefly, protein content in cell culture media was determined by a colorimetric assay (DC Protein Assay, Bio-Rad, Italy); 100 μg of total proteins per sample (final volume of 200 μL of Tris-buffered saline (TBS)) was spotted onto a nitrocellulose membrane using a Bio-Dot SF apparatus (Bio-Rad, Italy). After blocking for 1 h with 5% skimmed milk in TBST (TBS containing 0.05% Tween-20), pH 8, membranes were incubated for 1 h at room temperature in a monoclonal antibody to COL-I (1:1000 in TBST) (Sigma, Italy), to COL-III (1:2000 in TBST) (Sigma, Italy) and to MMP-1 (1 μg/ml in TBST, Millipore). After washing with TBST, membranes were incubated in HRP-conjugated rabbit anti-mouse serum for 1 h (1 : 6000 in TBST to detect COL-I and COL-III or 1 : 40,000 in TBST to detect MMP-1, respectively) (Sigma, Italy). Immunoreactive bands were revealed by the Opti-4CN substrate or Amplified Opti-4CN substrate (Bio-Rad, Italy) and quantified by densitometric scanning (UVBand, Eppendorf, Italy).

2.8. SDS-Zymography. Serum-free cell culture media were mixed 3 : 1 with sample buffer (containing 10% SDS), as previously described [16, 17]. Five μg of total protein per sample was run under nonreducing conditions without heat denaturation on 10% polyacrylamide gel (SDS-PAGE) copolymerized with 1 mg/mL of type I gelatin at 4°C. After SDS-PAGE, the gels were washed twice in a renaturing buffer

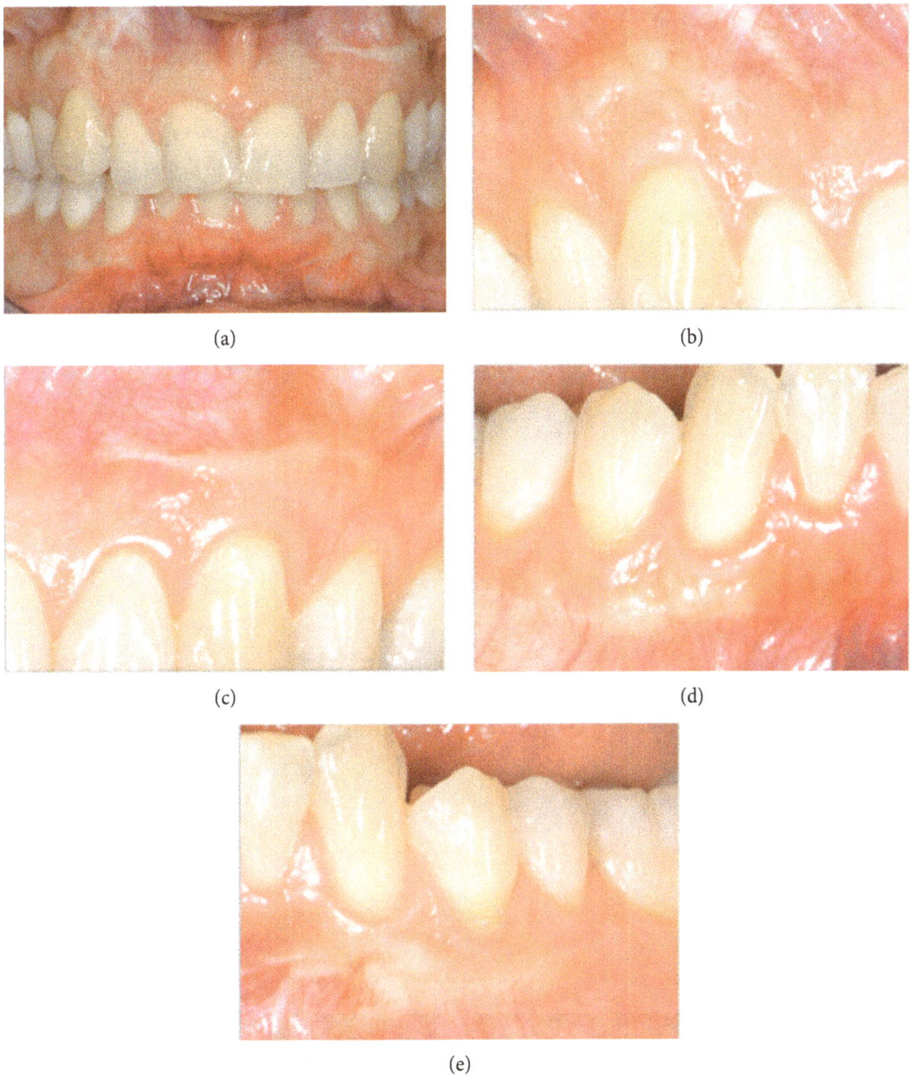

FIGURE 2: Clinical situation 4 years after the last surgical intervention. In the absence of gingival overgrowth, formation of thin scars is visible.

(2.5% Triton X-100, Tris-HCl 50 mM) for 30 min each and incubated overnight in a substrate buffer at 37°C (Tris-HCl 50 mM, $CaCl_2$ 5 mM, NaN_3 0.02%, pH 7.5). After staining the gels with Coomassie Brilliant Blue R-250, MMP gelatinolytic activity was detected as clear bands on a blue background. Bands were quantified by densitometric scanning (UVBand, Eppendorf, Italy).

2.9. Statistical Analysis. Data, expressed by mean ± standard deviation (SD), were analyzed by t-test. p values less than 0.05 were considered significant.

3. Results

3.1. Clinical Outcomes. From a clinical point of view, in the last follow-up visit, after 4 years from the last surgical intervention, no exostosis or gingival overgrowth formations could be observed (Figure 2) and we recorded a high degree of satisfaction with the treatment by the patient. However, scars, where surgeries were performed, were visible and clearly distinguishable from the surrounding tissues. Palpation did not reveal any overgrowth of soft or hard tissue.

3.2. Histological Analysis. Light microscopy analysis of hematoxylin and eosin-stained samples revealed that tissue integrity and structure were maintained in healthy and overgrown tissues (Figures 3(a) and 3(b)). The lining squamous-stratified epithelium was orthokeratinized, displaying a normal structure and normal thickness of the *stratum corneum* in both healthy and overgrown tissues. The dense irregular connective tissue was characterized by well-organized collagen fibers and an extracellular matrix with blood vessels normally distributed and without any inflammatory infiltrates. Sirius red staining specifically stained collagen fibers, densely packed in an irregular array, and revealed that the healthy and overgrown gingivae displayed a similar collagen content and arrangement (Figures 3(c) and 3(d)). The presence of connective papillary projections throughout the epithelium was also evident. The analysis of Sirius Red-stained sections under polarized light

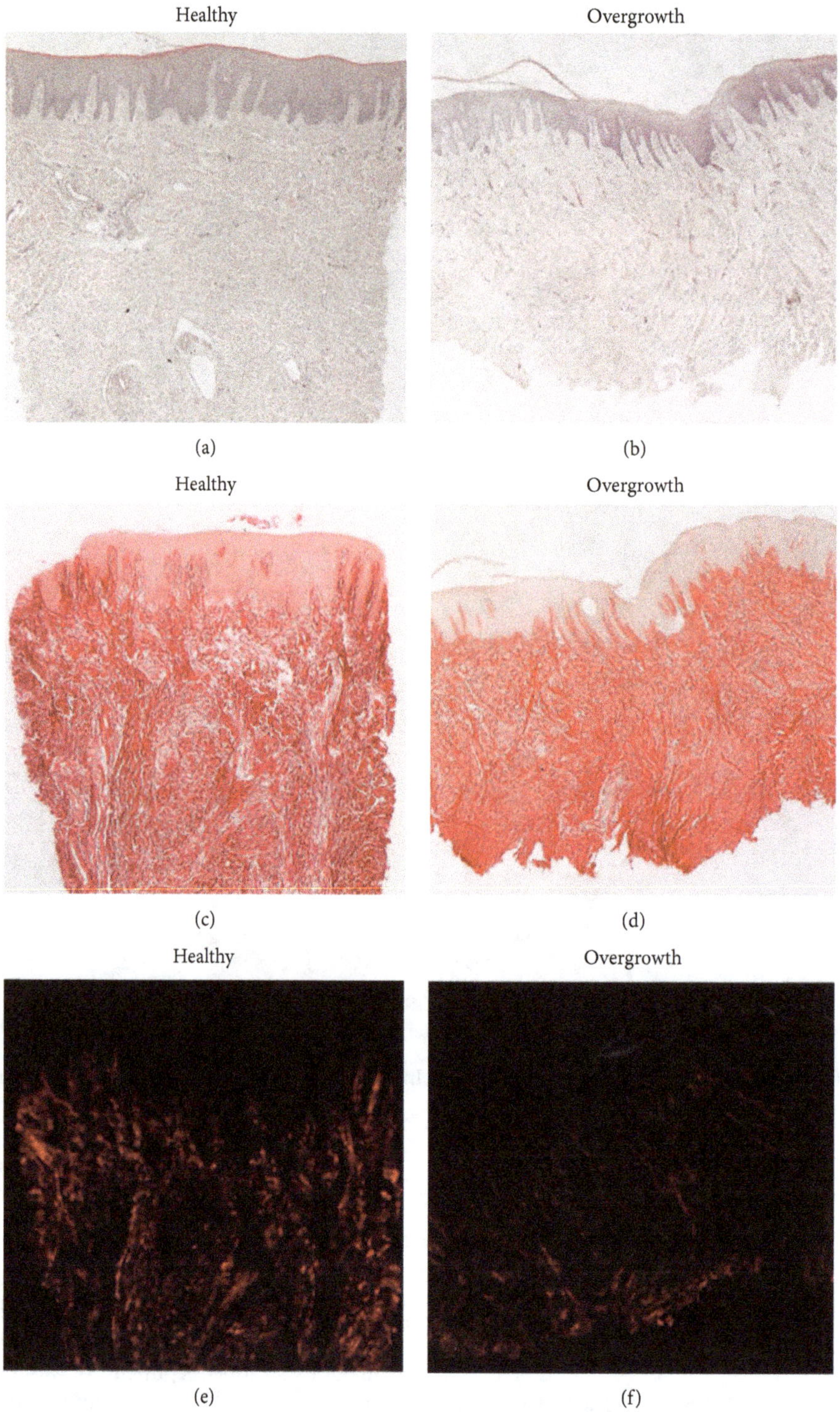

FIGURE 3: Micrographs showing the healthy and overgrown gingivae. (a-b) Hematoxylin and eosin staining reveals the morphological structure of the epithelium and of the connective tissue. (c-d) Sirius Red staining stains in red the collagen fibers of the connective tissue. (e-f) Polarized light performed on Sirius Red-stained samples shows birefringence relative to collagen fiber arrangement and maturation. Original magnification: 20x.

allowed detecting some qualitative differences in the epithelium and in the lamina propria of the healthy and overgrown gingivae. The healthy epithelium was totally lacking birefringence, while the overgrown gingiva showed a thin and not uniform birefringent layer in the superficial portion. The connective tissue was also analyzed under polarized light. According to Junqueira et al., under polarized light, the collagen matrix is stained from green to yellow to orange-red depending on the orientation of the collagen bundles and the maturation of collagen [15]. Specifically, the newly secreted and less mature collagen is stained in green while the mature collagen is stained in orange-red. Healthy gingiva

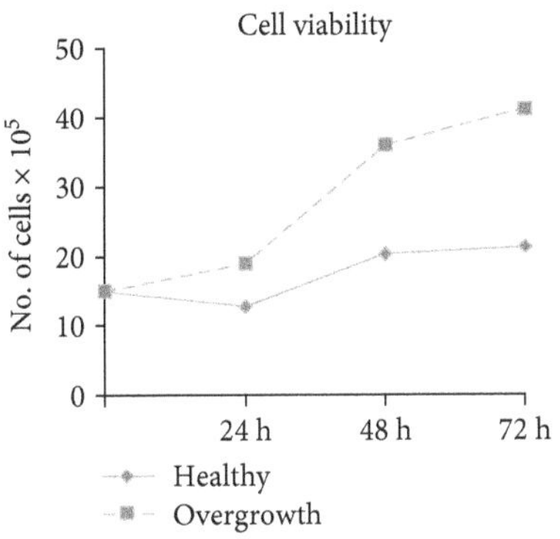

FIGURE 4: Cell proliferation. Growth curves showing cell viability in fibroblasts from healthy and overgrown gingivae after 24, 48, and 72 h.

appeared red under polarized light (Figure 3(e)). By contrast, red birefringence was less evident in the overgrown gingiva and the connective tissue was stained green to yellow, suggesting that the collagen was less mature (Figure 3(f)).

3.3. Cell Viability. Growth curves have shown that fibroblasts from the healthy and overgrowth gingivae exhibited a different proliferation rate at the considered time points. Fibroblasts from the overgrown gingiva tended to increase proliferation after 24, 48, and 72 h (Figure 4).

3.4. Collagen Turnover. The histological findings were supported by the analysis of collagen turnover. Collagen content in gingival fibroblast supernatants revealed that fibroblasts from the overgrown gingiva synthesized and secreted higher COL-I ($p < 0,01$, $p < 0,05$, and $p = 0,066$ vs. healthy gingiva after 24, 48, and 72 h, respectively) and COL-III protein levels ($p = 0,08$, $p = 0,09$, and p ns vs. healthy gingiva after 24, 48, and 72 h, respectively) (Figures 5(a) and 5(b)).

Gene expression for LOX resulted to be strongly upregulated in fibroblasts from the overgrown gingiva ($p < 0.005$ vs. healthy at 72 h) (Figure 5(c)).

Collagen degradation pathways were assayed by slot blot, real-time PCR, and SDS-zymography. MMP-1 levels tended to increase in fibroblasts obtained from the overgrown gingiva ($p < 0,05$, $p = 0,06$, and $p = 0,073$ vs. healthy gingiva after 24, 48, and 72 h, respectively) (Figures 6(a) and 6(b)). The expression of TIMP-1 mRNA, the main inhibitor of MMP-1, was unchanged after 24 and 48 h but strongly increased in fibroblasts from the overgrown gingiva after 72 h ($p < 0,001$) (Figure 6(c)). MMP-2 activity was characterized by a pattern concordant with MMP-1 protein levels ($p < 0,05$, $p < 0,05$, and p ns vs. healthy gingiva after 24, 48, and 72 h, respectively) (Figures 7(a) and 7(b)).

3.5. FAK Gene Expression. Gene expression analysis for FAK revealed similar mRNA levels in both experimental conditions after 24 and 48 h and a tendency towards upregulation in fibroblasts from the overgrown gingiva after 72 h ($p = 0.066$) (Figure 8).

4. Discussion

Alteration of the oral mucosa wounding affecting this patient suggests a possible relationship between keloid development and exostosis formation. To evaluate this association, we decided to analyze the healthy and overgrown gingivae overlying the exostosis of the same patient. According to the clinical observations, traumatism produced during the surgery seems to be relevant to the occurrence of relapses [1, 3].

Histological analysis revealed that the epithelium of the overgrown gingiva exhibited a normal general structure but showed an evident birefringence of the stratum corneum. We hypothesize that the mechanical stimulus exerted by the exostosis on the overlying gingiva resulted in a more compact stratum corneum, containing dense birefringent keratin bundles.

Collagen is the main component of the gingival dense irregular connective tissue. The histological analysis of the healthy and overgrown gingivae revealed a similar collagen content, as shown by Sirius Red staining. Polarized light microscopy revealed qualitative differences in collagen content, as the overgrown gingiva presented green-yellow coloration, while the healthy gingiva was stained in red, indicating that the collagen in the overgrown gingiva is less mature and therefore more susceptible to degradation by MMPs.

In order to understand the mechanisms responsible for this difference, we analyzed collagen turnover pathways in cultured gingival fibroblasts from the healthy and overgrown gingivae at the molecular level.

Collagen content is determined by the finely regulated dynamic balance between its synthesis and degradation by MMPs. MMP-1 begins collagen degradation breaking down the native triple helical region of interstitial collagens into characteristic 3/4- and 1/4-collagen degradation fragments, also known as gelatins [18], that can be further degraded to complete the digestion by less specific proteinases such as MMP-2 [19, 20]. MMP activity is regulated at the posttranslational level by TIMPs, inhibiting their activation and their activity [21]. Our results show that COL-I, the main component of gingival connective tissue, and COL-III protein levels were increased in supernatants of gingival fibroblasts from the overgrown gingiva. Moreover, an increased proliferation of fibroblasts obtained from the overgrown gingiva was observed. The apparent inconsistency between the morphological analysis, showing a similar collagen content, and increased collagen protein levels secreted by cultured fibroblasts obtained from the overgrown gingiva can be explained by analyzing the collagen degradation pathways. In fact, the observed concomitant increased MMP-1 and MMP-2 protein levels suggest an increased collagen turnover rate in fibroblasts from the overgrown gingiva. Consequently, increased collagen secretion in the overgrown gingiva is concomitant and paralleled with the increase in its degradation, resulting in a similar collagen content at the steady state in the connective tissue, as observed at the histological level. According to this suggestion, we can hypothesize that the observed TIMP-1 upregulation can be induced as a response to the MMP-1 overexpression, in order to balance it.

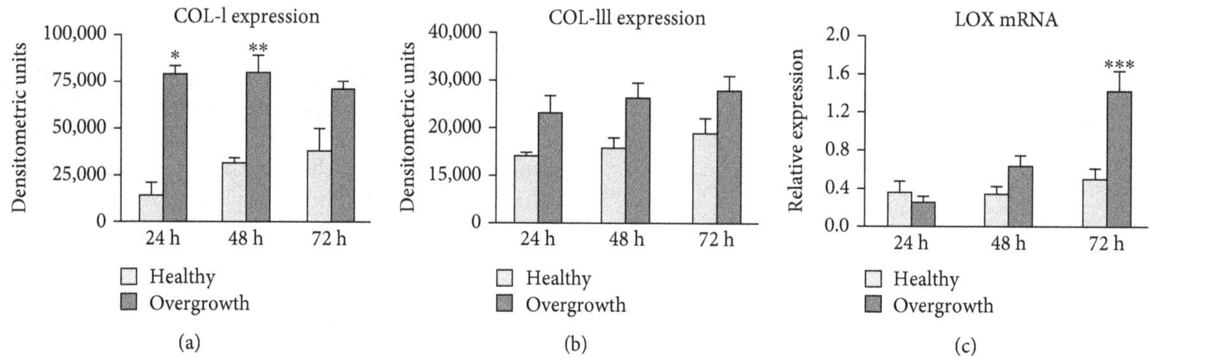

FIGURE 5: Collagen expression and maturation. Bar graphs showing COL-I (a) and COL-III (b) protein levels assessed by slot blot in cell culture supernatants of fibroblasts from healthy and overgrown gingivae. (c) Bar graphs showing LOX mRNA levels in fibroblasts from healthy and overgrown gingivae. GAPDH gene expression was used as internal control for normalization. Data are mean ± SD for samples run in duplicate. $^{*}p < 0.01$, $^{**}p < 0.05$, and $^{***}p < 0.005$.

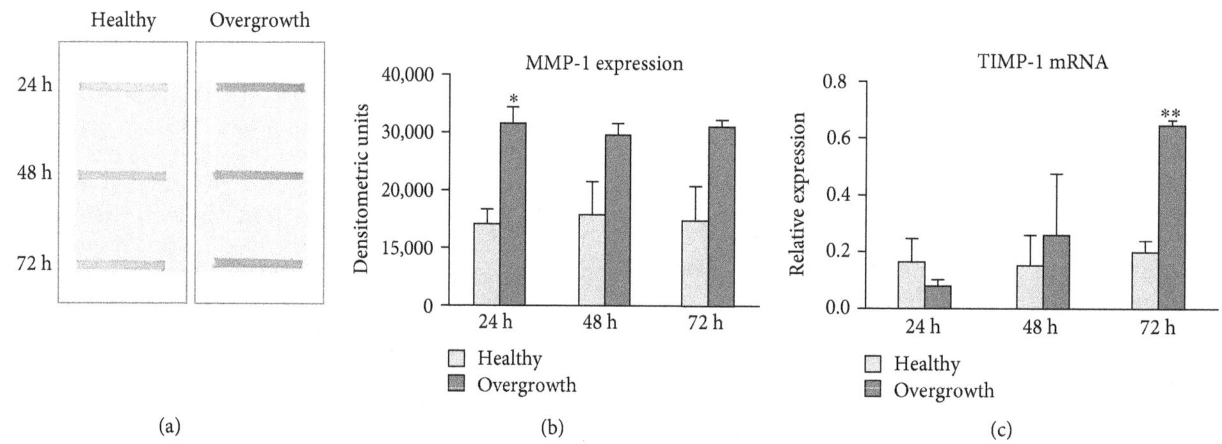

FIGURE 6: MMP-1 and TIMP-1 expression. (a) Representative slot blot showing MMP-1 levels in serum-free cell culture supernatants of fibroblasts from healthy and overgrown gingivae. Immunoreactive bands were quantified by densitometric scanning as described in Materials and Methods. (b) Bar graphs showing MMP-1 protein levels analyzed by slot blot. Data are expressed as densitometric units and are mean ± SD for samples run in duplicate. (c) Bar graphs showing TIMP-1 gene expression after normalization on GAPDH mRNA levels. Data are expressed as mean ± SD for samples run in triplicate. $^{*}p < 0.05$ and $^{**}p < 0.001$.

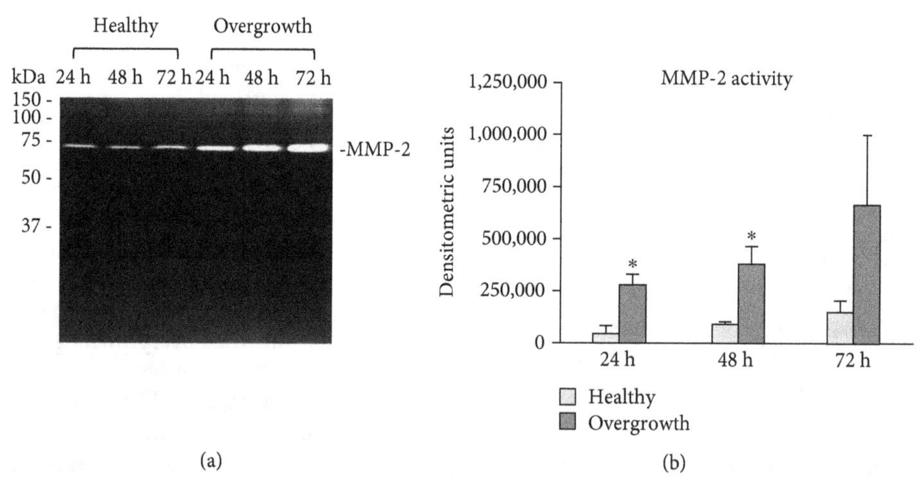

FIGURE 7: MMP-2 activity. (a) Representative SDS-zymography and (b) bar graphs showing MMP-2 activity in serum-free cell culture supernatants of fibroblasts from healthy and overgrown gingivae after densitometric analysis of immunoreactive and lytic bands. Data are expressed as densitometric units and are mean ± SD for samples run in duplicate. $^{*}p < 0.05$.

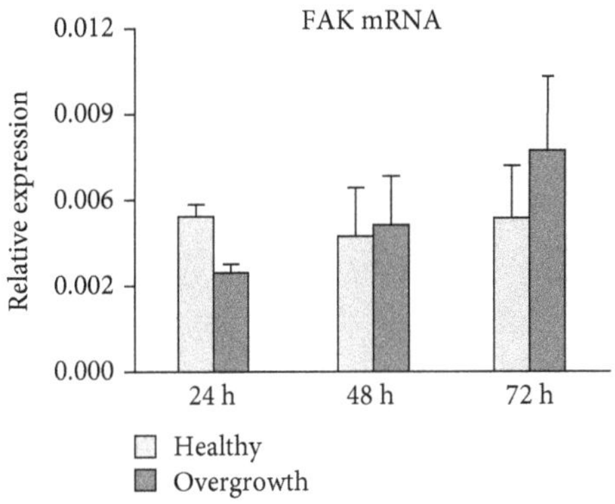

FIGURE 8: FAK mRNA levels. Bar graphs showing FAK mRNA levels after normalization on GAPDH gene expression. Data are expressed as mean ± SD for samples run in triplicate.

Newly synthesized collagen undergoes cross-linking, an important requirement for collagen maturation that provides collagen fibril stabilization and an increased tensile strength [22, 23]. Here, we show that LOX is strongly and significantly increased in fibroblasts from the overgrown gingiva, pointing to an increased collagen cross-linking activity induced by the exostosis.

The increased collagen turnover in fibroblasts from the overgrown gingiva could be therefore responsible for the differences revealed by the histological analysis. In fact, the exostosis could trigger a more rapid collagen turnover, consistent with the qualitative differences observed by polarized microscopy. However, in fibroblasts from the overgrown gingiva, LOX is significantly induced, suggesting that the newly secreted collagen in overgrown gingiva could undergo an increased cross-linking and maturation. Overexpression of LOX is very likely an adaptive response to avoid an excess collagen degradation in the gingiva, and it could favor collagen deposition in the gingival connective tissue covering the exostosis.

Collagen turnover rates can be affected by drugs as well as mechanical stimulation. Previous studies have shown that mechanical loading stimulates extracellular matrix (ECM) protein production by promoting the release of growth factors, such as TGF-β1, FGF, and PDGF [24]. Mechanical loading of cells has also been shown to modulate ECM turnover by regulating the expression and activity of MMPs [25–27]. Finally, mechanical loading interacts with growth factors and cytokines to regulate ECM homeostasis in various tissues [27–31]. We feel that our hypothesis of the role of exostosis as a triggering stimulus that influences gingival fibroblast activity is strengthened by the observations of gingival overgrowth exclusive to exostosis sites. Multiple exostoses were observed, each one covered by a gingival overgrowth lesion.

These suggestions are consistent with the tensegrity model described by Ingber, referring to a model of tensional integrity based on a network of structures that mechanically stabilize themselves using tensile prestress [32, 33]. According to this model, the whole structure is placed in a state of isometric tension that makes it strong, resilient, and immediately responsive to external mechanical stresses. The tensegrity model, referred to cells, led to the concept that mechanical forces would be sensed by cells using their cytoskeleton. In fact, a connection between cytoskeleton in the cell cytoplasm and the surrounding ECM is provided by the transmembrane proteins, integrins, working as mechanoreceptors, and finds its most useful application in understanding cellular mechanotransduction [34]. Integrins, mediating the attachment of cells to the ECM, are transmembrane proteins that provide a bridge through which forces can be transmitted between the inside and the outside of the cells. In fact, their extracellular domain binds to ECM components, whereas its cytoplasmic domain links various intracellular proteins interposed between actin filaments and integrin, forming focal adhesion complexes [35]. Mechanotransduction, the process that transforms mechanical stimuli into chemical signals, involves mechanosensory units integrated in the cell membrane that transduce mechanical signals into a biochemical response through force-dependent changes, important for regulation of global functions of the cell. Our data, showing a tendency to an increased gene expression of FAK, one of the components of the focal adhesions acting as a mechanoresponsive apparatus, is consistent with this hypothesis. In fact, an increase in focal adhesions as a response to mechanical stimulation elicited by the exostoses could be considered an adaptive response of gingival fibroblasts.

According to this model, we can consider gingival fibroblasts as cells using tensegrity architecture for their organization. This suggestion is supported by several studies that investigated the expression of ECM proteins in fibroblasts embedded in collagen gels under stretched and relaxed conditions, showing that the fibroblasts in the collagen adopted a synthetic phenotype characterized by their ability to synthesize matrix proteins and inhibit matrix degradation [36].

In this study, only one case of gingival overgrowth has been examined and we are aware that additional cases could advance and confirm our hypotheses; unfortunately, cases of multiple exostoses are very infrequent and this is the only case that came to our attention to date. Nevertheless, the association between exostoses and gingival overgrowth is strengthened by the presence of the overgrowths exclusively in the connective tissue covering each exostosis.

Our hypothesis is consistent with data previously reported [1, 3], showing a relationship between exostosis and FGG; these studies suggest that exostosis could be a rare side effect of FGG as a consequence of the periosteal traumatism during site preparation that induces the activation of osteoprogenitor cells. The clinical history of the patient revealed that the exostosis was formed after a surgical procedure that, very likely, triggered this mechanism inducing the exostosis, leading to the gingival overgrowth (Figure 9).

Our results suggest that exostosis could represent a mechanical stimulus stretching the overlying connective tissue and triggering a synthetic phenotype in gingival fibroblasts that, in turn, increase their activity in collagen turnover and maturation pathways. The effect of this stimulation seems responsible for the qualitative differences observed in the gingival connective tissue, thus affecting its biological and biomechanical properties. From a clinical

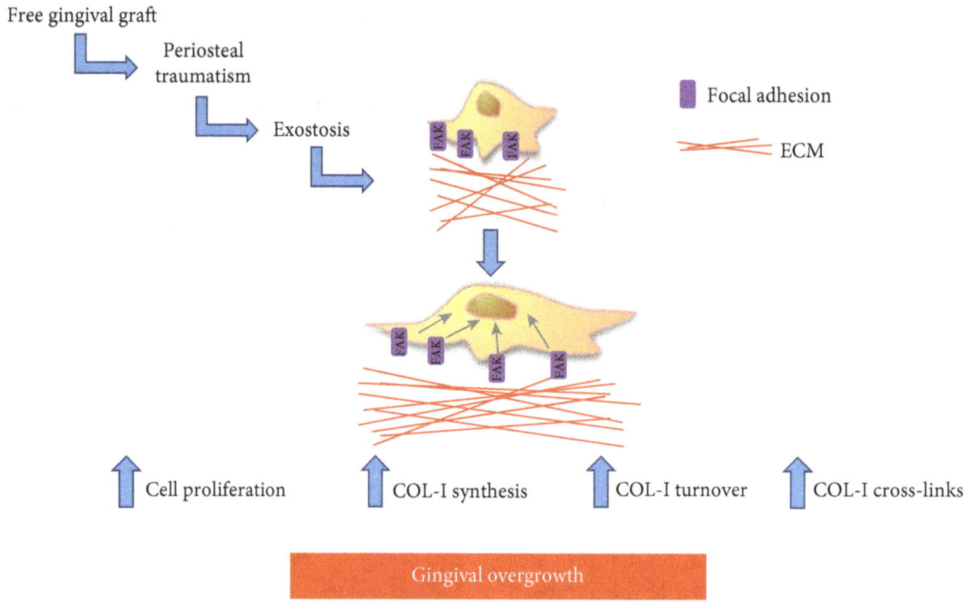

FIGURE 9: Diagram representing and summarizing the key events that could contribute to the development of gingival overgrowth covering the exostoses.

point of view, the results of this study suggest that the surgical removal of such lesions, which is the only possible treatment, should be performed using minimally invasive surgical techniques to avoid traumatizing the periosteal tissues and triggering the mechanisms that can lead to gingival overgrowth. This procedure can be successful in the eradication of the exostosis with minimal relapses. A cautious use of drugs interfering with gingival collagen turnovers, such as cyclosporine A, anticonvulsants, and calcium antagonists is also advised.

Authors' Contributions

Luca Francetti and Claudia Dellavia contributed equally to this work.

Acknowledgments

We thank Nataliya Khomchyna for the English editing of the manuscript.

References

[1] L. A. Chambrone and L. Chambrone, "Bony exostoses developed subsequent to free gingival grafts: case series," *British Dental Journal*, vol. 199, no. 3, pp. 146–149, 2005.

[2] R. E. Robinson, "The free mucosal graft in the edentulous mouth," *Journal of the California Dental Association*, vol. 43, no. 6, pp. 552–556, 1967.

[3] A. R. C. Pack, W. M. Gaudie, and A. M. Jennings, "Bony exostosis as a sequela to free gingival grafting: two case reports," *Journal of Periodontology*, vol. 62, no. 4, pp. 269–271, 1991.

[4] T. H. Morton Jr and E. Natkin, "Hyperostosis and fixed partial denture pontics: report of 16 patients and review of literature," *The Journal of Prosthetic Dentistry*, vol. 64, no. 5, pp. 539–547, 1990.

[5] W. C. Daniels, "Subpontic osseous hyperplasia: a five-patient report," *Journal of Prosthodontics*, vol. 6, no. 2, pp. 137–143, 1997.

[6] K. B. Frazier, P. S. Baker, R. Abdelsayed, and B. Potter, "A case report of subpontic osseous hyperplasia in the maxillary arch," *Oral Surgery, Oral Medicine, Oral Pathology, Oral Radiology, and Endodontology*, vol. 89, no. 1, pp. 73–76, 2000.

[7] E. A. Pechenkina and R. A. Benfer Jr, "The role of occlusal stress and gingival infection in the formation of exostoses on mandible and maxilla from Neolithic China," *HOMO*, vol. 53, no. 2, pp. 112–130, 2002.

[8] J. J. Echeverria, M. Montero, D. Abad, and C. Gay, "Exostosis following a free gingival graft," *Journal of Clinical Periodontology*, vol. 29, no. 5, pp. 474–477, 2002.

[9] W. M. Siegel and J. R. Pappas, "Development of exostoses following skin graft vestibuloplasty: Report of a case," *Journal of Oral and Maxillofacial Surgery*, vol. 44, no. 6, pp. 483-484, 1986.

[10] A. K. Hegtvedt, B. C. Terry, E. J. Burkes, and S. R. Patty, "Skin graft vestibuloplasty exostosis," *Oral Surgery, Oral Medicine, Oral Pathology*, vol. 69, no. 2, pp. 149–152, 1990.

[11] A. J. Corsair, V. J. Iacono, and S. S. Moss, "Exostosis following a subepithelial connective tissue graft," *Journal of the International Academy of Periodontology*, vol. 3, no. 2, pp. 38–41, 2001.

[12] A. Efeoglu and K. Demirel, "A further report of bony exostosis occurring as a sequela to free gingival grafts," *Periodontal clinical investigations: official publication of the Northeastern Society of Periodontists*, vol. 16, no. 1, pp. 20–22, 1994.

[13] C. A. Czuszak, G. E. Tolson, V. L. Kudryk, B. S. Hanson, and M. A. Billman, "Development of an Exostosis Following a Free Gingival Graft: Case Report," *Journal of Periodontology*, vol. 67, no. 3, pp. 250–253, 1996.

[14] F. J. Otero-Cagide, D. L. Singer, and J. N. Hoover, "Exostosis Associated With Autogenous Gingival Grafts: A Report of 9 Cases," *Journal of Periodontology*, vol. 67, no. 6, pp. 611–616, 1996.

[15] L. C. U. Junqueira, G. Bignolas, and R. R. Brentani, "Picrosirius staining plus polarization microscopy, a specific method for collagen detection in tissue sections," *The Histochemical Journal*, vol. 11, no. 4, pp. 447–455, 1979.

[16] N. Gagliano, C. Moscheni, C. Dellavia et al., "Effect of cyclosporin A on human gingival fibroblast collagen turnover in relation to the development of gingival overgrowth: an in vitro study," *Biomedicine & Pharmacotherapy*, vol. 58, no. 4, pp. 231–238, 2004.

[17] N. Gagliano, F. Costa, G. M. Tartaglia et al., "Effects of aging and cyclosporin a on collagen turnover in human gingiva," *The Open Dentistry Journal*, vol. 3, no. 1, pp. 219–226, 2009.

[18] T. Sakai and J. Gross, "Some properties of the products of reaction of tadpole collagenase with collagen," *Biochemistry*, vol. 6, no. 2, pp. 518–528, 1967.

[19] J. F. Woessner Jr, "Matrix metalloproteinases and their inhibitors in connective tissue remodeling," *The FASEB Journal*, vol. 5, no. 8, pp. 2145–2154, 1991.

[20] K. Brew, D. Dinakarpandian, and H. Nagase, "Tissue inhibitors of metalloproteinases: evolution, structure and function," *Biochimica et Biophysica Acta (BBA) - Protein Structure and Molecular Enzymology*, vol. 1477, no. 1-2, pp. 267–283, 2000.

[21] G. Murphy, F. Willenbrock, T. Crabbe et al., "Regulation of matrix metalloproteinase activity," *Annals of the New York Academy of Sciences*, vol. 732, no. 1 Inhibition of, pp. 31–41, 1994.

[22] M. Yamauchi and M. Shiiba, "Lysine hydroxylation and cross-linking of collagen," *Methods Mol Biol*, vol. 446, pp. 95–108, 2008.

[23] M. Yamauchi and M. Sricholpech, "Lysine post-translational modifications of collagen," *Essays In Biochemistry*, vol. 52, pp. 113–133, 2012.

[24] M. Skutek, M. Griensven, J. Zeichen, N. Brauer, and U. Bosch, "Cyclic mechanical stretching modulates secretion pattern of growth factors in human tendon fibroblasts," *European Journal of Applied Physiology*, vol. 86, no. 1, pp. 48–52, 2001.

[25] J. M. Archambault, M. K. Elfervig-Wall, M. Tsuzaki, W. Herzog, and A. J. Banes, "Rabbit tendon cells produce MMP-3 in response to fluid flow without significant calcium transients," *Journal of Biomechanics*, vol. 35, no. 3, pp. 303–309, 2002.

[26] M. Tsuzaki, D. Bynum, L. Almekinders, J. Faber, and A. J. Banes, "Mechanical loading stimulates ecto-ATPase activity in human tendon cells," *Journal of Cellular Biochemistry*, vol. 96, no. 1, pp. 117–125, 2005.

[27] N. von Offenberg Sweeney, P. M. Cummins, Y. A. Birney, J. P. Cullen, E. M. Redmond, and P. A. Cahill, "Cyclic strain-mediated regulation of endothelial matrix metalloproteinase-2 expression and activity," *Cardiovascular Research*, vol. 63, no. 4, pp. 625–634, 2004.

[28] A. J. Banes, M. Tsuzaki, J. Yamamoto et al., "Mechanoreception at the cellular level: the detection, interpretation, and diversity of responses to mechanical signals," *Biochemistry and Cell Biology*, vol. 73, no. 7-8, pp. 349–365, 1995.

[29] L. J. Bonassar, A. J. Grodzinsky, A. Srinivasan, S. G. Davila, and S. B. Trippel, "Mechanical and physicochemical regulation of the action of insulin-like growth factor-I on articular cartilage," *Archives of Biochemistry and Biophysics*, vol. 379, no. 1, pp. 57–63, 2000.

[30] M. Jin, G. R. Emkey, P. Siparsky, S. B. Trippel, and A. J. Grodzinsky, "Combined effects of dynamic tissue shear deformation and insulin-like growth factor I on chondrocyte biosynthesis in cartilage explants," *Archives of Biochemistry and Biophysics*, vol. 414, no. 2, pp. 223–231, 2003.

[31] M. Murata, L. J. Bonassar, M. Wright, H. J. Mankin, and C. A. Towle, "A role for the interleukin-1 receptor in the pathway linking static mechanical compression to decreased proteoglycan synthesis in surface articular cartilage," *Archives of Biochemistry and Biophysics*, vol. 413, no. 2, pp. 229–235, 2003.

[32] D. E. Ingber, "Tensegrity and mechanotransduction," *Journal of Bodywork and Movement Therapies*, vol. 12, no. 3, pp. 198–200, 2008.

[33] D. E. Ingber, N. Wang, and D. Stamenovic, "Tensegrity, cellular biophysics, and the mechanics of living systems," *Reports on Progress in Physics*, vol. 77, no. 4, article 046603, 2014.

[34] D. Ingber and J. D. Jamieson, "Cells as tensegrity structures: architectural regulation of histodifferentiation by physical forces tranduced over basement membranes," in *Gene expression during normal and malignant differentiation*, L. C. Andersson, C. G. Gahmberg, and P. Ekblom, Eds., Academic Press, Orlando, FL, USA, 1985.

[35] M. J. Reed, N. S. Ferara, and R. B. Vernon, "Impaired migration, integrin function, and actin cytoskeletal organization in dermal fibroblasts from a subset of aged human donors," *Mechanisms of Ageing and Development*, vol. 122, no. 11, pp. 1203–1220, 2001.

[36] D. Kessler, S. Dethlefsen, I. Haase et al., "Fibroblasts in mechanically stressed collagen lattices assume a "synthetic" phenotype," *Journal of Biological Chemistry*, vol. 276, no. 39, pp. 36575–36585, 2001.

12

A Successful Esthetic Approach of Gingival Depigmentation using Microneedling Technique and Ascorbic Acid (Vitamin C)

Diana Mostafa[1] **and Shaden M. Alotaibi**[2]

[1]*Clinical Periodontology Department, Faculty of Dentistry, Alexandria University, Alexandria, Egypt*
[2]*Preventive Dental Sciences, Vision colleges for dentistry and Nursing, Riyadh, Saudi Arabia*

Correspondence should be addressed to Diana Mostafa; dr.dianamostafa@gmail.com

Academic Editor: Giuseppe Alessandro Scardina

A gingival depigmentation is a periodontal plastic procedure that is performed in order to remove melanocytic pigmentation. A variety of different modalities have been proposed for removing hyperpigmentation involving surgical scraping, gingival autograft, cryotherapy, electrosurgery, and lasers. However, the microneedling technique is a nonsurgical procedure that creates microholes to facilitate the penetration of topical medications across the connective tissues. *Case Description.* A healthy female patient aged 25 years with a pigmented gingiva seeking gingival depigmentation. On examination, a dark brown ribbon of hyperpigmentation was observed within the mandibular attached gingiva. The case was diagnosed as physiological moderate gingival pigmentation (pigmentation index score = 3). The patient was interested in achieving aesthetic results with minimally invasive, nonexpensive procedures. Based on the patient's concerns, the microneedling technique using vitamin C was suggested and consented. We used a dermapen device to microneedle the gingiva until bleeding pinpoints were observed; then, topical ascorbic acid was applied. After 3 days, our outcomes revealed an excellent aesthetic pink gingival appearance. *Conclusions and Practical Implications.* Compared to other minimally invasive techniques, our technique is less expensive and more risk-free. Our novel technique of using dermapen and topical ascorbic acid has shown promising results to our case which gives new perspectives for its application in gingival depigmentation.

1. Introduction

Since perioaesthetics have become a major demand in dentistry, treatment protocols should not only address functional and biological problems but also establish harmony between white and pink (teeth and gingiva). A typical macroanatomical feature of healthy gingiva is its pink colour which diverges into various shades depending on the degree of keratinization, the thickness of the gingiva, the degree of vascularization, reduction of haemoglobin, and the presence of melanocytic cells [1].

Hyperpigmented gingiva is caused by a wide range of external or internal influences. It is maybe due to physiological or pathological factors, which cause the excessive deposition of melanin granules in melanocytes in the basal and suprabasal layers of the epithelium [2]. Gingival hyperpigmentation can cause a cosmetic problem that may have an adverse psychological impact on patients, especially those with short lips and high smile lines. However, gingival pigmentation (GP) tends to be more prominent among dark-skinned individuals. It is more likely to be observed in the anterior area than the posterior, and the mandible is more commonly affected than the maxilla. The degree of GP is affected by melanocyte activity, melanosomes number, dispersion degree, and degradation of the pigment [1, 2].

Gingival hyperpigmentation was classified according to melanin index by Hanioka et al. [3] into three classes; class 0 indicates no pigmentation, class 1 represents solitary units of pigmentation in papillae only, and class 2 displays a continuous ribbon of gingival pigmentation (GP). In addition, the oral pigmentation index was introduced by Dummett and Gupta in 1971 [4] as scores for GP according to its colour degree; score 1 is given to pink gingiva (no pigmentation), score 2 indicates light brown pigmentation (mild

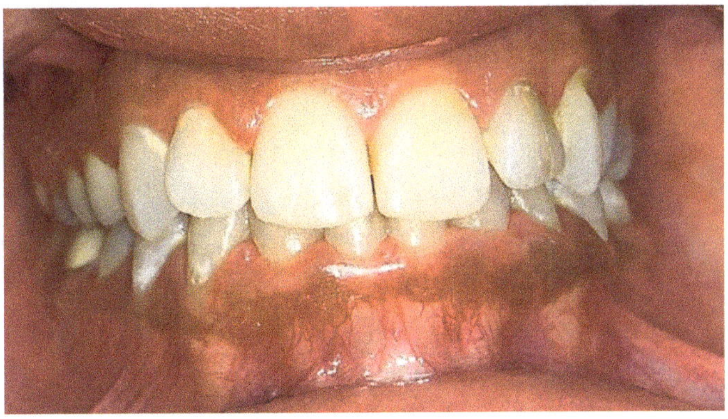

Figure 1: Preoperative picture of moderate gingival pigmentation.

pigmentation), score 3 represents medium brown or mixed brown pink and brown pigmentation (moderate pigmentation), and score 4 indicates deep brown or bluish-black pigmentation (heavy pigmentation). In 2017, the American Academy of Periodontology and the European Federation of Periodontology proposed a new classification of periodontal and peri-implant diseases [5] in which gingival colour alterations are diagnosed as "gingival pigmentations" and it was classified into melanoplakia, smoker's melanosis, drug-induced pigmentations, and amalgam tattoo.

Gingival depigmentation (GD) is considered a periodontal plastic procedure whereby melanocytic pigmentation is removed. A variety of different modalities have been proposed for removing hyperpigmentation involving bur abrasion, surgical scraping, gingival autograft, cryotherapy, electrosurgery, and laser [6]. In addition, some studies suggest that ascorbic acid (vitamin C) could be used to treat gingival pigmentation [7].

However, the microneedling (MN) technique is a non-surgical procedure that is known as collagen induction therapy involving repetitive punctures on the skin. In dermatology, MN has been utilized considerably in recent years as it is an effective, simple, economical, well-tolerated, and cosmetically and therapeutically beneficial procedure [8]. The MN serves to separate the cells instead of cutting through forming microconduits which increases the skin's permeability and blood flow into the epidermis. This process facilitates the penetration of topical medications across the stratum corneum layer. Besides, growth factors are produced promoting the regeneration of collagen and elastin [8, 9].

However, ascorbic acid (AA) has been demonstrated as a water-soluble antioxidant and an essential nutrient for collagen biosynthesis [10]. It plays a role in immunomodulation as well as the elimination of the hyperpigmented spots [11] by interacting with the copper ions at the tyrosinase active site and inhibiting the activity of the enzyme tyrosinase, thereby diminishing melanin production [10].

While many clinical investigations have been documented, on the effectiveness of the MN technique in treating scars and wrinkles, promoting skin rejuvenation, and managing pigmentation disorders [8, 12–14], scarce dental studies have been conducted on its application in the oral cavity. For the current case, we utilized the MN technique using dermapen to enhance the absorption of topical AA (vitamin C) into pigmented gingival mucosa.

2. Aim of the Study

The purpose of the study was to assess the performance of the microneedling technique using dermapen with topical ascorbic acid paste on gingival depigmentation.

3. Case Description

A healthy 25-year-old female patient complained of aesthically unappealing dark colour in the lower front gum area (Figure 1). According to her detailed history, hyperpigmentation was evident from birth, which implied physiological hyperpigmentation. In addition, it was reported that the patient had never taken any medications or been diagnosed with any systemic conditions which would affect the gingival colour. Besides, her family and social histories were insignificant. According to her, she had never smoked or been exposed to second-hand smoke. Furthermore, her complaint had not been addressed in an oral setting previously.

4. Clinical Findings and Diagnostic Assessment

On clinical examination, no abnormalities were identified extraorally. Intraoral examination revealed a minimal accumulation of plaque and supragingival calculus, indicating an acceptable level of oral hygiene. She had an average plaque index of 0.8 and an average gingival index of 1 with no bleeding upon probing. Neither clinical attachment loss nor radiographic bone loss was determined. There was only mild marginal gingival inflammation accompanied by rolled margins and blunted interdental papillae.

A dark brown ribbon of hyperpigmentation was noticed within the gingival mucosa of the mandibular arch confined to the attached gingiva region from right to left 2nd premolars (Figure 1). The case was diagnosed as physiological moderate gingival pigmentation (pigmentation index score = 3) according to the Dummett-Gupta Oral Pigmentation Index [4] with extended ribbon-like melanin pigmentation (melanin index class 2).

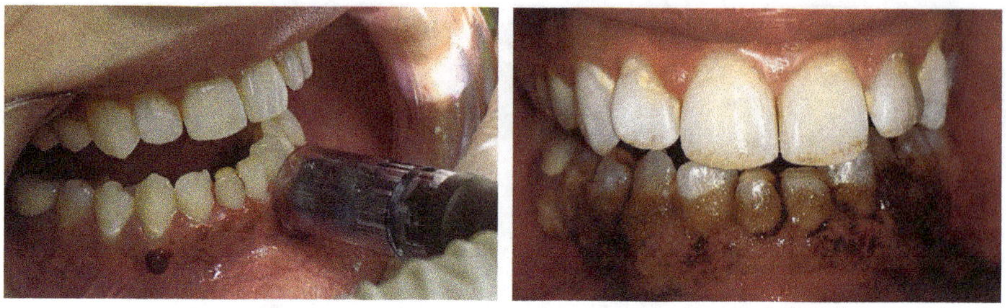

FIGURE 2: Microneedling technique using dermapen and ascorbic acid (vitamin C) application.

5. Therapeutic Intervention

The patient was most concerned about achieving aesthetic results with minimally invasive, nonexpensive procedures. In light of the patient's concerns, the MN technique was suggested. The patient was provided with a detailed explanation of this off-label procedure, its instructions, and potential complications. Informed consent was established as well as permission for this off-label procedure, photos, and publication.

As a preliminary routine, supragingival scaling was performed and oral hygiene instructions were provided by the dental hygienist. We subsequently scheduled the procedure and performed it aseptically. Local anaesthesia 2% lignocaine (1 : 80,000 adrenaline) was administered by infiltration technique in the mandibular region. To microneedle the gingival mucosa, we used a dermapen device model M8 with 24 microneedles arranged in rows, which was adjusted with 1.5 mm depth at the 6th mode speed of 700 cycles/min. The dermapen was used in intermittent motion on the sextant gingival area for 30-40 seconds/tooth. When bleeding pinpoints were observed on all areas of pigmented gingiva, the gingival mucosa was irrigated with a saline solution and sterile gauze was applied to dry the area. Then, topical AA powder (1000 mg/ml) was mixed with saline in a small glass dish forming a paste. The mixed slurry paste was applied to the gingival mucosa using for 10 minutes as shown in Figure 2. The treated area was left without dressing. Our patient was instructed to refrain from drinking acidic or hot beverages for 24 hours and to not brush her lower teeth for one day to avoid any mechanical trauma to the gingiva. Following the procedure, neither mouthwashes nor medications were prescribed for her. The photos were taken before, during, and at follow-up appointments until 6 months.

6. Clinical Follow-Up and Outcomes

One day after the procedure, the attached gingiva exhibited an increase in volume and an alteration in texture as well as the appearance of white and red-coloured areas, indicating tissue inflammation (Figure 3(a)). Neither pain nor tenderness was reported, and only discomfort sensation was experienced. On the third day, all of these findings diminished resulting in the pink appearance of the gingiva (Figure 3(b)). The same procedure was performed after 2 weeks, resulting in same the postoperative tissue inflammation which diminished on the 3rd day of the second application. Clinical outcomes showed complete disappearance of gingival pigmentation. Generally, after the first and second application, healing was normal and satisfactory providing excellent aesthetic results where the pigmentation index score decreased to zero with reduction of melanin index (class 0) as presented in Figures 3(c) and 3(d). After the 6th month of the follow-up period, repigmentation of the gingiva was detected showing light brown solitary pigmented areas as depicted in Figure 4.

7. Discussion

Although the GP does not exhibit any medical concerns, patients frequently complain of "black gums" seeking cosmetic solutions. In this case presentation, the patient was diagnosed with physiological pigmentation based on the negative history of any pathological cause, since the physiologic pigmentation is probably genetic in nature.

GD is considered a periodontal plastic procedure whereby the gingival hyperpigmentation is removed or reduced through various techniques such as scalpel scraping, bur abrasion, free gingival graft, cryosurgery, electrosurgery, and laser [6]. In the present case, we achieved GD by a novel technique using microneedling and topical AA. It is a minimally invasive, well-tolerated, safe, not expensive, and less time-consuming procedure.

To our knowledge, this is the first study to introduce NM with AA in gingival depigmentation. Nevertheless, there was a study done by Ozsagir et al. [15] who compared the use of i-PRF alone or in combination with microneedling for gingival augmentation. They concluded that after 6 months, the group using i-PRF combined with microneedling showed a statistically significant increase in gingival thickness compared to the group using only i-PRF.

Although, the FDA has legally authorized microneedling devices to improve the appearance of facial acne scars, facial wrinkles, and abdominal scars in patients aged 22 years or older, these devices are still considered as off-label procedures for oral use. However, there are various types of MN devices including dermaroller, dermastamp, and dermapen. Unlike other MN devices, dermapen is the only device that can be applied intraorally due to its small size, changeable head. This increases the accessibility inside the mouth and makes it easy to be used for a larger number of patients. This device is a wireless electric device with automated features that allow the operator to modify the speeds, pressures, and depth of penetration, thus reducing the probability of operator-related side effects.

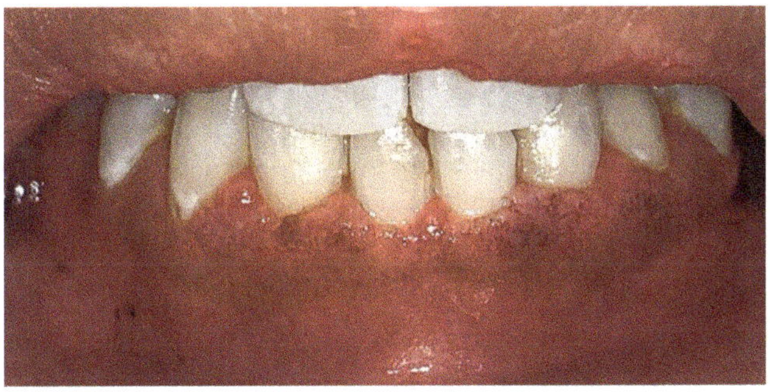

(a) Immediately after microneedling and ascorbic acid application

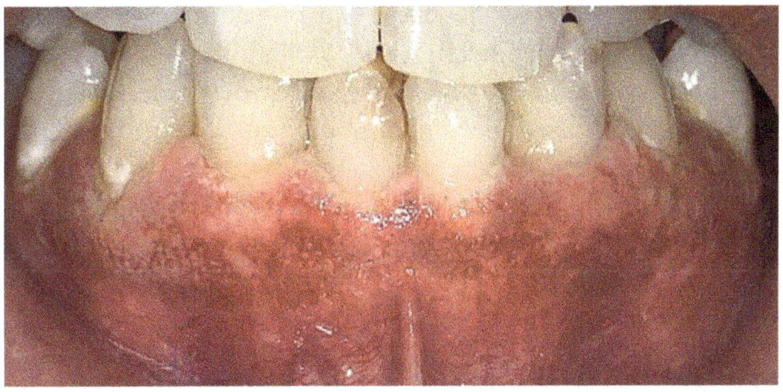

(b) After one day of the procedure

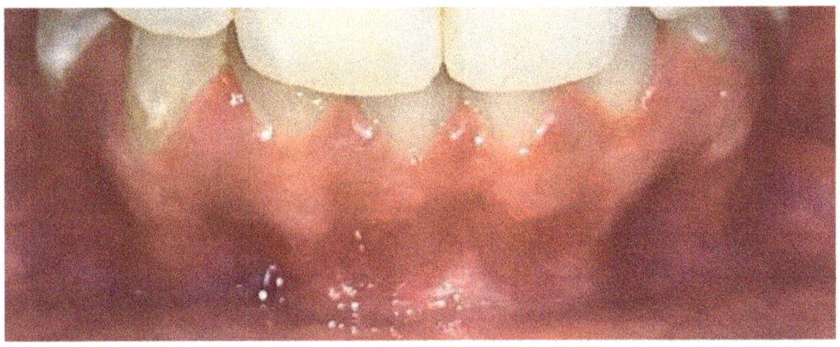

(c) After 3 days of the procedure

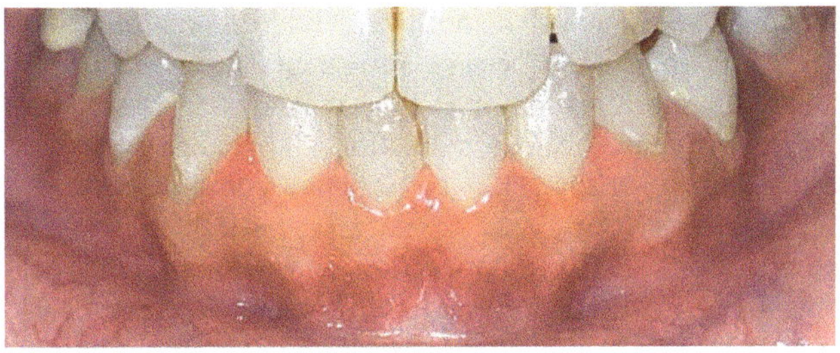

(d) After 3 months

FIGURE 3: (a–d) Postoperative pictures of gingival depigmentation.

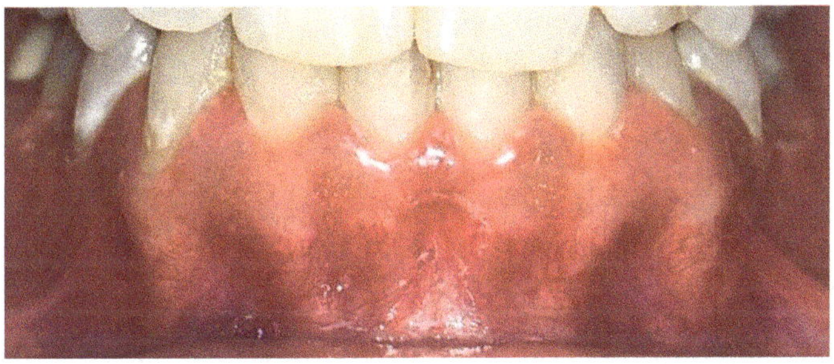

FIGURE 4: Recurrence of gingival pigmentation started after 6 months.

In the present study, the patient agreed and signed explicit written consent for this off-label procedure being used as a part of research. During the procedure, it was necessary to generate precise bleeding pinpoints by MN to achieve optimal results [16]. These microholes allow the therapeutic medication to penetrate easily into the connective tissues, stimulating new collagen production and affecting melanocytes [8].

Then, we used topical AA as a therapeutic medication that was reported to be effective in reducing melanogenesis directly and thus promoting depigmentation, because melanin acts as a reservoir for reactive oxygen species (ROS), Cu, and calcium within the cells. Following AA entry into the target tissue, it binds to melanin causing a deficiency of ROS, Cu, and Ca, resulting in the reduction in melanin production [17]. As to say that AA affects melanocyte function rather than the number, as opposed to other approaches relying on the destruction of melanocytes.

Our outcomes revealed excellent aesthetic results, and these were in agreement with Yussif et al. [18] who used intraepithelial injections of 1-1.5 ml AA (200-300 mg) in the gingival mucosa and reported that its direct delivery reduced pigmentation incidence scores and area of pigmentation. As well as comparing injectable AA to conventional scalpel depigmentation by Yussif et al. [19] in 2019 who concluded that injecting AA into pigmented cells presented comparable results to conventional surgery.

Furthermore, our findings were consistent with the results of Shimada et al. [20] who applied topical vitamin C gel to the gingiva and concluded that AA inhibited melanin pigmentation. However, a study made by El-Mofty et al. [21] stated that intramucosal AA injections were better and more efficacious than topical AA gels for GD.

Following the first day of the procedure, the gingiva showed an increase in volume and a change in texture with white and red-coloured areas representing gingival inflammation, oedema, and irritation. These results were corresponding with numerous clinical studies in dermatology which revealed that the MN technique can cause postoperative transit oedema and erythema that resolves usually after 1-3 days [22–25].

In contrast to any other depigmentation procedure, the patient was able to see these excellent aesthetic results after 3 days (Figure 3). However, healing after scalpel depigmentation takes 7-10 days, and other procedures take more than 2 weeks to heal [26, 27]. In addition, a dressing is not necessary after the procedure since microholes are created without perfused bleeding and heal quickly, unlike scalpel depigmentation where the gingiva should be covered with dressing as it leaves denuded connective tissue and heals by secondary intention [5]. Moreover, a free gingival graft can be used for GD, but it involves a second surgical site (donor site) and it has unaesthetic colour matching [28].

Compared to other minimally invasive techniques, our technique poses less risk of complications and is less expensive. However, lasers are considered easy, fast, and efficient modalities that have hemostasis and decontamination effects, but they are expensive and tissues heal within 1-2 weeks [29, 30]. Additionally, electrosurgery has been reported to cause heat accumulation and undesired tissue destruction, and it takes 5-14 days for complete healing [31]. While cryosurgery may cause postoperative swelling and increase soft tissue destruction as well as difficulty in controlling the depth and freezing duration, also it takes 3-4 weeks for complete keratinization [26].

Pigment recurrence is described as a spontaneous and recurrent process that occurs within 24 hours up to 8 years following the depigmentation procedure which poses a challenge to a dentist [28]. Methods of treatment, number of recall periods, genetic and ethnic factors, tobacco consumption, and hormonal factors influence the gingival repigmentation [32]. It has been hypothesized that the rate of melanin formation is higher in darker individuals [33]. Also, gingival pigmentation is more in the anterior gingiva than posterior ones which have been attributed to sunlight exposure [34]. Many authors [35–37] who used surgical technique showed early recurrence of pigmentation after 15-56 days of follow-up periods. However, the majority of the available literature has shown a lower recurrence rate for cryosurgery and lasers [38]. Nakamura et al. [39] described repigmentation after 24 months after laser depigmentation. Additionally, previous studies [40–43] have reported gingival pigmentation recurrence after 12-48 months following cryosurgery depigmentation.

In our case report, repigmentation was observed after 6 months (Figure 4). This might be due to the proliferation of melanocytes and their migration to the depigmented area [27]. These recurrence findings vary from those of Sheel et al. [44] who used scalpel depigmentation along with the monthly local application of AA, which gave positive aesthetic results, but recurrence was observed after 9 months. This may be related to the amount of AA that gingival tissues are exposed to.

However, our procedure is well tolerated by patients and can be repeated from time to time for more aesthetic results.

8. Conclusions

Clinical experience, affordability, and personal preferences should be considered when selecting a technique for treating gingival hyperpigmentation. Our novel technique of using dermapen and topical ascorbic acid in the treatment of gingival pigmentation showed promising results, which gives new perspectives for its application. Although our technique is a simple and safe GD method, it should be performed cautiously; otherwise, tissue destruction and gingival recession may result. Our results were limited to this particular case. Therefore, the present findings should be confirmed in future randomized controlled clinical trials, including histological analysis.

Consent

Patient consent for publication was obtained.

Authors' Contributions

DM contributed to conceptualization, manuscript writing and editing, and clinical work. SA contributed to conceptualization, manuscript preparation, and writing.

References

[1] C.-R. Yuri, "Gingival melanosis:, a review of diagnosis and treatment criteria," *Odontoestomatología*, vol. 21, no. 33, pp. 54–61, 2019.

[2] Y. Çiçek and U. Ertaş, "The normal and pathological pigmentation of oral mucous membrane: a review," *The Journal of Contemporary Dental Practice*, vol. 4, no. 3, pp. 76–86, 2003.

[3] T. Hanioka, K. Tanaka, M. Ojima, and K. Yuuki, "Association of melanin pigmentation in the gingiva of children with parents who smoke," *Pediatrics*, vol. 116, no. 2, pp. e186–e190, 2005.

[4] C. O. Dummet and G. Barens, "Oromucosal pigmentation: an updated literary review," *Journal of Periodontology*, vol. 42, no. 11, pp. 726–736, 1971.

[5] P. Corteillini and N. F. Bissada, "Mucogingival conditions in the natural dentition: narrative review, case definitions, and diagnostic considerations," *Journal of Clinical Periodontology*, vol. 45, pp. S190–S198, 2018.

[6] A. Thangavelu, S. Elavarasu, and P. Jayapalan, "Pink esthetics in periodontics - gingival depigmentation: a case series," *Journal of Pharmacy & Bioallied Sciences*, vol. 4, Suppl 2, pp. S186–S190, 2012.

[7] R. M. Sanadi and R. S. Deshmukh, "The effect of vitamin C on melanin pigmentation - a systematic review," *J Oral Maxillofac Pathol.*, vol. 24, no. 2, pp. 374–382, 2020.

[8] C. Iriarte, O. Awosika, M. Rengifo-Pardo, and A. Ehrlich, "Review of applications of microneedling in dermatology," *Clinical, Cosmetic and Investigational Dermatology*, vol. - Volume 10, pp. 289–298, 2017.

[9] A. Singh and S. Yadav, "Microneedling: advances and widening horizons," *Indian Dermatology Online Journal*, vol. 7, no. 4, pp. 244–254, 2016.

[10] J. Velisek and K. Cejpek, "Biosynthesis of food constituents: vitamins, water-soluble vitamins, part 2 – a review," *Czech Journal of Food Sciences*, vol. 25, pp. 49–64, 2008.

[11] S. J. Padayatty and M. Levine, "Vitamin C: the known and the unknown and Goldilocks," *Oral Diseases*, vol. 22, no. 6, pp. 463–493, 2016.

[12] M. T. McCrudden, E. McAlister, A. J. Courtenay, P. González-Vázquez, T. R. Raj Singh, and R. F. Donnelly, "Microneedle applications in improving skin appearance," *Experimental Dermatology*, vol. 24, no. 8, pp. 561–566, 2015.

[13] F. Al Qarqaz and A. Al-Yousef, "Skin microneedling for acne scars associated with pigmentation in patients with dark skin," *Journal of Cosmetic Dermatology*, vol. 17, no. 3, pp. 390–395, 2018.

[14] J. W. Jung, W. O. Kim, H. R. Jung, S. A. Kim, and Y. W. Ryoo, "A face-split study to evaluate the effects of microneedle radiofrequency with Q-switched Nd: YAG laser for the treatment of melasma," *Annals of Dermatology*, vol. 31, no. 2, pp. 133–138, 2019.

[15] Z. B. Ozsagir, E. Saglam, B. Sen Yilmaz, J. Choukroun, and M. Tunali, "Injectable platelet-rich fibrin and microneedling for gingival augmentation in thin periodontal phenotype: a randomized controlled clinical trial," *Journal of Clinical Periodontology*, vol. 47, no. 4, pp. 489–499, 2020.

[16] A. Gowda, B. Healey, H. Ezaldein, and M. Merati, "A systematic review examining the potential adverse effects of microneedling," *The Journal of Clinical and Aesthetic Dermatology*, vol. 14, no. 1, pp. 45–54, 2021.

[17] T. H. Tsai, C. J. Huang, W. H. Wu, W. C. Huang, J. H. Chyuan, and P. J. Tsai, "Antioxidant, cell-protective, and anti-melanogenic activities of leaf extracts from wild bitter melon (Momordica charantia Linn var abbreviata Ser) cultivars," *Botanical Studies*, vol. 55, no. 1, p. 78, 2014.

[18] N. M. Yussif, S. O. Zayed, S. A. Hasan, and S. S. Sadek, "Evaluation of injectable vitamin C as a depigmenting agent in physiologic gingival melanin hyperpigmentation: a clinical trial," *Rep Opinion*, vol. 8, pp. 113–120, 2016.

[19] N. M. Yussif, A. R. Abdel Rahman, and E. Elbarbary, "Minimally invasive non-surgical locally injected vitamin C versus the conventional surgical depigmentation in treatment of gingival hyperpigmentation of the anterior esthetic zone: a prospective comparative study," *Clinical Nutrition Experimental*, vol. 24, pp. 54–65, 2019.

[20] Y. Shimada, H. Tai, A. Tanaka et al., "Effects of ascorbic acid on gingival melanin pigmentation in vitro and in vivo," *Journal of Periodontology*, vol. 80, no. 2, pp. 317–323, 2009.

[21] M. El-Mofty, S. Elkot, A. Ghoneim, D. Yossri, and O. M. Ezzatt, "Vitamin C mesotherapy versus topical application for gingival hyperpigmentation: a clinical and histopathological study," *Clinical Oral Investigations*, vol. 25, no. 12, pp. 6881–6889, 2021.

[22] S. Yadav and S. Dogra, "A cutaneous reaction to microneedling for postacne scarring caused by nickel hypersensitivity," *Aesthetic Surgery Journal*, vol. 36, no. 4, p. NP168–170, 2016.

[23] S. Dogra, S. Yadav, and R. Sarangal, "Microneedling for acne scars in Asian skin type: an effective low cost treatment modality," *Journal of Cosmetic Dermatology*, vol. 13, no. 3, pp. 180–187, 2014.

[24] T. M. Leheta, R. M. Abdel Hay, R. A. Hegazy, and Y. F. El Garem, "Do combined alternating sessions of 1540 nm nonablative fractional laser and percutaneous collagen induction with trichloroacetic acid 20% show better results than each individual modality in the treatment of atrophic acne scars? A randomized controlled trial," *The Journal of Dermatological Treatment*, vol. 25, no. 2, pp. 137–141, 2014.

[25] M. R. Al-Naggar, A. S. Al-Adl, A. R. Rabie, M. R. Abdelkhalk, and M. L. Elsaie, "Intralesional bleomycin injection vs microneedling-assisted topical bleomycin spraying in treatment of plantar warts," *Journal of Cosmetic Dermatology*, vol. 18, no. 1, pp. 124–128, 2019.

[26] K. Almas and W. Sadiq, "Surgical treatment of melanin-pigmented gingiva: an esthetic approach," *Indian Journal of Dental Research*, vol. 13, no. 2, pp. 70–73, 2002.

[27] R. Kathariya and A. R. Pradeep, "Split mouth de-epithelization techniques for gingival depigmentation: a case series and review of literature," *J Indian Soc Periodontol.*, vol. 15, no. 2, pp. 161–168, 2011.

[28] S. A. Mokeem, "Management of gingival hyperpigmentation by surgical abrasion: report of three cases," *Saudi Dental Journal*, vol. 18, pp. 162–166, 2006.

[29] P. Atsawasuwan, K. Greethong, and V. Nimmanon, "Treatment of gingival hyperpigmentation for esthetic purposes by Nd: YAG laser: report of 4 cases," *Journal of Periodontology*, vol. 71, no. 2, pp. 315–321, 2000.

[30] H. Tal, D. Oegiesser, and M. Tal, "Gingival depigmentation by erbium: YAG laser: clinical observations and patient responses," *Journal of Periodontology*, vol. 74, no. 11, pp. 1660–1667, 2003.

[31] M. J. Oringer, Ed., *Electrosurgery in Dentistry*, W.B. Saunders Co, Philadelphia, 2nd ed. edition, 1975.

[32] R. Hegde, A. Padhye, S. Sumanth, A. Jain, and N. Thukral, "Comparison of surgical stripping; erbium-doped: yttrium, aluminum, and garnet laser; and carbon dioxide laser techniques for gingival depigmentation: a clinical and histologic study," *Journal of Periodontology*, vol. 84, no. 6, pp. 738–748, 2013.

[33] R. E. Billingham, "Dendritic cells in pigmented human skin," *Journal of Anatomy*, vol. 83, no. 2, pp. 109–115, 1949.

[34] R. B. Raut, M. A. Baretto, F. S. Mehta, M. K. Sanjana, and K. L. Shourie, "Gingival pigmentation: its incidence amongst the Indian adults," *JAIDA*, vol. 26, pp. 9-10, 1954.

[35] T. M. Ginwalla, B. C. Gomes, and B. R. R. Verma, "Surgical removal of gingival pigmentation (a preliminary study)," *Journal of the Indian Dental Association*, vol. 38, no. 6, pp. 147–50 passim, 1966.

[36] T. K. Pal, K. K. Kapoor, C. C. Parel, and K. Mukherjee, "Gingival melanin pigmentation – a study on its removal for esthetic," *J Indian Soc of Periodontology*, vol. 3, pp. 52–54, 1994.

[37] C. O. Dummett and T. E. Bolden, "Post surgical clinical repigmentation of the gingiva," *Oral Surgery, Oral Medicine, Oral Pathology, Oral Radiology, and Endodontics*, vol. 16, no. 3, pp. 353–365, 1963.

[38] D. S. Alasmari, "An insight into gingival depigmentation techniques: the pros and cons," *Int J Health Sci (Qassim).*, vol. 12, no. 5, pp. 84–89, 2018.

[39] Y. Nakamura, M. Hossain, K. Hirayama, and K. Matsumoto, "A clinical study on the removal of gingival melanin pigmentation with the CO2 laser," *Lasers in Surgery and Medicine.*, vol. 25, no. 2, pp. 140–147, 1999.

[40] L. Jokar, M. Bayani, H. Hamidi, M. Keivan, and S. Azari-Marhabi, "A comparison of 940 nm diode laser and cryosurgery with liquid nitrogen in the treatment of gingival physiologic hyperpigmentation using split mouth technique: 12 months follow up," *J Lasers Med Sci.*, vol. 10, no. 2, pp. 131–138, 2019.

[41] A. R. S. Shirazi, A. M. Taghavi, and F. Khorakian, "Treatment of gingival physiologic pigmentation in adolescent using cryosurgery technique with liquid nitrogen: one year follow up," *Journal of Cosmetic Dermatology*, vol. 33, pp. 331–342, 2010.

[42] C.-J. Yeh, "Cryosurgical treatment of melanin-pigmented gingiva," *Oral Surgery, Oral Medicine, Oral Pathology, Oral Radiology, and Endodontics*, vol. 86, no. 6, pp. 660–663, 1998.

[43] T. Haim, L. Jacob, and K. Avital, "Cryosurgical depigmentation of the gingiva - a case report," *Journal of Clinical Periodontology*, vol. 14, no. 10, pp. 614–617, 1987.

[44] V. Sheel, P. Purwar, J. Dixit, and P. Rai, "Ancillary role of vitamin C in pink aesthetics," *BML Case Reports*, vol. 2015, no. -jun08 1, p. bcr2014208559, 2015.

13

A Modified Bilaminar Technique with the use of a Fibrin-Fibronectin System for a Single Gingival Recession: A Case Report with a Follow-Up of 3 Years

Michele Perelli,[1] Paolo Giacomo Arduino ,[2] Mario Semenza,[3] Roberto Abundo,[1] and Hector Sarmiento[4]

[1]*Indipendent Researcher, Turin, Italy*
[2]*Department of Surgical Sciences, CIR-Dental School, University of Turin, Turin, Italy*
[3]*Indipendent Researcher, Sant'Angelo Lodigiano, Italy*
[4]*Indipendent Researcher, New York City, USA*

Correspondence should be addressed to Paolo Giacomo Arduino; paologiacomo.arduino@unito.it

Academic Editor: Samir Nammour

This case report described a modified bilaminar technique for treating a single gingival recession. Patient presented a gingival recession in a maxillary canine. Tooth was in a buccally prominent position and soft keratinized tissue apical to the recession was reduced but still present. A split-full-split thickness trapezoidal flap was designed. Root's surface was prepared with curettes. Epithelial-connective tissue graft was harvested from the palate with reduced dimension. After deepithelialization, the graft was placed with a fibrin-fibronectin system at the maximum root coverage level, and the flap coronally advanced and sutured. At 3-year follow-up control, the free gingival margin was still stable at the postsurgery position, with a thicker biotype corresponding to the grafted area, with no probing and a suitable aesthetic result.

1. Introduction

Gingival recession consists in the apical shift of the free gingival margin with the consequent exposure of the cementum enamel junction and the root surface [1]. This gingival loss may determine aesthetic problems, as well as dental hypersensitivity, noncarious cervical lesions, or radicular caries.

Different authors have reported a relationship between the inflammatory state of the marginal soft tissue and the amount of keratinized soft tissue, demonstrating the need of a minimum quantity of such tissue to permit a proper plaque control [2, 3]. In addition, patients' aesthetic concerns, and their perception, have currently increased, and different surgical techniques have been developed to reach root coverage (complete when is possible) and to increase keratinized marginal soft tissue [4–7]. Among them, both coronally advanced flap (CAF) [8–10] and connective tissue graft (CTG) [11–15] have shown suitable and predictable results. Different studies have demonstrated how the addition of a CTG to a coronally advanced flap (called "bilaminar technique") may act as a flap stabilizer thickening of the marginal soft tissue, resulting in a more predictable and stable result of root coverage especially in the long-term follow-up [16, 17]. Since the first reported bilaminar technique [12], various surgical approaches have been proposed to reduce graft dimension, patient palatal discomfort, and morbidity in the second surgical area.

Aim of this case report was to describe a modified bilaminar technique, with a reduced mesiodistal dimension of the CTG and bonded to the radicular dentin by means of a

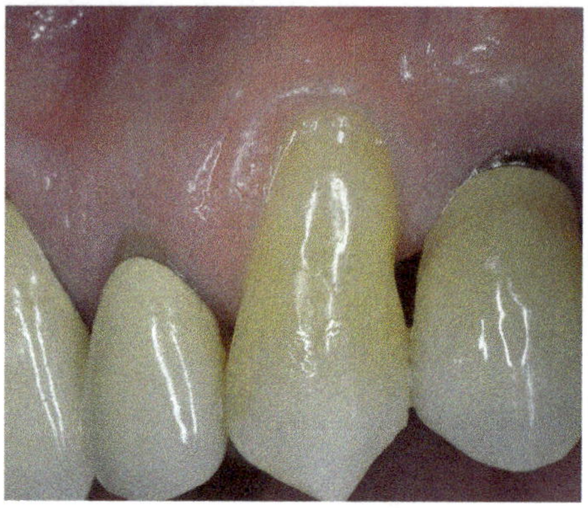

Figure 1: Left maxillary canine presenting a RT2 gingival defect.

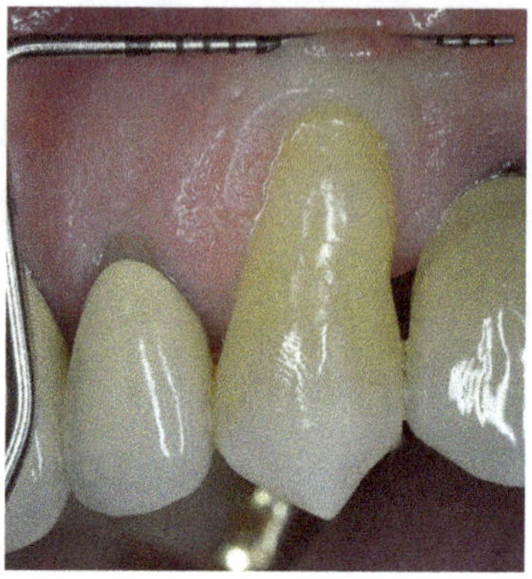

Figure 3: A minimum amount of keratinized tissue apical to the recession is still present.

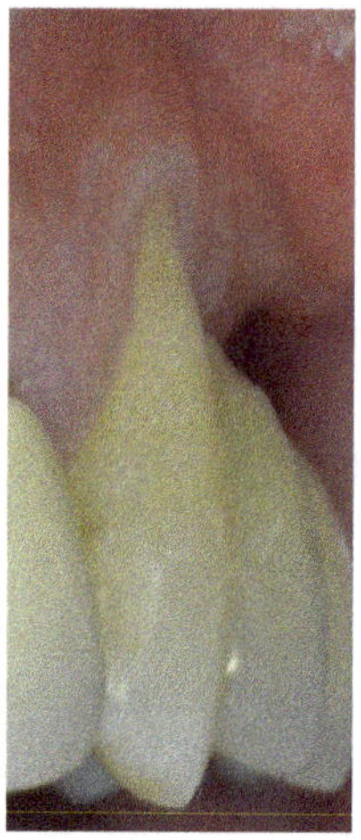

Figure 2: Lateral view: noncarious cervical lesion with composite restoration is evident (note the radicular concavity).

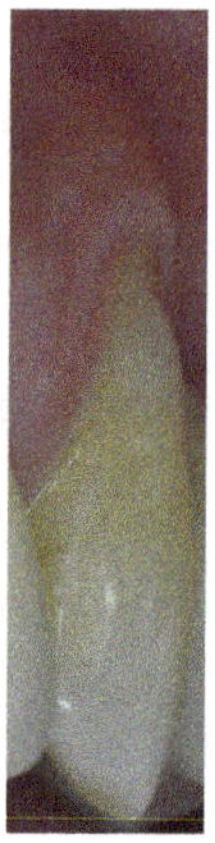

Figure 4: The composite restoration is reshaped at the maximum root coverage level.

fibrin-fibronectin system. Over a follow-up period of 3 years, this technique has demonstrated to be effective in reaching a good root coverage, a marginal soft tissue stability and an increased connective volume.

2. Case Presentation

A 53-year-old male, not smoker, presenting a recession type 2 (RT2) gingival defect [18] in correspondence of the maxillary left canine, was referred for a periodontal evaluation (Figures 1 and 2). His main complaint was tooth hypersensitivity and scar of losing all the gingival support. He did not present any medical contraindication for periodontal surgery. The treatment plane was aimed at partial root coverage and marginal soft tissue augmentation. After signing a tailored written consent, he firstly received a nonsurgical periodontal therapy, including oral hygiene instructions and supra- and subgingival scaling, by an experienced dental hygienist. Patient was also instructed about oral hygiene maintenance at home; instructions included modified Bass technique with soft brushes, in order not to damage soft marginal tissue. At 1-month control, the full-mouth bleeding score (FMBS) and the full-mouth plaque score (FMPS) indexes were both ≤25%.

Tooth #23 was in a buccal prominent position, also presenting a cervical restoration in good maintenance. Adherent keratinized tissue apical to the recession was still present with small but still adequate thickness and high to perform a CAF (Figure 3). In accordance with Stefanini and coworkers [19], considering the interdental clinical attachment loss and the soft tissue loss, combined with the buccal malposition of the root, a CAF together with a CTG was planned.

After local anaesthesia, using articaine with adrenaline (1 : 100.000), the maximum root coverage (MRC) [20] was determined, and the present cervical restoration was shortened and smoothed at that level (Figure 4).

The amount of gingival recession, plus 1 mm distance, was reported buccally and vertically from the top of the mesial and distal anatomical papillae, and at this level, a horizontal bleeding line of 3 mm was done with the top of the mini 15-c blade. From the angular point of such bevelled incision slightly divergent, two split thickness incisions were performed reaching the mucogingival junction (Figure 5). Afterwards, with the blade parallel to the oral mucosa, two split thickness surgical papillae were elevated, starting laterally and going out from the marginal sulcus. Split thickness surgical papillae ended when the coronal part of the free gingival margin was reached. With a proper elevator inserted

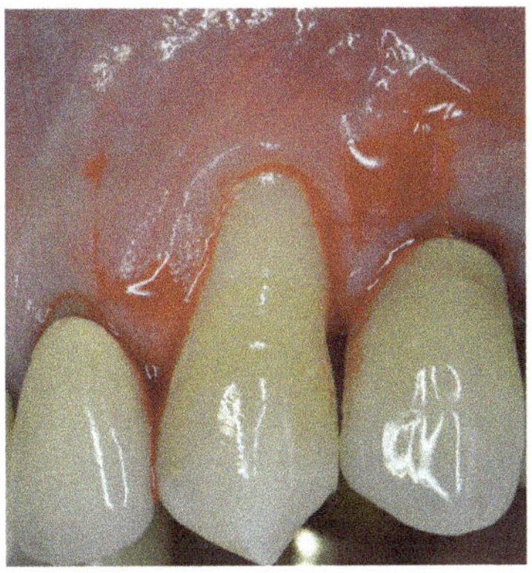

FIGURE 5: A trapezoidal flap is designed with vertical releasing incisions arriving just at the mucogingival junction.

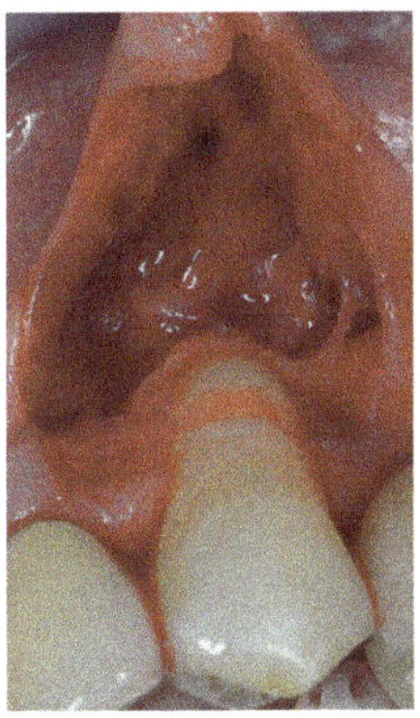

FIGURE 6: Two horizontal releasing incision are done: one deep, parallel to the bone crest and one, more extended, more superficial parallel to the oral mucosa (note the elasticity of the mucosa).

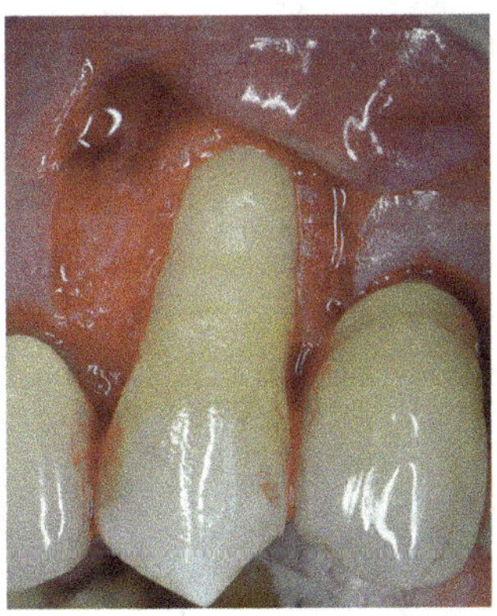

FIGURE 7: Root surface is treated with curettes and anatomical papillae deepithelialized.

into the sulcus, a full thickness central flap was elevated, exposing 3 mm of bone crest, apically to the anatomical root dehiscence. With a Gracey's minicurette root, the surface apical to the MRC was gently treated, removing the contaminated cementum. Then, a first deep horizontal releasing incision with the blade parallel to the bone crest was performed. After a second, more extended superficial horizontal incision was performed with the blade parallel to the oral mucosa, in order to mobilize the flap thanks to mucosa's elasticity, without cutting deeper structure, reducing in such way the possible bleeding and swelling (Figure 6). The anatomical papillae were deepithelialized (Figure 7). Anaesthesia was reinforced into the palate, and an epithelial-connective tissue graft was harvested. The dimension of the graft was 4 mm in height and in length, and the mesiodistal dimension was 1.5 mm exceeding in both side the avascular root surface in the area corresponding the MRC (Figure 8). The donor site was filled with a collagen sponge, and a compressive suture was performed reducing bleeding and stabilizing the sponge. Graft was gently de-epithelized with a blade. After washing the root surface with physiological solution, the fibrin fibronectin glue (Tisseel VH ®, Baxter, U.S.A.) was applied with two drops on the side of the graft facing the dental surface and the graft was immediately positioned on the root at the established level and maintained in such position with a slight finger pressure for 5 minutes (Figures 9 and 10). Then, after gently checking the stability of the graft, the flap was coronally advanced and sutured. Sutures started from the apical part of the vertical releasing incisions with circle point catching the periosteum when movable mucosa was laterally present. Finally, a sling suture, suspended around the cingulum was done, suturing the surgical papillae to the corresponding anatomical papillae (Figure 11).

The patient received antibiotic therapy, consisting of 1 g of amoxicillin plus clavulanic acid, starting from 1 day before surgery, twice a day, for 6 days; ibuprofen 600 mg was also prescribed to be taken twice a day for 2 days after surgery, then only if needed, and chlorhexidine spray to be used 3 times daily for 15 days.

Healing period was uneventful. After 15 days, sutures were removed and both surgical areas appeared in good status (Figures 12 and 13). Patient was instructed not to brush for other 20 days, reducing chemically plaque accumulation; then, for the first month, it was possible to brush with an ultrasoft toothbrush, later using the classic soft toothbrush. He was enrolled in a supportive nonsurgical periodontal therapy every six months. At 3-year follow-up, free gingival margin was stable at MRC level, no buccal probing was recorded, and marginal soft tissue texture and blending were equivalent to the adjacent tissues. In addition, gingival thickness graft improved during these years, creating a good connective tissue protection to the underlying periodontal structures as well as a natural emergency profile of the anatomical crown (Figures 14 and 15).

3. Discussion

Coronally advanced flap with the addition of a subepithelial connective tissue graft has demonstrated to be effective in covering the root at the MRC, providing optimal clinical and aesthetic results [21, 22].

To the best of our knowledge, this surgical technique has never been reported. This modified, simplified bilaminar technique could enable clinicians to achieve several targets: to reduce the dimension of the palatal graft (the length particularly), to simplify the graft stabilization without using sutures, and to possibly promote an effective adhesion

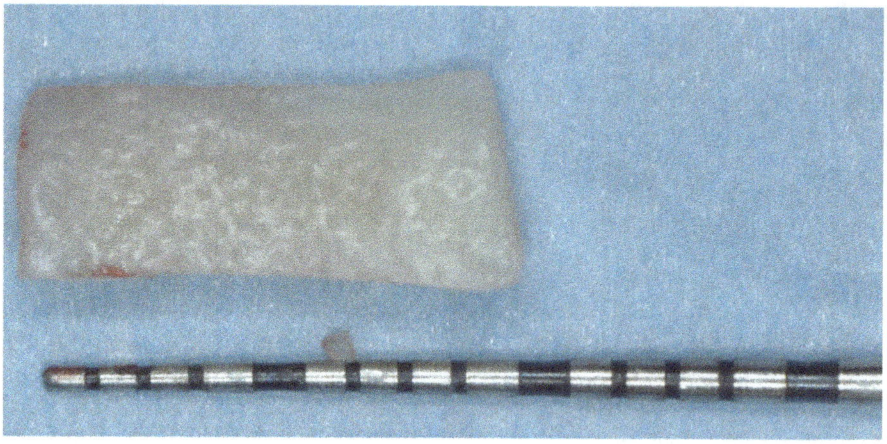

FIGURE 8: An epithelial-connective tissue graft is harvested. The height is 4 mm, and the length corresponds to the root width plus 3 mm.

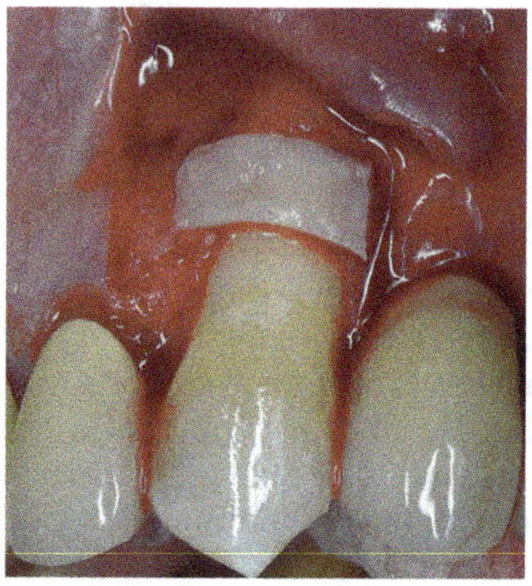

FIGURE 9: The connective tissue graft is attached with the fibrin-fibronectin glue to the root at the MRC level.

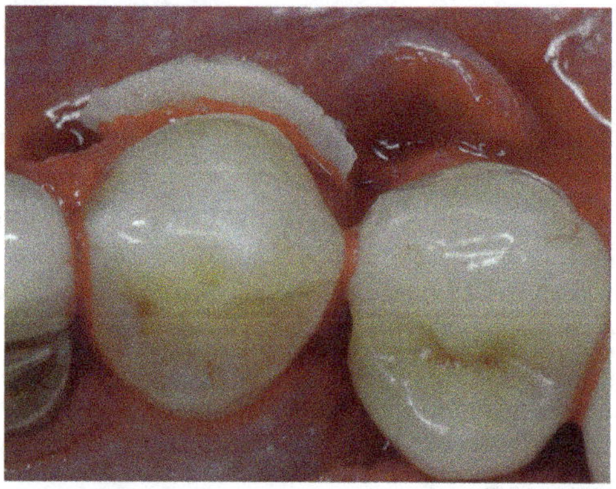

FIGURE 10: Note the thickness of the CTG bonded to the root.

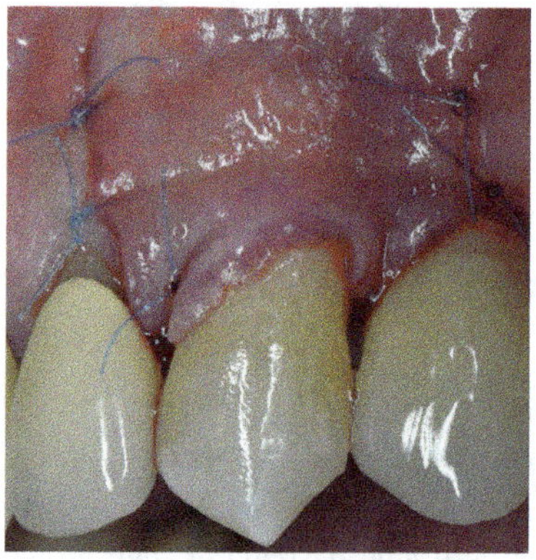

FIGURE 11: The flap has been coronally advanced and sutured.

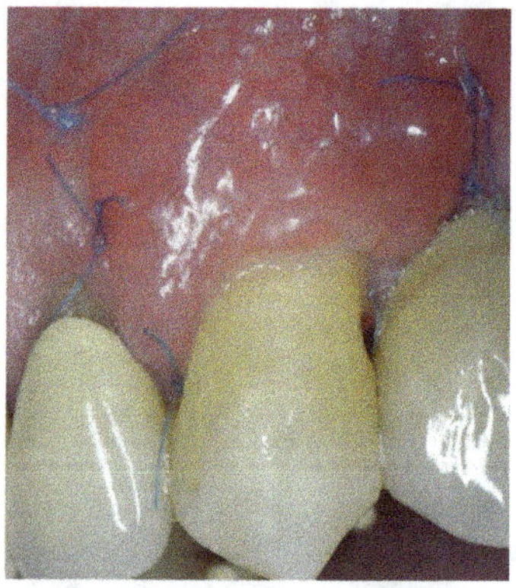

FIGURE 12: Healing of the flap after 15 days, at sutures removal.

between the graft's connective tissue and the connective fibres in the dentin tubules. The proposed natural healing could determine the soft tissue thickness augmentation as well as the root coverage maintenance.

In this 3-year follow-up, we have noticed a proper tissue's augmentation, together with the reestablishment of the natural emergency profile of the affected tooth crown, similar to the goals usually obtained with the conventional technique, but in a simpler and possible more biological manner. Traditionally, the graft is sutured to the split thickness anatomical papillae or the adjacent recipient split area. Ideally, even if it is well positioned on the root, the graft is not very attached to the exposed root but just stretched on it. The fibrin-fibronectin human glue used have demonstrated to allow a real biological, chemical, and physical attachment with the collagen present in the dentin tubules, consequently improving the stability of the coagulum [23]. In addition, bonding the graft is much easier than suturing it. Thanks to these

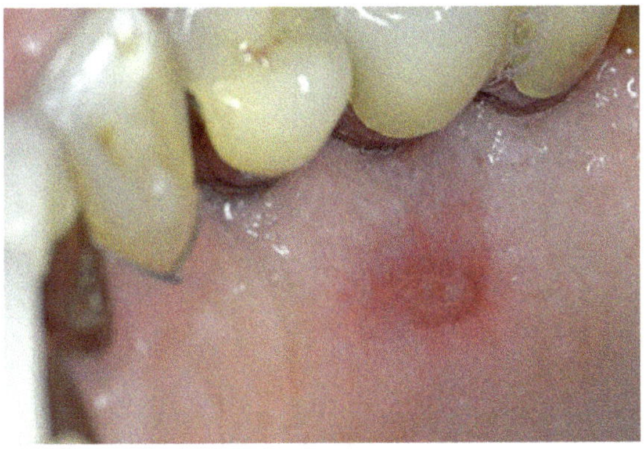

Figure 13: Palatal donor site healing after 15 days.

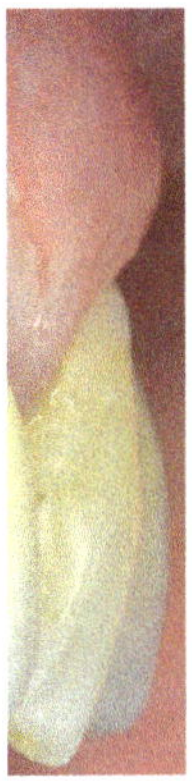

Figure 14: 3-year lateral view (note the thickness of the soft tissue corresponding to the grafted area).

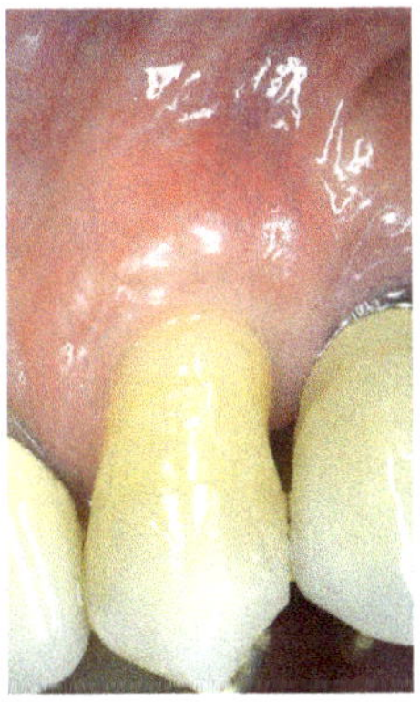

Figure 15: 3-year buccal view (note the stability of the gingival margin, the partial root coverage achieved and the aesthetic blending of the area).

aspects, graft could have reduced dimension; it was 4 mm in height, and as reported in literature, there is no need to harvest graft covering the apical bone crest or all the radicular exposure in such a case [17]. In fact, in the original described technique, graft covering adjacent bone areas acted as an obstacle form blood supply between the flap and the recipient bed. This aspect could sometimes influence to early graft exposure and to obtain not appropriate aesthetic results [24]. The mesiodistal extension is also shortened. In case of sutures, 3 mm interproximal exceeding root exposure was recommended. In this case report, the dimension was reduced of the 50% (1.5 mm in each side), shortening the global length of 3 mm.

The abovementioned peculiarities improved the adaptation of the surgical papillae to anatomical, optimizing vascular exchange without interfering the healing and avoiding the post-op look of papillae too big implementing the aesthetic result in medium-term follow-up.

The adjunct of the fibrin-fibronectin glue to this bilaminar modified technique has demonstrated to be effective in reaching a proper graft stability, providing prompt clinical attachment and no mobility on the root, and reducing its length with fewer healing area of the palatal donor site. These advantages should be confirmed by a larger sample of patients, but they seem promising in terms of patient satisfaction and clinical results.

References

[1] J. Wennstrom, "Mucogingival surgery," *Proceedings of the 1st European Workshop on Periodontology*, N. P. Lang and T. Karring, Eds., , pp. 193–209, Quintessence, London, 1994.

[2] L. Chambrone and D. N. Tatakis, "Periodontal soft tissue root coverage procedures: a systematic review from the AAP regeneration workshop," *Journal of Periodontology*, vol. 86, no. 2-s, pp. S8–S51, 2015.

[3] N. P. Lang and H. Löe, "The relationship between the width of keratinized gingiva and gingival health," *Journal of Periodontology*, vol. 43, no. 10, pp. 623-627, 1972.

[4] H. E. Grupe and R. F. Warren Jr., "Repair of gingival defects by a sliding flap operation," *Journal of Periodontology*, vol. 27, no. 2, pp. 92–95, 1956.

[5] J. P. Bernimoulin, B. Luscher, and H. R. Muhlemann, "Coronally repositioned periodontal flap. Clinical evaluation after one year," *Journal of Clinical Periodontology*, vol. 2, no. 1, pp. 1–13, 1975.

[6] E. P. Allen and P. D. Miller Jr., "Coronal positioning of existing gingiva: short term results in the treatment of shallow marginal tissue recession," *Journal of Clinical Periodontology*, vol. 60, no. 6, pp. 316–319, 1989.

[7] J. M. Nabers, "Free gingival grafts," *Periodontics*, vol. 4, no. 5, pp. 243–245, 1966.

[8] M. Del Pizzo, G. Zucchelli, F. Modica, R. Villa, and C. Debernardi, "Coronally advanced flap with or without enamel matrix derivative for root coverage: a 2-year study," *Journal of Clinical Periodontology*, vol. 32, no. 11, pp. 1181–1187, 2005.

[9] M. De Sanctis and G. Zucchelli, "Coronally advanced flap: a modified surgical approach for isolated recession-type defects: three-year results," *Journal of Clinical Periodontology*, vol. 34, no. 3, pp. 262–268, 2007.

[10] L. Tavelli, S. Barootchi, F. Cairo, G. Rasperini, K. Shedden, and H. L. Wang, "The effect of time on root coverage outcomes: a network meta-analysis," *Journal of Dental Research*, vol. 98, no. 11, pp. 1195–1203, 2019.

[11] H. C. Sullivan and J. H. Atkins, "Free autogenous gingival grafts. I. Principles of successful grafting," *Periodontics*, vol. 6, no. 3, pp. 121–129, 1968.

[12] P. B. Raetzke, "Covering Localized Areas of Root Exposure Employing the "Envelope" Technique," *Journal of Periodontology*, vol. 56, no. 7, pp. 397–402, 1985.

[13] R. J. Harris, "The connective tissue and partial thickness double pedicle graft: a predictable method of obtaining root coverage," *Journal of Periodontology*, vol. 63, no. 5, pp. 477–486, 1992.

[14] A. L. Allen, "Use of the supraperiosteal envelope in soft tissue grafting for root coverage. II. Clinical results," *The International Journal of Periodontics & Restorative Dentistry*, vol. 14, no. 4, pp. 302–315, 1994.

[15] G. Zucchelli, C. Clauser, M. de Sanctis, and M. Calandriello, "Mucogingival versus guided tissue regeneration procedures in the treatment of deep recession type defects," *Journal of Periodontology*, vol. 69, no. 2, pp. 138–145, 1998.

[16] M. Roccuzzo, M. Bunino, I. Needleman, and M. Sanz, "Periodontal plastic surgery for treatment of localized gingival recessions. A systematic review," *Journal of Clinical Periodontology*, vol. 29, pp. 178–194, 2002.

[17] G. Zucchelli, C. Amore, N. M. Sforza, L. Montebugnoli, and M. de Sanctis, "Bilaminar techniques for the treatment of recession-type defects. A comparative clinical study," *Journal of Clinical Periodontology*, vol. 30, no. 10, pp. 862–870, 2003.

[18] F. Cairo, M. Nieri, S. Cincinelli, J. Mervelt, and U. Pagliaro, "The interproximal clinical attachment level to classify gingival recessions and predict root coverage outcomes: an explorative and reliability study," *Journal of Clinical Periodontology*, vol. 38, no. 7, pp. 661–666, 2011.

[19] M. Stefanini, M. Marzadori, S. Aroca, P. Felice, M. Sangiorgi, and G. Zucchelli, "Decision making in root-coverage procedures for the esthetic outcome," *Periodontology 2000*, vol. 77, no. 1, pp. 54–64, 2018.

[20] G. Zucchelli, T. Testori, and M. de Sanctis, "Clinical and anatomical factors limiting treatment outcomes of gingival recession: a new method to predetermine the line of root coverage," *Journal of Periodontology*, vol. 77, no. 4, pp. 714–721, 2006.

[21] L. Chambrone, M. A. S. Ortega, F. Sukekava et al., "Root coverage procedures for treating single and multiple recession-type defects: an updated Cochrane systematic review," *Journal of Periodontology*, vol. 90, no. 12, pp. 1399–1422, 2019.

[22] F. Cairo, S. Barootchi, L. Tavelli et al., "Esthetic- and Patient-Related Outcomes Following Root Coverage Procedures: A Systematic Review and Network Meta-Analysis," *Journal of Clinical Periodontology*, 2020.

[23] J. G. Caton, A. M. Polson, G. P. Prato, E. G. Bartolucci, and C. Clauser, "Healing after application of tissue-adhesive material to denuded and citric acid-treated root Surfaces," *Journal of Periodontology*, vol. 57, no. 6, pp. 385–390, 1986.

[24] R. J. Harris, "The connective tissue with partial thickness double pedicle graft: the results of 100 consecutively-treated defects," *Journal of Periodontology*, vol. 65, no. 5, pp. 448–461, 1994.

14

Necrotizing Ulcerative Gingivitis, a Rare Manifestation as a Sequel of Drug-Induced Gingival Overgrowth: A Case Report

Marah Damdoum[1] **Sudhir Rama Varma**[1,2] **Mohamed A. Jaber**[1,2] **and Manjusha Nambiar**[3]

[1]*Department of Clinical Sciences, College of Dentistry, Ajman University, Ajman, UAE*
[2]*Centre of Medical and Biomedical Allied Health Sciences Research, Ajman University, Ajman, UAE*
[3]*Department of Periodontics, Sri Rajiv Gandhi College of Dental Sciences and Hospital, Banguluru, Karnataka State 560032, India*

Correspondence should be addressed to Marah Damdoum; marahdamdoum@gmail.com and Sudhir Rama Varma; s.varma@ajman.ac.ae

Academic Editor: Ronald S. Brown

Purpose. The purpose of this case report is to present a rare case of amlodipine-induced gingival overgrowth with a secondary formation of necrotizing ulcerative gingivitis involving the upper and lower arches of a 68-year-old female patient with a chief complaint of "swollen gums and pain on mastication which has been recurring for the past 5 years." *Materials and Methods.* The treatment plan of this case was divided according to quadrants of the mouth. Each week, one quadrant was surgically excised, and the remaining quadrants were observed for any changes. The gingival overgrowths were excised using a 15 blade, and debris/plaque was removed with Gracey curettes. *Results.* Although full-mouth exodontia was performed, the patient unfortunately suffered with recurrences in GO. These results are suggestive of idiopathic causes of GO. *Conclusion.* Careful examination, physician referrals, and biopsy to rule out any specific anomalies and to assist in proper diagnosis are followed by sequential management of the case results in productive outcomes.

1. Introduction

Drug-induced gingival overgrowth (DIGO) manifests as a result of drug interactions mainly produced by anticonvulsants [1], immunosuppressants [2], and calcium channel blockers [3]. Several factors including age, sex, genetic predisposition, systemic diseases, hormonal imbalances, congenital disorders, poor oral hygiene, and local plaque/debris may influence the relationship of these drugs to gingival overgrowth [4]. Gingival overgrowths can affect speech, mastication, and esthetics, and there are various methods of treatment for excising the excess tissue [5]. These overgrowths can be classified according to their size and location and graded between grade 0 and grade III [6] (Table 1). The pharmacological action of each drug is different; however, they all act similarly to secondary tissue receptors by creating enlargements in the gingival tissue. The exact mechanism of these gingival overgrowths in association to drugs is not fully understood, and there are many hypotheses and theories related to DIGO [7–11]. Drug-induced gingival overgrowth is typically detected after 3 months of drug consumption [12]. Clinical features of DIGO could be localized or generalized and may range from mild to severe enlargements of the marginal and papillary gingiva [13]. The anterior region of the mouth is more affected than the posterior region and is more pronounced on the facial surfaces than the palatal/lingual surfaces [14]. DIGO cannot be prevented in susceptible patients but it can be tolerated by regular periodontal therapy and plaque control [15]. The current case report presents a rare case of necrotizing ulcerative gingivitis as a secondary reaction to amlodipine-induced gingival overgrowth.

2. Pathophysiology

The mechanism of gingival overgrowth and its contributory mechanism with relation to fibroblastic proliferation are varied. A theory of genetic predisposition was earlier postulated by Seymour et al. in 1996 [3]. The inflammatory changes

Table 1: Bokenkamp and Bohnhorst, 1994 classification.

Grade	Clinical findings
Grade 0	No signs of gingival overgrowth
Grade I	Gingival hyperplasia confined to interdental papilla
Grade II	Hyperplasia of interdental papilla and marginal gingiva
Grade III	Gingival hyperplasia covering at least three quarters of tooth crowns

and responses of gingival fibroblasts coupled with connective tissue matrix proliferation exemplify the fibroblastic characterization with relation to the various drugs responsible for this change [16]. Another theory postulated that bacterial plaque was responsible for gingival inflammation. The drugs responsible for gingival overgrowth causes an increased production of glycosaminoglycans. The drugs further reduce folate uptake in the cellular matrix. Reduced folate uptake results in decreased synthesis of matrix metalloproteinases which is responsible for conversion of collagenase precursor into mature collagenase, resulting in a matrix and connective tissue build up. The bacterial plaque when present causes the inflammatory component, thus completing the cycle [17].

3. Case Report

This case presents a 68-year-old female patient with a chief complaint of swollen gums and pain on mastication which has been recurring for the past 5 years. According to the patient, she started taking amlodipine 5 mg/day 7 years ago and started experiencing enlargements of the gingiva 5 years ago. She stopped taking amlodipine for 6 months and claims the enlargements improved. However, her physician recommended that she continue taking amlodipine 10 mg/day due to her uncontrolled hypertension. Medical history was taken in which the patient reported having diabetes mellitus type II and hypercholesterolemia for the past 8 years. She takes a series of drugs for her medical conditions (Table 2). She has been hypertensive for the past 7 years and has been taking amlodipine since then. She stopped amlodipine 2 years ago for 6 months due to gingival overgrowths; however, amlodipine had to be continued due to her uncontrolled hypertension.

On taking dental history, it was found that she underwent multiple gingivectomies in the past with recurrence every few months. During previous episodes, the patient had described the condition as similar to the one presented currently with excruciating pain and pus discharge. Furthermore, the patient described the treatment advised as "gum shaping by the doctor". From patient's explanations, it was assumed that the clinical picture matched the current situation, and a history of NUG could have been prevalent at that time period.

The patient presented with a dental history that includes thick deposits of calculus and plaque on all remaining teeth with fibrous, nodular, hard gingival overgrowths extending to most of the clinical crown in the anterior and posterior parts of the maxillary and mandibular arches (Figure 1). The overgrowths can be classified as grade III according to Bokenkamp's 1994 classification for gingival overgrowth [6] (Table 1). Additionally, a yellowish-white pseudomembranous slough was found covering the interdental papilla in the mandibular left area (Figure 2). Radiographically, bone loss can be observed around the teeth and implants; however, clinically, the implants are not mobile as submerged (Figure 3). Abrasion of the teeth can be observed indicating parafunctional habits, as the patient had given a history of clenching which was consciously done and also from her family member, that patient was a bruxer and exhibited grinding at night. This also confirmed our diagnosis as stage 4, grade C periodontitis, currently unstable.

3.1. Sequence of Treatment. The treatment plan of this case was divided according to quadrants of the mouth. Each week, one quadrant was surgically treated with the overgrown gingival tissue being excised, and the mobile teeth were extracted. The decision to extract her teeth was from a multidisciplinary point of view involving a periodontist and prosthodontist, as salvaging the remaining teeth was challenging and time consuming with hopeless prognosis. Since the overgrowths affected mastication, speech, and esthetics, a surgical approach (i.e., gingivectomy) was utilized with local anesthesia being administered. The gingival overgrowths were excised using a 15 blade; plaque and calculus were removed with Gracey curettes (Dentsply, USA). After every gingivectomy, azithromycin-xithrone (Amoun Egypt) 500 mg, diclofenac-rofenac (Bin Sina, UAE) 50 g sachet, along with chlorhexidine mouthwash (Curasept, UK), were prescribed. Surgical excision began in quadrant 4, which was the least affected quadrant. An external bevel incision gingivectomy was performed along with scaling and root surface debridement. The gingiva was sutured with silk (Black Braided, size 4-0, 19 cm, Teleflex, USA). At one-week surgical postop, the following was noted: the gingiva in the mandibular right quadrant was healing within normal limits. The gingiva in the mandibular left quadrant was edematous, fibrous, hemorrhagic, and painful swellings which had purulent exudate (Figure 2). An external bevel incision gingivectomy was done along with extraction of #33, #34, #35, and 45 due to extensive grade III mobility (Figures 4 and 5). The mobile teeth were diagnosed as stage 4 grade C periodontitis, currently unstable (AAP Classification, 2017). Apical curettage was performed, and copious irrigation with saline was done. Simple interrupted sutures were placed with silk. Placement of a periodontal pack along with oral hygiene reinforcement instructions was given. During the follow-up visit the following week, healing was uneventful for the most part with slight regression of gingival overgrowth. Poor oral hygiene can be observed along the

TABLE 2: Drugs taken by the patient.

Name of the drug	Dosage	Duration	Pharmacological action	Medical condition
Gliclazide	60 mg	8 years	Sulfonylureas	Diabetes mellitus type II
Bisoprolol hemifumarate	2.5 mg	1 year	Nonselective beta blocker	Heart murmurs
Perindopril arginine	5 mg	1 year	ACE inhibitor	Hypertension
Amlodipine besylate	10 mg	7 years	Calcium channel blocker	Hypertension
Rosuvastatin	10 mg	8 years	HMG-CoA reductase inhibitor	Hypercholesterolemia

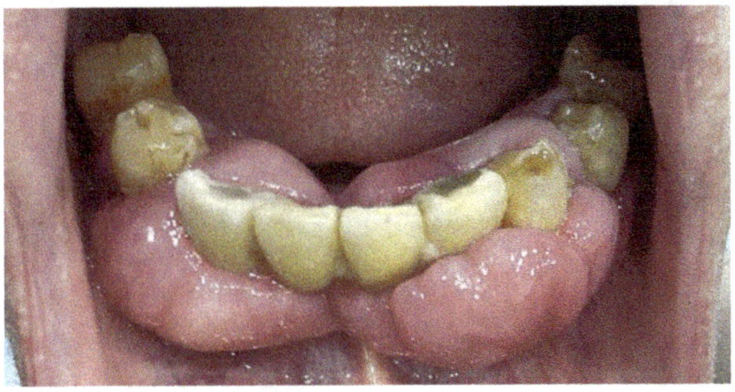

FIGURE 1: Fibrous, nodular, hard gingival overgrowths extending to most of the clinical crown in the anterior and posterior parts of the mandibular arch.

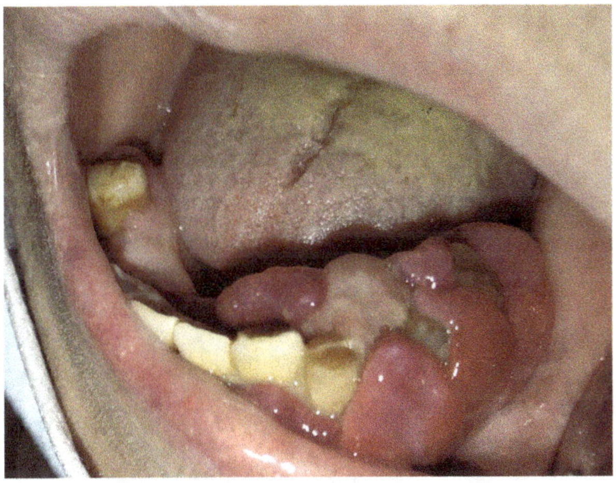

FIGURE 2: Yellowish-white pseudomembranous slough was found covering the interdental papilla in the mandibular left area.

sutures which were surrounded by plaque and debrıs (Figure 6). For the maxillary arch, an external bevel incision gingivectomy was done, and extraction of #11, #21, and #12 was done due to grade III mobility (Figures 7–9).

During the follow-up visits, the maxillary arch presented with signs of inflammation, pus, and exudates around the teeth and sutures (Figure 10). There also seemed to be recurrence of gingival overgrowth around the implant-retained 4 unit bridge in the anterior mandible (Figure 11). The bridge was removed, and implants remained submerged in the alveolar bone. After bridge removal, azithromycin was prescribed as reported in earlier literature about its efficiency in treating DIGO [18]. During a 2-week follow-up, recurrence of GO was identified in all quadrants. The patient

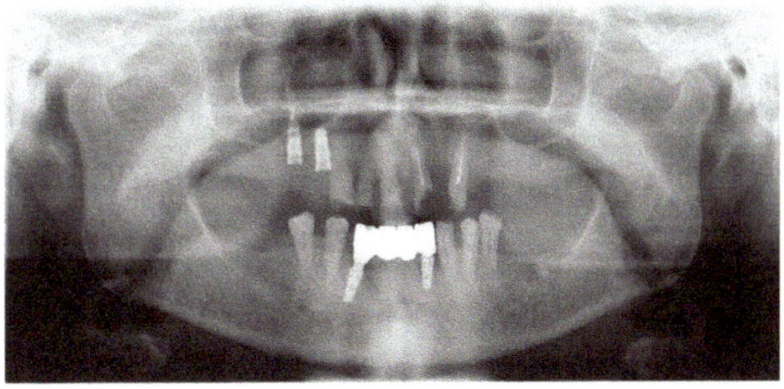

FIGURE 3: Panoramic radiograph presenting bone loss around teeth and lower 4-unit implant-retained bridge.

was referred to a cardiologist for a follow-up and possible substitution of amlodipine. Perindopril indapamide (a thiazide-like diuretic) was recommended by the cardiologist as an alternative. The remaining drugs consumed by the patient continued normally. During the first recall visit after complete exodontia and drug substitution, the patient presented with recurrence in the upper and lower arches. Since gingival overgrowth did not subside after complete exodontia and drug substitution, it can be assumed that the submerged implants in the lower anterior region and upper right posterior region could be the cause for this recurrence. Treatment modalities were further contemplated with regard to removal of the submerged implants; however, after clinical and radiographic assessment, it was further decided to retain the implants and to put the patient on follow-up to see if there was a possibility of recurrence. The patient was put on a strict oral hygiene plan and maintenance recall phase every 2 months.

4. Results

This case report presents a rare case of nonhealing AIGO with a secondary NUG reaction. Two biopsies were taken to confirm the diagnosis in which both biopsies revealed chronic inflammatory processes. For AIGO-associated conditions, there are a range of treatment modalities that clinicians can explore. The proposed modes of treatment in the literature include nonsurgical and surgical drug modification and periodontal therapies. For the current case, all of these modalities were performed, and biopsies were done to confirm NUG as a manifestation of DIGO. Although full-mouth exodontia was performed, the patient unfortunately suffered with recurrences in GO. These results are suggestive of idiopathic causes of GO.

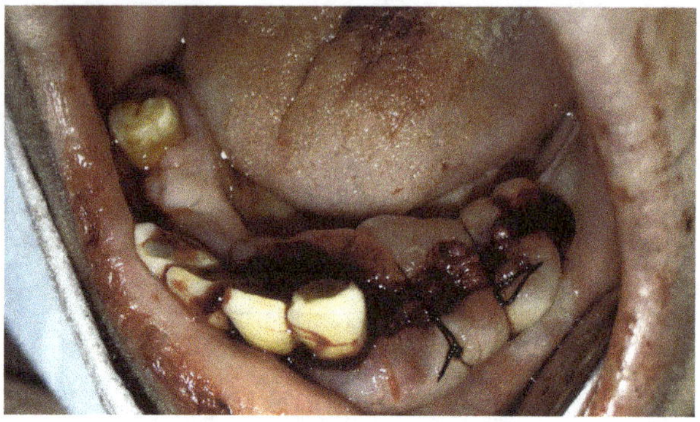

Figure 4: External bevel incision gingivectomy of the lower left quadrant and exodontia of #33, #34, and #35.

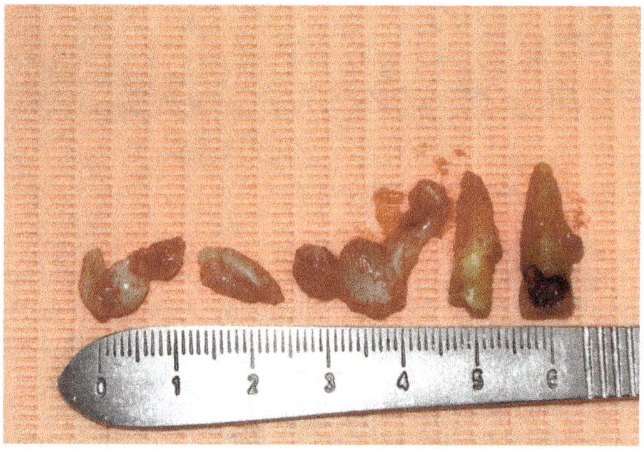

Figure 5: Gingiva removed from the lower left quadrant and extracted teeth (#33, #34, and #35).

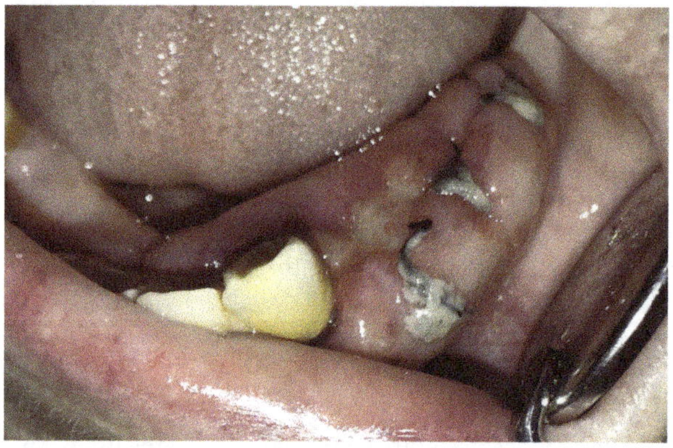

Figure 6: 1 week after surgical excision of the lower left quadrant.

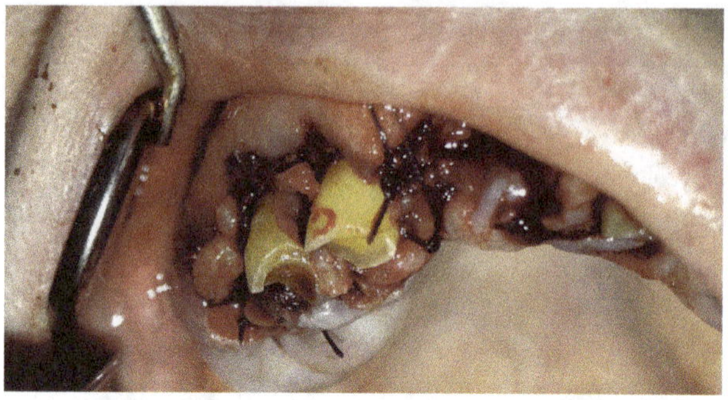

Figure 7: External bevel gingivectomy of the upper right quadrant.

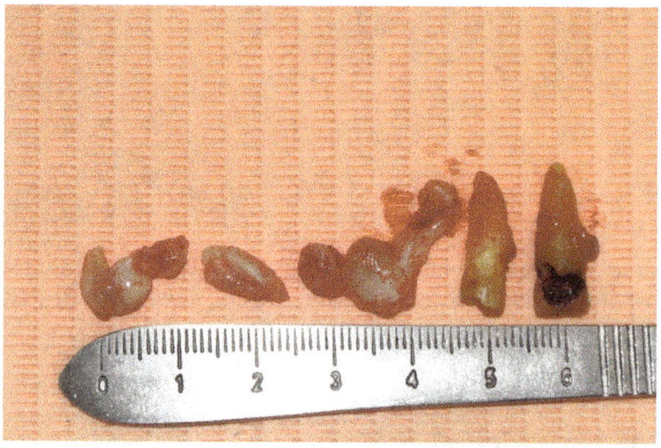

Figure 8: Gingiva removed from the upper left quadrant and extracted teeth (#11 and #21).

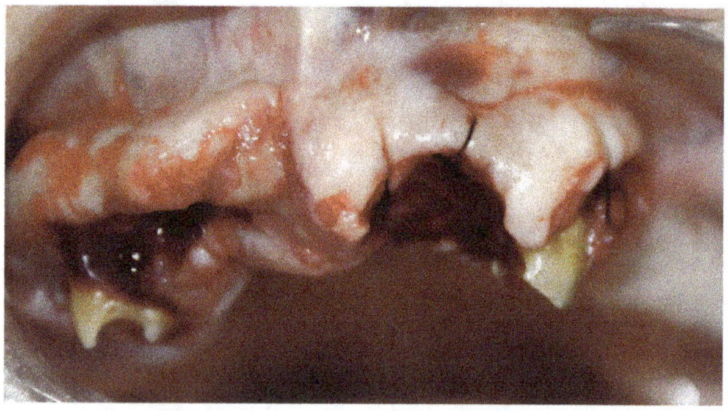

Figure 9: External bevel gingivectomy of the upper left quadrant.

5. Discussion

5.1. Oral Hygiene. Some studies say oral hygiene and local factors like plaque and calculus can affect the severity of gingival overgrowth; however, it is not a requirement for DIGO [4, 19]. A crosssectional study done in 1973 tested the association between dilantin-induced gingival overgrowth and oral hygiene. The study did not show that oral hygiene was statistically significant in the formation of gingival hyperplasia [4]. Seymour et al. reported in 2000 that most of the evidence to support a relationship between bacterial plaque and gingival overgrowth has been derived from crosssectional studies, and it is not clear whether plaque is a contributory factor or a consequence of the gingival changes [4]. A 2015 case report by Mathur et al. took a nonsurgical approach to their DIGO case. They reported that "there appears to be three significant factors which are important for the expression of these gingival changes, notably drug variables, plaque-induced inflammatory changes in gingival tissue, and genetic factors which determine the heterogeneity of the fibroblasts" [19]. The gingival overgrowths subsided after periodontal therapy, and no surgical intervention was needed. In a 2020 case report by Uppal et al., they

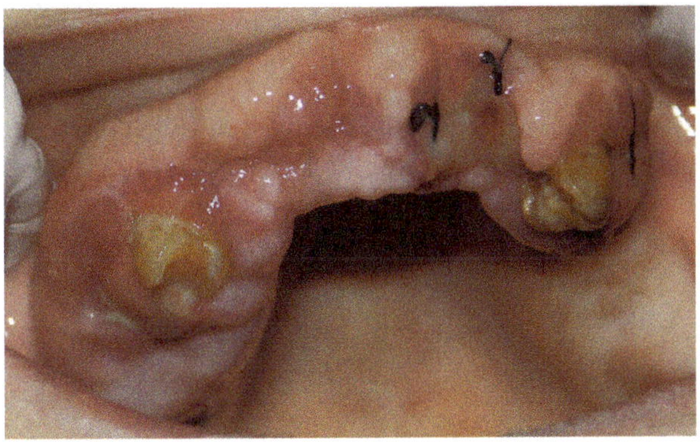

FIGURE 10: Recall after 2 weeks of surgical intervention of maxillary arch. Pus and exudates were observed around teeth and sutures. Full exodontia was done for the remaining teeth in the upper arch.

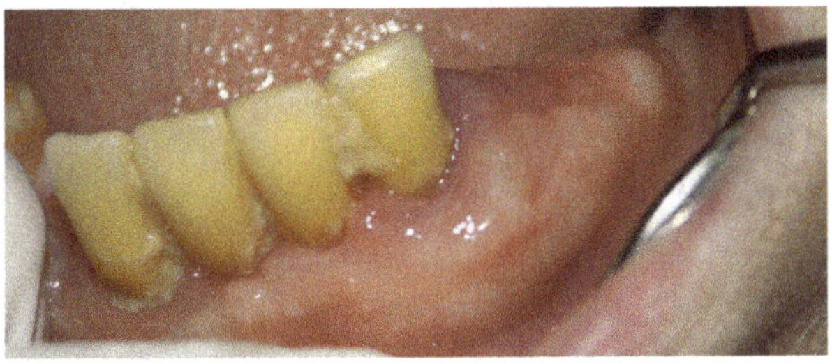

FIGURE 11: 1 month recall after surgical intervention of the mandibular arch. Recurrence was presented, and full-mouth exodontia was done for the lower arch.

report a case of DIGO that was treated nonsurgically through a periodontal approach first and report that "as the enlargement did not subside after drug substitution and phase 1 therapy, surgical phase was planned further" [20]. There is definitely an unclear definition as to whether oral hygiene plays a role in DIGO, but regardless, patient education on oral hygiene and maintenance is crucial in every treatment plan.

5.2. Histopathology. For this case, a biopsy was sent with a gross description of the tissue sample; it consisted of two pieces of gray white to brown tissue measuring $2.0 \times 0.8 \times 0.5$ cm and $1.5 \times 1.4 \times 0.8$ cm.

Microscopically, the histopathological sections show mucosa covered soft tissue with an area of ulceration along with granulation tissue. Subepithelial soft tissue is hyalinized and shows a dense infiltrate composed predominantly of plasma cells merged with a few lymphocytes, eosinophils, and neutrophils. These features are consistent with acute on chronic inflammatory processes. The predominance of inflammatory cells indicates that the gingival overgrowth was not only caused by a drug induction but rather by presence of a secondary condition as well. This secondary condition can be identified as necrotizing ulcerative gingivitis. In the literature, the histopathology of NUG has been identified as ulcerations with dense infiltrations of PMNs and plasma cells which is interpreted as an area of established chronic gingivitis on which the acute lesion became superimposed [2].

Our biopsy showed areas of ulcerations, predominance of plasma cells (indicating a chronic lesion), along with some PMNs. The signs and symptoms along with the histopathological review were suggestive of NUG as a secondary reaction to AIGO. A second biopsy was taken of healthy gingival tissue, to confirm our diagnosis of AIGO. The biopsy was received in a labelled container with patient identification and fixed in formalin, where multiple pieces are gray brown in color, irregular soft tissue, and measured in aggregate $1.5 \times 1 \times 0.2$ cm. All submitted in one cassette. The gingival biopsy revealed squamous epithelium hyperplasia with underlying chronic inflammation (Figures 12 and 13), consistent with a reactive process, and negative for hyperkeratosis and atypia. These reports are consistent with a secondary inflammatory reaction (NUG) as a manifestation of amlodipine-induced gingival overgrowth [21]. The current case is similar to a case report where DM type 2, hypercholesterolemia, and amlodipine for hypertension were of similar findings. The difference being the time frame for the presentation, in the current case, was nine months ago, while in the earlier reported literature, it had presented after three years of intake of the medication (amlodipine) [22]. Meanwhile, our patient has had GO for the past 5 years and experienced the changes in her gingiva almost instantly after switching back to amlodipine the second time. Interestingly, in the current case, a possible role of statins in the progression of GO could be attributed as seen from a previous study where statins and calcium channel blockers when prescribed together resulted in adverse effects, a predominant feature being GO [23].

5.3. Secondary Reactions. In our case, we reported necrotizing ulcerative gingivitis (NUG) as a secondary reaction to amlodipine-induced gingival overgrowth. In an earlier study by Vishnusdas et al., they reported a case involving amlodipine-induced gingival plasma cell granuloma, and the etiology is multifactorial, with a possible role of drug/cellular interaction playing a contributory role in the pathogenesis of this entity [24]. Another case report done in 2019 by Gulati et. al found an unusual plasma cell granuloma formation secondary to GO. This case report states that biopsies for unusual lesions should be comprehensively examined regardless of clinical appearance or treatment success rate in order to rule out neoplasms and plan for treatment accordingly [21]. For this case, a biopsy was sent with a gross description of the tissue sample, it consisted of two pieces of gray white to brown tissue measuring $2.0 \times 0.8 \times 0.5$ cm and $1.5 \times 1.4 \times 0.8$ cm. Microscopically, the histopathological sections show mucosa covered soft tissue with an area of ulceration along with granulation tissue. Subepithelial soft tissue is hyalinized and shows a dense infiltrate composed predominantly of plasma cells merged with a few lymphocytes, eosinophils, and neutrophils. These features are consistent with acute on chronic inflammatory processes. The predominance of inflammatory cells indicates that the gingival overgrowth was not only caused by a drug induction, but rather by presence of a secondary condition as well. This secondary condition can be identified as necrotizing ulcerative gingivitis. In the literature, the histopathology of NUG

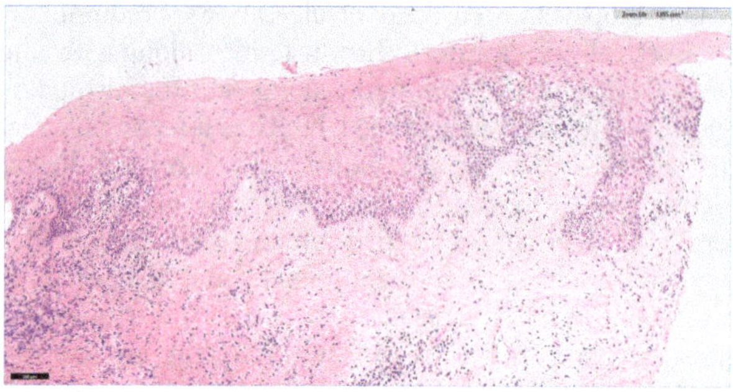

FIGURE 12: Histopathological slide of gingival biopsy revealed squamous epithelium hyperplasia with underlying chronic inflammation.

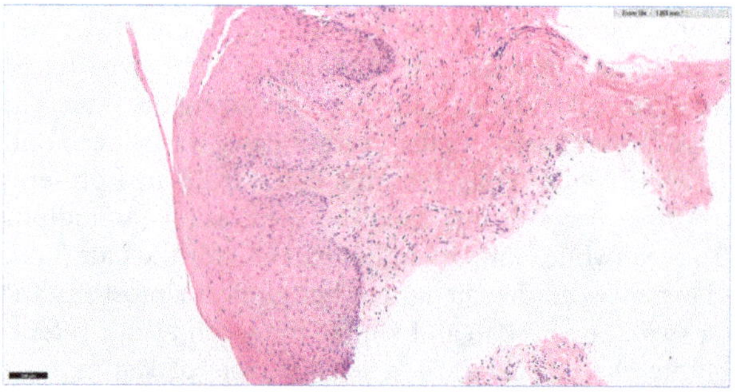

FIGURE 13: Histopathological slide of gingival biopsy revealed squamous epithelium hyperplasia with underlying chronic inflammation.

has been identified as ulcerations with dense infiltrations of PMNs and plasma cells which is interpreted as an area of established chronic gingivitis on which the acute lesion became superimposed [2]. Our biopsy showed areas of ulcerations, predominance of plasma cells (indicating a chronic lesion), along with some PMNs. The signs and symptoms along with the histopathological review were suggestive of NUG as a secondary reaction to AIGO. A second biopsy was taken of healthy gingival tissue, to confirm our diagnosis of AIGO. The biopsy was received in a labelled container with patient identification and fixed in formalin, where multiple pieces are gray brown in color, irregular soft tissue, and measured in aggregate $1.5 \times 1 \times 0.2$ cm. All submitted in one cassette. The gingival biopsy revealed squamous epithelium hyperplasia with underlying chronic inflammation (Figures 12 and 13). Consistent with a reactive process. Negative for hyperkeratosis and atypia. These reports are consistent with a secondary inflammatory reaction (NUG) as a manifestation of amlodipine-induced gingival overgrowth.

The current case is similar to a case report where DM type 2, hypercholesterolemia, and amlodipine for hypertension were of similar findings. The difference being the time frame for the presentation, in the current case, was nine months ago, while in the earlier reported literature, it had presented after three years of intake of the medication (amlodipine) [22]. Meanwhile, our patient has had GO for the past 5 years and experienced the changes in her gingiva almost instantly after switching back to amlodipine the second time. Interestingly, in the current case, a possible role of statins in the progression of GO could be attributed as seen from a previous study where statins and calcium channel blockers when prescribed together resulted in adverse effects, a predominant feature being GO [23].

6. Conclusion

DIGO related to calcium channel blockers, immunosuppressants, and anticonvulsants in the past reported clinical presentations concluded by clinicians as rare entities. The case presented in our study shows the possible effects of amlodipine-induced GO and the challenges dentists can face in the management of this condition. Careful examination, physician referrals, and biopsy to rule out any specific anomalies and to assist in proper diagnosis are followed by sequential management of the case results in productive outcomes.

Abbreviations

DIGO: Drug-induced gingival overgrowth
AIGO: Amlodipine-induced gingival overgrowth
GO: Gingival overgrowth
NUG: Necrotizing ulcerative gingivitis
PMN: Polymorphonuclear cells.

References

[1] J. L. Cebrian, M. Chamorro, J. Arias, and E. Gomez, "Extreme phenytoin-induced gingival hyperplasia. Presentation of two cases," *Medicina oral, Patología Oral y Cirugía Bucal*, vol. 3, no. 4, pp. 237–240, 1998.

[2] J. Eggerath, H. English, and J. W. Leichter, "Drug-associated gingival enlargement: case report and review of aetiology, management and evidence-based outcomes of treatment," *Journal of the New Zealand Society of Periodontology*, vol. 88, pp. 7–14, 2005.

[3] R. A. Seymour, J. S. Ellis, J. M. Thomason, S. Monkman, and J. R. Idle, "Amlodipine-induced gingival overgrowth," *Journal of Clinical Periodontology*, vol. 21, no. 4, pp. 281–283, 1994.

[4] R. A. Seymour, J. S. Ellis, and J. M. Thomason, "Risk factors for drug-induced gingival overgrowth," *Journal of Clinical Periodontology: Review article*, vol. 27, no. 4, pp. 217–223, 2000.

[5] M. Mavrogiannis, J. S. Ellis, J. M. Thomason, and R. A. Seymour, "The management of drug-induced gingival overgrowth," *Journal of Clinical Periodontology*, vol. 33, no. 6, pp. 434–439, 2006.

[6] A. Bökenkamp, B. Bohnhorst, C. Beier, N. Albers, G. Offner, and J. Brodehl, "Nifedipine aggravates cyclosporine A-induced gingival hyperplasia," *Pediatric Nephrology*, vol. 8, no. 2, pp. 181–185, 1994.

[7] W. A. Border and N. A. Noble, "Transforming growth factor beta in tissue fibrosis," *The New England Journal of Medicine*, vol. 331, pp. 1286–1292, 1994.

[8] R. S. Brown, P. Sein, R. Corio, and W. K. Bottomley, "Nitrendipine-induced gingival hyperplasia: First case report," *Oral*

Surgery, Oral Medicine, and Oral Pathology, vol. 70, no. 5, pp. 593–596, 1990.

[9] S. J. Das and I. Olsen, "KeratinocytE growth factor is upregulated by the hyperplasia-inducing drug nifedipine," *Cytokine*, vol. 12, no. 10, pp. 1566–1569, 2000.

[10] A. Nyska, M. Shemesh, H. Tal, and D. Dayan, "Gingival hyperplasia induced by calcium channel blockers: Mode of action," *Medical Hypotheses*, vol. 43, no. 2, pp. 115–118, 1994.

[11] C. J. van der Vleuten, M. A. Trijbels-Smeulders, and P. C. van de Kerkhof, "Telan-giectasia and gingival hyperplasia as side-effects of amlodipine (Norvasc) in a 3-year-old girl," *Acta Dermato-Venereologica*, vol. 79, no. 4, pp. 323-324, 1999.

[12] R. Livada and J. Shiloah, "Calcium channel blocker-induced gingival enlargement," *Journal of Human Hypertension*, vol. 28, no. 1, pp. 10–14, 2014.

[13] R. I. Marshall and P. M. Bartold, "Medication induced gingival overgrowth," *Oral Diseases*, vol. 4, no. 2, pp. 130–151, 1998.

[14] M. G. Newman, H. Takei, P. R. Klokkevold, and F. A. Carranza, *Carranza's Clinical Periodontology*, Elsevier Health Sciences, 2011.

[15] J. Y. Kim, S. H. Park, K. S. Cho et al., "Mechanism of azithromycin treatment on gingival overgrowth," *Journal of Dental Research*, vol. 87, no. 11, pp. 1075–1079, 2008.

[16] A. A. Agrawal, "Gingival enlargements: differential diagnosis and review of literature," *World Journal of Clinical Cases*, vol. 3, no. 9, pp. 779–788, 2015.

[17] A. Dongari-Bagtzoglou and Research, Science and Therapy Committee, American Academy of Periodontology, "Drug-associated gingival enlargement," *Journal of Periodontology-Periodontics*, vol. 75, no. 10, pp. 1424–1431, 2004.

[18] L. A. Klar, "Gingival hyperplasia during dilantin-therapy; a survey of 312 patients," *Journal of Public Health Dentistry*, vol. 33, no. 3, pp. 180–185, 1973.

[19] S. Mathur, R. K. Khatri, R. Mathur, R. Srivastava, and B. P. Nag, "Drug induced gingival overgrowth: a rare case report," *Journal of Clinical and Diagnostic Research: JCDR*, vol. 9, no. 1, pp. ZD31–ZD33, 2015.

[20] J. Uppal, H. Trivedi, N. D. Gupta, and A. Bey, "Periodontal management of severe periodontitis and generalized gingival enlargement in a patient with chronic renal failure," *Journal of Indian Society of Periodontology*, vol. 24, no. 3, pp. 284–288, 2020.

[21] R. Gulati, M. S. Ratre, S. Khetarpal, and M. Varma, "A case report of a gingival plasma cell granuloma in a patient on anti-hypertensive therapy: diagnostic enigma," *Frontiers in Dentistry*, vol. 16, no. 2, pp. 144–148, 2019.

[22] K. Smitha, "Amlodipine-induced gingival overgrowth in a patient with uncontrolled type 2 diabetes mellitus with hypercholesterolemia: a case report," *Clinical Advances in Periodontics*, vol. 2, no. 2, pp. 115–122, 2012.

[23] G. G. Missouris, R. G. Kalaitzidis, F. P. Cappuccio, and G. A. MacGregor, "Gingival hyperplasia caused by calcium channel blockers," *Journal of Human Hypertension*, vol. 14, no. 2, pp. 155-156, 2000.

[24] Z. Sameer, B. Shriram, K. Rekha, and B. Vishnudas, "Amlodipine induced plasma cell granuloma of the gingiva: a novel case report," *Journal of Natural Science, Biology, and Medicine*, vol. 5, no. 2, p. 472, 2014.

15

Bone Regeneration in Vertical Osseous Defect in Periodontitis Patients using Bovine Colostrum

P. L. Ravishankar,[1] Preethikaa Guruprasath,[1] Padmaja Vangipuram,[1] Jasmine Vaidya,[1] G. Visithiriyan,[1] A. Thirumal Raj,[2] Shilpa Bhandi,[3] Shankargouda Patil,[4] and Snehashish Ghosh[5]

[1]*Department of Periodontics, SRM Kattankulathur Dental College, Potheri, 603203, Tamil Nadu, India*
[2]*Department of Oral Pathology and Microbiology, Sri Venkateswara Dental College and Hospital, Chennai 600130, India*
[3]*Department of Restorative Dental Science, Division of Operative Dentistry, College of Dentistry, Jazan University, Jazan 45142, Saudi Arabia*
[4]*Department of Maxillofacial Surgery and Diagnostic Sciences, Division of Oral Pathology, College of Dentistry, Jazan University, Jazan 45142, Saudi Arabia*
[5]*Department of Oral Pathology, College of Medical Sciences, Bharatpur, Nepal*

Correspondence should be addressed to Snehashish Ghosh; drsnehashishop@gmail.com

Academic Editor: Samir Nammour

Background. The treatment plan for periodontitis may include both nonsurgical and surgical phases. During surgical procedures, bone grafts and barrier membranes were used after degranulation in order to achieve healing. Colostrum is one of the materials that is composed of bioactive components which has either osteoinductive or regenerative potential. *Aim.* The aim of the present study is to evaluate the effectiveness of bovine colostrum as bone regeneration material in periodontitis. *Case Description.* Clinical periodontal parameters, including probing depth (PD), clinical attachment level (CAL), bleeding on probing (BOP), and plaque index (PI), were evaluated. Patients who were diagnosed with localised periodontitis were selected. Three patients presenting vertical defect at buccal sites were treated with bovine colostrum. Following nonsurgical treatment, flap surgery was performed using bovine colostrum. After 6 months, favourable clinical and radiographical improvements were obtained. *Conclusion.* All cases showed reduction in PD; these findings suggest that the bovine colostrum could favour periodontal regeneration. The clinical significance is that bovine colostrum is cost effective and easily available and enhances bone regeneration. It can therefore be used as an alternative to bone grafts during periodontal surgery.

1. Introduction

Periodontal disease can be localised or generalised. Unlike common perception, periodontitis cases are not restricted to the elderly population [1]. Cases have been recorded at adolescence and are characterised by interproximal attachment loss of the first molar and/or incisors, absence of inflammation, a deep probing depth, and progressive bone resorption. In many cases, plaque is insignificant in comparison to the amount of damage it causes, which can be largely attributed to the bacteria such as *Aggregatibacter actinomycetemcomitans* (*A.a*) and *Porphyromonas gingivalis* (*P.g*). Secondary clinical symptoms include diastema development between incisors with distolabial migration, mobility of the affected teeth, sensitivity of the denuded root, deep dull radiating jaw pain, and periodontal abscess lymph node enlargement [2].

In younger patients with a higher rate of bone loss, a well-planned treatment strategy and, in some cases, a more intensive treatment approach are required to prevent future periodontal deterioration and restore as much periodontal attachment as feasible [3]. Periodontal surgical therapy allows for access to bone abnormalities, allowing for osseous resection, recontouring, and other procedures such as regeneration. To rebuild the periodontal structures that have been destroyed, many regenerative procedures like bone grafting, GTR, and tissue engineering have been used [1].

The initial milk produced after the birth of the calf is known as bovine colostrum (BC). BC is necessary for the new-born calf's nutritional and immunological support, growth, and development. It is made by the dairy industry in powder form, and it is offered commercially to potentially aid in health and immunological support. This powder is mixed with water and consumed orally. It has been shown to have bioactive components including immunoglobulins and growth factors, as well as oligosaccharides, antimicrobials, and immune-regulating factors [4].

Although bone grafts are considered an ideal material for regeneration, they are relatively expensive. In contrary, bovine colostrum is cost-effective and has been effectively used postendodontic surgery to treat periapical defects [5]. Thus, bovine colostrum powder (immune strong, B colostrum, an Ayurveda proprietary drug from India) was employed during periodontal surgery to fill the bone deficiency in the present case series. The present case series was aimed at evaluating the effectiveness of bovine colostrum as bone regeneration material in vertical osseous defect of periodontitis patients in a relatively younger age group.

2. Case Description

2.1. Case 1. A 32-year-old female patient visited our department with complaint of pain in the right lower back tooth region for the past 2 months. The patient was in good health. The patient has undergone extraction before 3 months. In respect to the mandibular right first molar, probing depth of 10 mm, grade II tooth mobility, suppuration and bleeding on probing, and gingival irritation were all noted. In relation to 46, a periapical radiograph was taken (Figure 1). Radiolucency extending from middle one-third of the distal aspect of the root of 46 to middle one-third of the root of the mesial aspect of the root of 47 is suggestive of vertical bone defect. Periodontal damage was manifested by deep infrabony deformities. The patient got root planing at 1-week intervals after full-mouth scaling. Systemic antibiotics were recommended. After three weeks of phase I therapy, the flap surgery was performed. A full-thickness mucoperiosteal flap was reflected with sulcular incision and interdental incision from the distal aspect of 45 till the mesial aspect of 47. Debridement of granulation tissue was done followed by sterile saline irrigation. The required amount of bovine colostrum (immune strong, B colostrum, an Ayurveda proprietary drug from India) was taken in a sterile Dappen dish and adapted to the defect in powder form. The GTR membrane was placed, and suturing was done using 3-0 silk thread (Figure 2). After the surgery, the patient was given postoperative instructions and medications. At 3 months, clinical measures were taken with a manual periodontal probe. Clinical benefits were shown in measurements. The afflicted areas' PD has dropped to a maximum of 4 mm. Six months after therapy, radiographs revealed that the bone defects had been filled (Figure 2).

2.2. Case 2. A 28-year-old male patient visited our department with complaint of mobile teeth. The patient was in good health. The patient had dental history of restoration done before 5 months. In respect to the mandibular right first molar, probing depth of 11 mm, grade II tooth mobility, and the presence of suppuration and bleeding on probing and gingival inflammation were noted. A periapical radiograph in relation to 46 was taken. Deep infrabony defects were observed in relation to 46. The patient got root planing at 1-week intervals after full-mouth scaling. Systemic antibiotics were recommended. After three weeks of phase I therapy, the flap surgery was performed. A full-thickness mucoperiosteal flap was reflected with sulcular incision and interdental incision from the distal aspect of 45 till the mesial aspect of 47. Debridement of granulation tissue was done followed by sterile saline irrigation. The required amount of bovine colostrum was taken in a sterile Dappen dish, mixed with saline and made into dough form, and adapted to the defect. The GTR membrane was placed, and suturing was done using 3-0 silk thread (Figure 3). After the surgery, the patient was given postoperative instructions and medications. The patient did not report back for review.

2.3. Case 3. A 35-year-old female patient visited our department for regular dental check-up. The patient had medical history of hypothyroidism, and she was under medication for the past three years. This was the patient's first visit to the dentist. In respect to the mandibular left first molar, PD of 9 mm, grade I tooth mobility, bleeding on probing, and gingival inflammation were noted. A periapical radiograph in relation to 36 was taken. Radiolucency extending from the distal aspect of the root of 35 to the mesial aspect of the root of 36 and also extending from the distal aspect of the root of 36 to the mesial aspect of the root of 37 is suggestive of vertical bone defect. Deep infrabony defects were observed in relation to 35 and 36. The patient got root planing at 1-week intervals after full-mouth scaling. Systemic antibiotics were recommended. After three weeks of phase I therapy, the flap surgery was performed. A full-thickness mucoperiosteal flap was reflected with sulcular incision and interdental incision from the distal aspect of 35 till the mesial aspect of 37. Debridement of granulation tissue was done followed by sterile saline irrigation. The required amount of bovine colostrum was taken in a sterile Dappen dish and adapted to the defect in powder form. The GTR membrane was placed, and suturing was done using 3-0 silk thread (Figure 4). After the surgery, the patient was given postoperative instructions and medications. At 3 months, clinical measures were taken with a manual periodontal probe. Clinical benefits were shown in measurements. The afflicted areas' PD has dropped to a maximum of 4 mm. Six months after therapy, radiographs revealed that the bone defects had been filled (Figure 5).

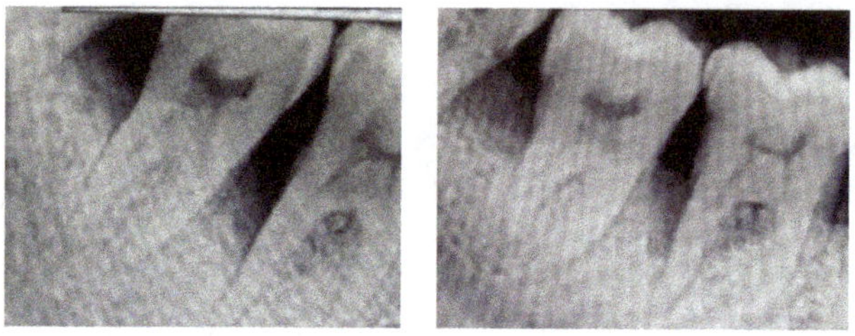

(a) (b)

FIGURE 1: Radiographic image: (a) preoperative and (b) postoperative.

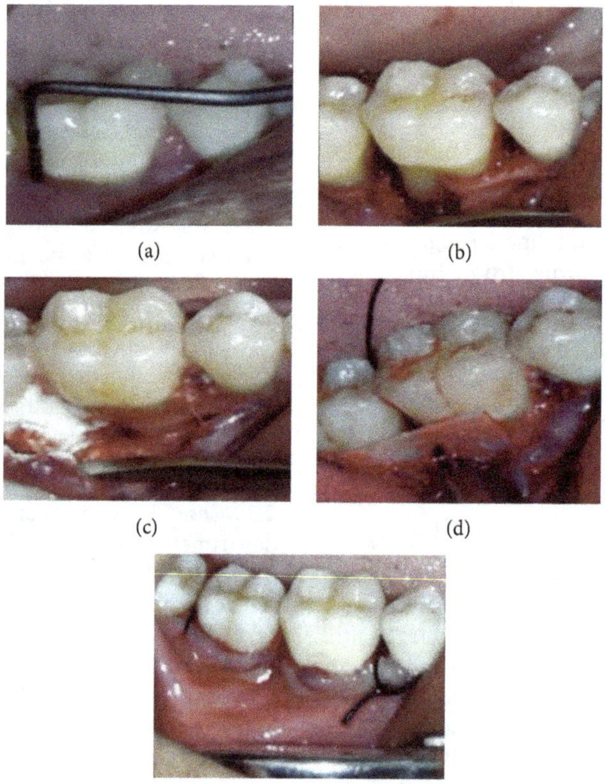

(a) (b) (c) (d) (e)

FIGURE 2: (a) PPD-10 mm. (b) Debridement done. (c) Placement of bovine colostrum. (d) GTR placement—suturing done.

3. Discussion

Periodontal disease is an inflammatory disorder that affects the tissues around the teeth as a result of dental plaque on the surface of the teeth. The breakdown of supporting tissues occurs as a result of the host-activated inflammatory response, which is usually triggered by gram-negative micro-organisms. Several regeneration approaches have been examined as a supplement to surgical therapy [6, 7].

Bovine colostrum is a nutritional supplement, and it has been shown that colostrum in oral care products boosts the natural defence system and improves periodontal repair [4]. Other clinical uses of bovine colostrum include improvement of oral hygiene in people with oral lichen planus and Sjogren's syndrome [8], dietary supplements in immunodeficiency-related diarrhoea, prophylaxis and treatment of infectious diseases caused by *Vibrio cholerae*, *Helicobacter pylori*, and rotavirus, and treatment of multiple sclerosis and gastrointestinal inflammation caused by non-steroidal anti-inflammatory drugs [9, 10].

Lactose, oligosaccharides, glycolipids, glycoproteins, and nucleotide sugars are all carbohydrates found in BC. It also contains about 7% fat, which is mostly made up of milk fat globules. BC is high in water-soluble vitamins and fat-soluble, both of which are important for a variety of biological activities, especially bone formation and antioxidant properties. Improved immune function and mental health have also been related to vitamin D [9, 11].

Colostrinin (also known as PRP or proline-rich polypeptide) is a naturally present blend of proline-rich polypeptides that have been demonstrated to assist in the reduction of excessive inflammatory responses. It contains Milk Fat

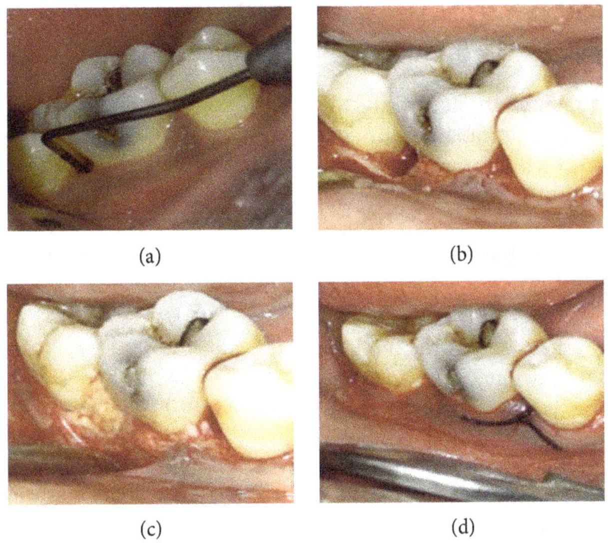

Figure 3: (a) PPD-10 mm. (b) Debridement done. (c) Placement of bovine colostrum. (d) Suturing done.

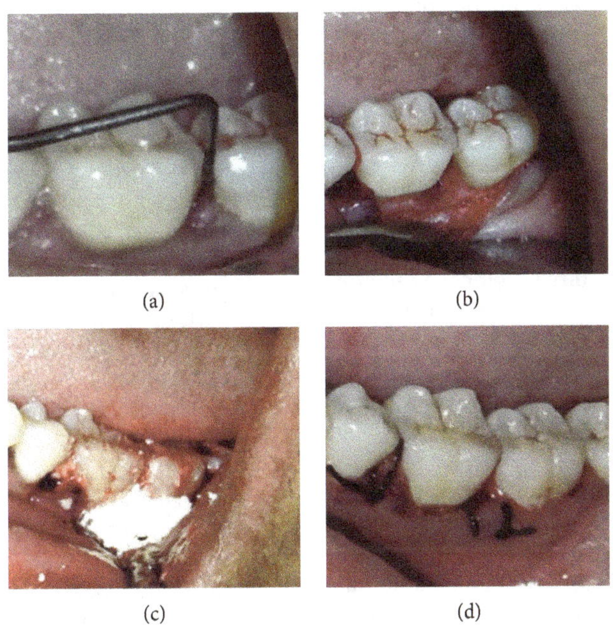

Figure 4: (a) PPD-10 mm. (b) Debridement done. (c) Placement of bovine colostrum. (d) Suturing done.

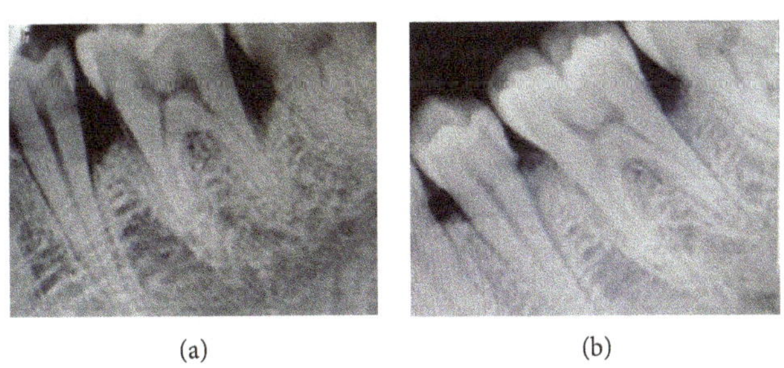

Figure 5: Radiographic image: (a) preoperative and (b) postoperative.

Globule-Epidermal Growth Factor 8 (MFG-E8) and also growth factors such as insulin-like growth factor, epidermal growth factor, transforming growth factor, platelet-derived growth factor, and vascular endothelial growth factor. MFG-E8 is a secreted protein that was shown to be a key part of the bovine colostrum milk. It improves phagocytosis' clearance of injured and apoptotic cells, stimulation of VEGF-mediated new vessel creation, and mucosal repair [4, 9–11].

An effective amount of bovine colostrum, according to the invention, has antibacterial or antimicrobial action in the oral cavity. Immunoglobulins, growth factors, lactoferrin, lysozyme, lactoperoxidase, cytokines and nucleosides, calcium, and phosphate are among the bioactive compounds found in it [5, 8, 12]. Bovine colostrum has been employed in periapical surgery and had achieved bone gain without any side effects [5]. Thus, based on the clinical success evidenced in the published literature, bovine colostrum powder was used in the current case series to fill the osseous defect.

Cases 1 and 3 had remarkable surgical healing. Clinical improvements were observed six months after treatment. The PD reduction was between 3 and 4 mm. There was no longer any suppuration, and there were no symptoms of gingival inflammation. The periapical radiographs taken 6 months following therapy revealed that the bone deficiencies had been filled and that the treatment outcome had remained stable. Although all sites showed similar clinical benefits, there were differences in the degree of radiological defect filling. This finding was in contrary to Veeramachaneni et al. [5] where bovine colostrum was used in the management of periapical lesion.

The bovine colostrum was used in powder form, and this may help in faster resorption of the material. This was in contrary to the study done by Bhaskar et al. [13] where they reported that larger particle size required prolonged time for resorption. Prior to therapy with bovine colostrum, a periapical radiograph was done to examine the bone defect. Colostrum appeared radiolucent at first, and the radiopacity gradually increased over time. This emphasises colostrum's ability to promote regeneration.

When compared to alternative bone grafts, bovine colostrum is less expensive. Growth factors included in bovine colostrum, including transforming growth factor, insulin-like growth factor, and epidermal growth factor, have been shown to aid in the regeneration and repair of numerous bodily tissues [5]. These same elements could have had a role in bone healing in these circumstances.

4. Conclusion

Based on the clinical and radiological findings of the 3 cases included in the present case series, there is preliminary evidence to suggest that colostrum-based treatment of bone deficiency following periodontal surgery had a beneficial effect. There are a few limitations in this case series. These include a lack of microbiological and histological evaluation. In addition, being a treatment-based report, a case series with 3 cases would not be sufficient to objectively assess the success of the treatment. Thus, considering the present case series as preliminary evidence, further large-scale multicentre randomized controlled trials are needed to validate the findings of the present report.

References

[1] N. Saroch, "Periobasics: a textbook of periodontics and implantology," in *India Sushruth Publ*, Sushrut Publications Private Limited, 2nd edition, 2017.

[2] M. Newman, H. Takei, P. Klokkevold, and F. Carranza, *Newman and Carranza's Clinical Periodontology E-Book*, Elsevier Heal, 2018.

[3] K. M. Lyons and I. Darby, "Interdisciplinary periodontics: the multidisciplinary approach to the planning and treatment of complex cases," *Periodontology 2000*, vol. 2017, no. 74, pp. 7–10, 2017.

[4] S. Ghosh and M. Iacucci, "Diverse immune effects of bovine colostrum and benefits in human health and disease," *Nutrients*, vol. 13, no. 11, p. 3798, 2021.

[5] C. Veeramachaneni, C. Gayathri, A. Kakani, and R. Mohini, "Use of bovine colostrum in periapical defects following surgical endodontics: two case reports," *Journal of Conservative Dentistry*, vol. 20, no. 5, pp. 374–377, 2017.

[6] A. Sculean, D. Nikolidakis, G. Nikou, A. Ivanovic, I. L. C. Chapple, and A. Stavropoulos, "Biomaterials for promoting periodontal regeneration in human intrabony defects: a systematic review," *Periodontology 2000*, vol. 2015, no. 68, pp. 182–216, 2015.

[7] Y.-D. Cho, K.-H. Kim, H.-M. Ryoo, Y.-M. Lee, Y. Ku, and Y.-J. Seol, "Recent advances of useful cell sources in the periodontal regeneration," *Current Stem Cell Research & Therapy*, vol. 14, no. 1, pp. 3–8, 2019.

[8] A. Pedersen, L. Andersen Torpet, J. Reibel, P. Holmstrup, and B. Nauntofte, "Oral findings in patients with primary Sjögren's syndrome and oral lichen planus - a preliminary study on the effects of bovine colostrum-containing oral hygiene products," *Clinical Oral Investigations*, vol. 6, no. 1, pp. 11–20, 2002.

[9] A. Arslan, M. Kaplan, H. Duman et al., "Bovine colostrum and its potential for human health and nutrition," *Frontiers in Nutrition*, vol. 8, 2021.

[10] M. Rathe, K. Müller, P. T. Sangild, and S. Husby, "Clinical applications of bovine colostrum therapy: a systematic review," *Nutrition Reviews*, vol. 72, no. 4, pp. 237–254, 2014.

[11] G. S. Kelly, "Bovine colostrums: a review of clinical uses," *Alternative Medicine Review*, vol. 8, no. 4, pp. 378–394, 2003.

[12] L. Elfstrand, H. Lindmark-Månsson, M. Paulsson, L. Nyberg, and B. Åkesson, "Immunoglobulins, growth factors and growth hormone in bovine colostrum and the effects of processing," *International Dairy Journal*, vol. 12, no. 11, pp. 879–887, 2002.

[13] S. N. Bhaskar, D. E. Cutright, M. J. Knapp, J. D. Beasley, B. Perez, and T. D. Driskell, "Tissue reaction to intrabony ceramic implants," *Oral Surgery, Oral Medicine, Oral Pathology*, vol. 31, no. 2, pp. 282–289, 1971.

16

Lateral Periodontal Cyst Treated with Enucleation and Guided Bone Regeneration: A Report of a Case and a Review of Pertinent Literature

Sundar Ramalingam,[1] **Yasser Fahad Alrayyes,**[2] **Khalid Buayjan Almutairi,**[2] **and Ibrahim O. Bello**[3]

[1]*Department of Oral and Maxillofacial Surgery, College of Dentistry, King Saud University, Riyadh 11545, Saudi Arabia*
[2]*Dental University Hospital, College of Dentistry, King Saud University, Riyadh 11545, Saudi Arabia*
[3]*Department of Oral Medicine and Diagnostic Sciences, College of Dentistry, King Saud University, Riyadh 11545, Saudi Arabia*

Correspondence should be addressed to Sundar Ramalingam; sundar.ksu@gmail.com

Academic Editor: Danyel E. Da Cruz Perez

Lateral periodontal cyst (LPC) is an uncommon developmental odontogenic cyst arising on the lateral surface of tooth roots. Commonly reported in mandibular canine-premolar or maxillary anterior regions, it presents as a well-circumscribed or tear drop-shaped radiolucency with a sclerotic border. Associated teeth are asymptomatic and vital, and roots may be displaced without resorption. Histopathologically, cystic lining resembles reduced enamel epithelium along with glycogen-rich clear cells and epithelial plaques. Unilateral variant of LPC has low recurrence and is managed by enucleation. A 43-year-old male patient reported with asymptomatic swelling in the left mandibular canine and first premolar region. Both teeth were vital, and radiographs revealed well-circumscribed radiolucency between the roots. Following consent, surgical enucleation and guided bone regeneration (GBR) with xenograft and resorbable collagen membrane were done under local anesthesia. The immediate postoperative period was uneventful, and complete bone fill of cystic cavity and healing of periodontal tissues was observed after a one-year follow-up. Histopathologic examination confirmed the diagnosis. LPC should be a differential diagnosis in cystic lesions lateral to the surface of a tooth and without any associated inflammation. Based on this case report, unicystic LPC can be successfully managed through surgical enucleation with GBR for better periodontal healing.

1. Introduction

Lateral periodontal cyst (LPC) is a relatively rare odontogenic pathology, representing about 0.4% of all odontogenic cysts [1–4]. It has been reported predominantly as an incidental finding and is a harmless entity characterized by an intraosseous, nonkeratinized, noninflammatory, and developmental odontogenic cyst of epithelial origin [2, 4, 5]. LPC is usually symptomless and is discovered during routine radiographic examination and occurs most frequently in the alveolar process of the mandibular canine and premolar regions, followed by the anterior maxilla [5]. Although it is commonly reported between the fourth to the seventh decades of life, cases have been reported in younger individuals too and it does not have a specific gender predilection [2]. Interestingly the epithelial cell of origin of LPC has been debated considerably [2]. Reports from the literature indicate a possible origin from either the rests of the dental lamina, reduced enamel epithelium, or rests of Malassez [3, 5, 6].

According to the World Health Organization (WHO) classification of odontogenic tumors and cysts (4th Edition, 2017), LPC is classified as an odontogenic cyst of developmental origin (Table 1) [7]. Clinically, LPC presents as an asymptomatic gingival swelling occurring on the facial aspect in between two teeth, and it should be differentiated from its soft tissue counterpart, the gingival cyst of adults (GCA), which presents as a blue fluctuant swelling [1, 5, 8]. Radiologically, they present as a well-circumscribed unilocular

Table 1: World Health Organization (WHO) classification of odontogenic tumors and cysts (4th Edition, 2017) [7].

Odontogenic tumors	Malignant tumors	Ameloblastic carcinoma Primary intraosseous carcinoma, NOS Sclerosing odontogenic carcinoma Clear cell odontogenic carcinoma Ghost cell odontogenic carcinoma Odontogenic carcinosarcoma Odontogenic sarcomas
	Benign epithelial origin tumors	Ameloblastoma, conventional (i) Ameloblastoma, unicystic type (ii) Ameloblastoma, extraosseous/peripheral type (iii) Metastasizing (malignant) ameloblastoma Squamous odontogenic tumor Calcifying epithelial odontogenic tumor Adenomatoid odontogenic tumor
	Benign mixed (epithelial-mesenchymal) origin tumors	Ameloblastic fibroma Primordial odontogenic tumor Odontoma (i) Compound type (ii) Complex type Dentinogenic ghost cell tumor
	Benign mesenchymal origin tumors	Odontogenic fibroma Odontogenic myxoma/myxofibroma Cementoblastoma Cemento-ossifying fibroma
Odontogenic cysts	Developmental origin cysts	Dentigerous cyst Odontogenic keratocyst Lateral periodontal and botryoid odontogenic cyst Gingival cyst Glandular odontogenic cyst Calcifying odontogenic cyst Orthokeratinized odontogenic cyst
	Inflammatory origin cysts	Radicular cyst Collateral inflammatory cyst

radiolucency with a sclerotic margin, in the alveolar process, in between the roots of vital teeth [5, 8]. While most LPCs are less than 1 cm in diameter, the uncommon botryoid variant may present as a larger and multilocular radiolucency, extending up to the periapical region [1, 5, 9]. Described for the first time in 1973, the botryoid odontogenic cyst (BOC) is associated with a greater risk of recurrence (30.1%), in comparison to LPC [9]. Based on reports available in the literature, BOC is known to affect patients in the fifth decade, with a slight preponderance towards females (53.5%) and more commonly in the mandible (83.3%) [4, 9]. Interestingly, LPC, BOC, and GCA have a common histogenetic origin and are classified as developmental odontogenic cysts as per WHO classification [4, 7]. It is reported that BOC arises from multiple foci of closely located epithelial rests, resulting in a multicystic lesion [4, 9]. Nevertheless, multiple, separate LPCs occurring in close proximity have also been reported by Siponen et al. [4].

Although untreated odontogenic cysts could cause root resorption in adjacent teeth, it has not been reported in association with LPC [1, 8]. Moreover, the associated teeth are usually vital unless they have been otherwise affected by dental caries or periodontitis [2]. Pain and tenderness, with or without cortical expansion in cases of LPC, have also been infrequently reported in the literature [1, 8]. LPCs are commonly differentially diagnosed as either a gingival cyst, an odontogenic keratocyst, or a residual cyst owing to their clinical and radiographic similarities [2, 5]. However, LPCs are histologically unique and are most frequently lined by a thin, nonkeratinizing layer of squamous or cuboidal epithelium, typically ranging from 1 to 3 cell layers in thickness and resembling the reduced enamel epithelium [2, 4, 5, 10, 11]. The epithelial cells in an LPC present with small, pyknotic nuclei and are occasionally separated by intercellular fluid [1, 4, 8]. In addition, focal plaques of epithelial thickenings in a fusiform or spindle-shaped pattern, along with glycogen-rich clear cells, have also been reported in the cystic lining [4, 10].

Treatment of LPC, which provided that the lesion is unilocular on radiological examination, is by conservative surgical enucleation and following up the patient over a period of six months to one year, in order to monitor for recurrence [1, 12]. Nevertheless, simple surgical enucleation is associated with a residual bone defect which could potentially affect the periodontal health of the associated teeth [10]. With the advent of tissue regeneration techniques in dentistry, several techniques including guided tissue regeneration (GTR) and guide bone regeneration (GBR) have been

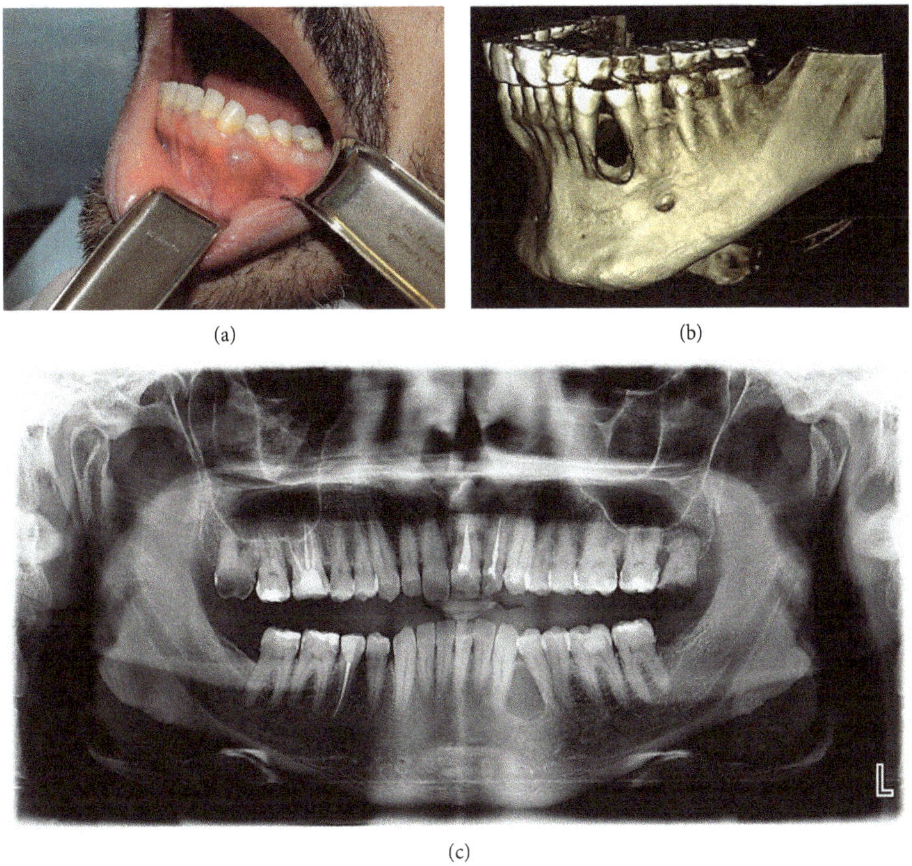

Figure 1: Preoperative clinical photograph and radiographs showing (a) circumscribed swelling in the attached gingiva in between the left mandibular canine (33) and premolar (34); (b) three-dimensional reconstructed cone beam computed tomography image of left mandible showing cystic lesion between roots of teeth 33 and 34, along with loss of buccal and lingual cortices; and (c) orthopantomograph showing well-circumscribed radiolucency with a sclerotic border in between roots of teeth 33 and 34, along with displacement of the roots.

reported for the treatment of bone defects, following enucleation of LPC [10, 13]. The technique of GBR, which has been reported with a considerable clinical success, involves placement of an osteoconductive scaffold within a bone defect and covering it with a resorbable or nonresorbable barrier membrane [14].

The aim of this paper is to present a case of LPC treated with surgical enucleation and primary bone defect repair using GBR with xenograft and resorbable collagen membrane, along with a recurrence-free follow-up period of one year. In addition, this case is being reported for the similarities in clinical and radiographic presentation between LPC and other odontogenic lesions and a proposed modality towards definitive treatment.

2. Case Presentation

A 43-year-old Saudi male patient reported to the oral surgery outpatient clinic at the College of Dentistry and Dental University Hospital, King Saud University, with a complaint of painless swelling in the left mandibular premolar region. Although the history revealed a presence of the swelling for more than one year without any associated symptoms, the patient preferred to obtain clinical consultation as he was concerned about the swelling. The patient had no previous history of dental treatment except for periodic oral prophylaxis and reported no systemic comorbidities.

2.1. Clinical and Radiographic Examination. Upon clinical examination, a well-circumscribed and fluctuant swelling, measuring about 9-12 mm in diameter, was observed at the junction of the buccal attached and free gingival margins in between the left mandibular canine (33) and premolar tooth (34) (Figure 1). The swelling was nontender, and there was no dental focus of infection or inflammation in the associated teeth. Similarly, no abnormalities were detected clinically in the lingual aspect of the left mandibular canine and premolar teeth. Both teeth 33 and 34 were vital upon testing with a cold stimulus and upon electric pulp testing. Extra oral examination revealed no clinically discernible asymmetry, swelling, or lymphadenopathy. Aspiration of the swelling with a large bore needle yielded clear fluid indicative of a cystic lesion and ruling out an abscess or vascular lesion.

Radiographic examination (orthopantomogram (OPG)) of the left mandibular body region revealed a well-circumscribed radiolucency, with a sclerotic border in between the roots of teeth 33 and 34. The radiolucency measured approximately 1.5 cm superior-inferiorly and 1.2 cm mesiodistally. Although the roots of the associated teeth (33 and 34) were displaced, there was no discernible

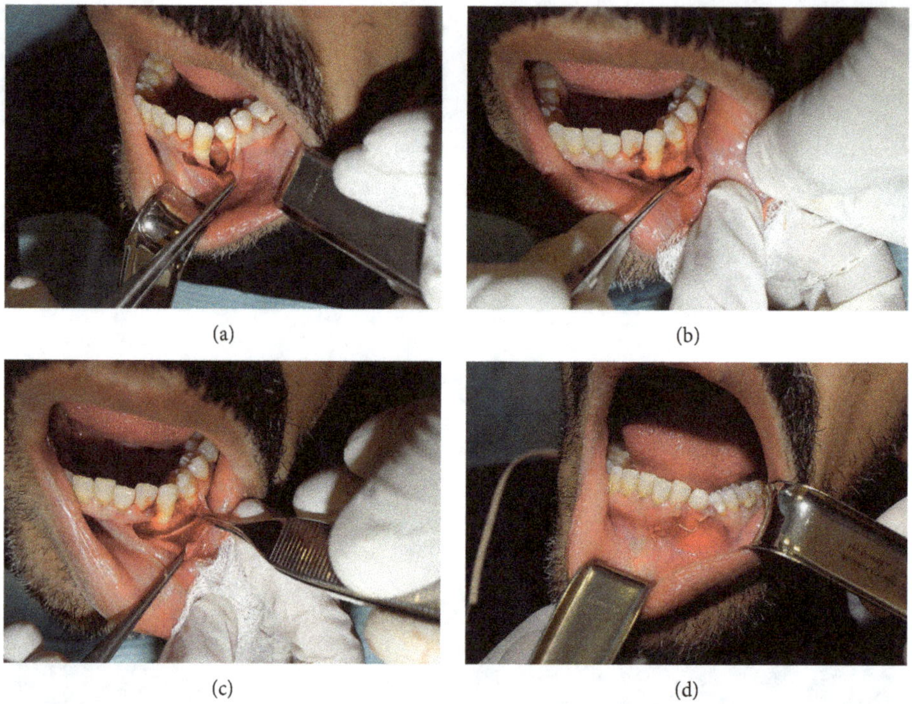

FIGURE 2: Intraoperative clinical photographs showing (a) mucoperiosteal flap elevation and visualization of the cyst in between roots of teeth 33 and 34; (b) identification and enucleation of the cystic lining; (c) grafting the cyst cavity with xenograft bone and placement of a resorbable collagen membrane; and (d) reapproximation of the mucoperiosteal flap and closure with resorbable sutures.

loss of the lamina dura in them. Cone beam computed tomography (CBCT) of the region of interest revealed a cystic lesion between the roots of the left mandibular canine and premolar, along with resorption of both the buccal and lingual cortical plates (Figure 1).

2.2. Surgical Procedure and Follow-Up. Based on a clinical and radiographic diagnosis of a lateral periodontal cyst, the patient was consented for enucleation and curettage of the cystic lesion and primary reconstruction of the defect site using guided bone regeneration. Following informed consent, under local anesthesia, the lesion was surgically approached through a gingival crevicular incision extending from tooth 32 to tooth 35. After mucoperiosteal flap elevation, an anterior vertical releasing incision was provided for optimum visualization and sharp dissection using a pair of scissors was done superficial to the cystic wall in order to separate the mucoperiosteal flap without compromising its integrity. While the cystic lesion was identified and enucleated in total, mild adhesions to the lingual mucoperiosteum were released through blunt dissection using the surgical curette (Figure 2).

Following enucleation and curettage, the cystic cavity was thoroughly irrigated with sterile normal saline. Clinical examination revealed a bony wall with intact mucoperiosteum on the lingual aspect, and there was no resorption of the roots of the tooth mesial and distal to the lesion. The residual defect left behind by the cystic lesion was then filled with a xenograft bone (Bio-Oss, Geistlich Pharma, Princeton, NJ, USA) soaked in sterile normal saline and covered by a resorbable collagen membrane (RCM) (Bio-Gide, Geistlich Pharma, Princeton, NJ, USA). The mucoperiosteal flap was reapproximated and closed with Vicryl 4-0 interrupted sutures (Polyglactin 910, ETHICON, Somerville, NJ, USA) (Figure 2). Postoperative radiographs revealed complete filling of the bone defect with graft material, and the patient was discharged with specific postoperative instructions and antibiotic and analgesic medication. The immediate postoperative period was uneventful, and the surgical wound healed remarkably well. Follow-up examinations at six months and one year after cyst enucleation and guided bone regeneration revealed no clinical or radiographic evidence of recurrence of the lesion. Moreover, teeth 33 and 34 were still vital during follow-up (Figure 3).

2.3. Histopathology Examination. The excised soft tissue specimen was immediately fixed in 10% neutral buffered formalin and was sent for histopathology examination (HPE). HPE of the excised specimen revealed a cystic lesion lined in most areas by a thin epithelial lining composed of one or two rows of cuboidal or flattened epithelial cells. Focal areas of epithelial thickenings, with a few duct-like spaces rimmed by cuboidal cells and areas of swirling orientation of the cells, were also noted. Occasional clear cells in the lining along with odontogenic epithelium in the cyst wall were also seen. Based on HPE and clinicoradiological correlation, a diagnosis of lateral periodontal cyst was established. Considering the low risk of recurrence associated with the lesion, it was decided to follow up the patient closely (Figure 4).

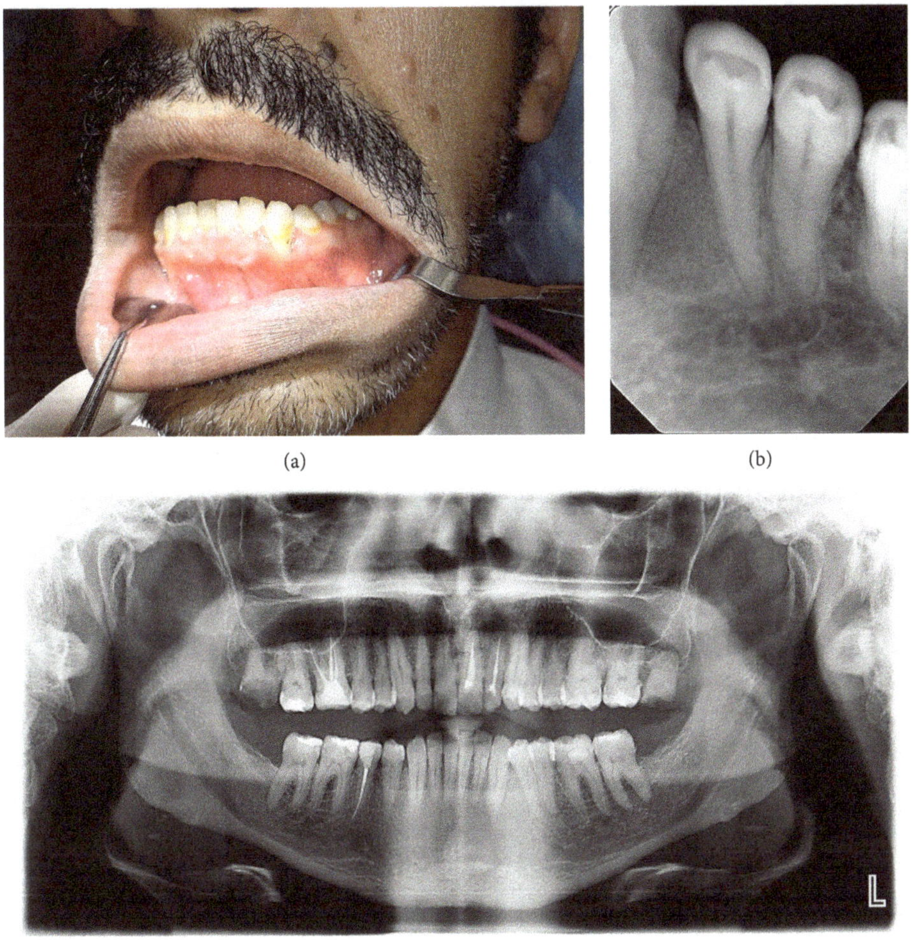

(a) (b)

(c)

FIGURE 3: Postoperative clinical photograph and radiographs at one-year follow-up showing (a) healthy gingiva and periodontium in between teeth 33 and 34; (b) periapical radiograph and (c) orthopantomograph showing no evidence of cyst recurrence and complete bone fill between roots of teeth 33 and 34.

3. Discussion

In this report, a case of LPC has been presented along with its corresponding clinical, radiographic, and histopathologic findings, in addition to its primary management with GBR. The first documented report of LPC in the literature was as early as 1958 by Standish and Shafer [15], who reported a series of five cases of LPC presenting in the mandibular canine-premolar region. LPC is an uncommon developmental odontogenic cyst which occurs in association with vital teeth and is usually reported as a coincidental finding during routine radiograph [2, 3]. Owing to its noninflammatory nature, it is asymptomatic until and unless the cystic lesion is secondarily infected [3]. In the present case report, the patient did not complain of any symptoms other than a painless swelling in the left mandibular canine-premolar (teeth 33 and 34) region, and the associated teeth were vital. In spite of a clinical swelling, the lesion was coherent with the classical clinical presentation of LPC, namely, asymptomatic swelling associated with vital teeth in the canine-premolar region in a middle-aged patient (Figure 1) [2, 3, 12]. Radiographically, the lesion presented as a well-circumscribed radiolucency surrounded by a sclerotic border and not encroaching upon the periodontal ligament space of the adjacent teeth (Figure 1). The above findings were in line with the radiographic presentation of LPC as reported in the literature [2, 3, 5, 12]. Based on the clinical and radiographic findings, a provisional diagnosis of LPC was considered and treatment was planned accordingly.

In spite of its distinguishing radiographic and clinical presentation, it is considered prudent enough to confirm the diagnosis of LPC through HPE [3]. The characteristic histopathological features of LPC include a nonkeratinized epithelial lining, 1-3 cell layers in thickness, resembling the odontogenic epithelium, along with epithelial plaques and glycogen-rich clear cells [4, 10, 11, 16, 17]. Although the collagen-rich connective tissue wall displays areas of hyalinization, there is no evidence of inflammatory cells [16, 17]. LPC was originally believed to arise from the epithelial rests in the periodontal ligament space, in the absence of any associated inflammatory stimulus [15]. Currently, it is reported to arise from the reduced enamel epithelium, remnants of

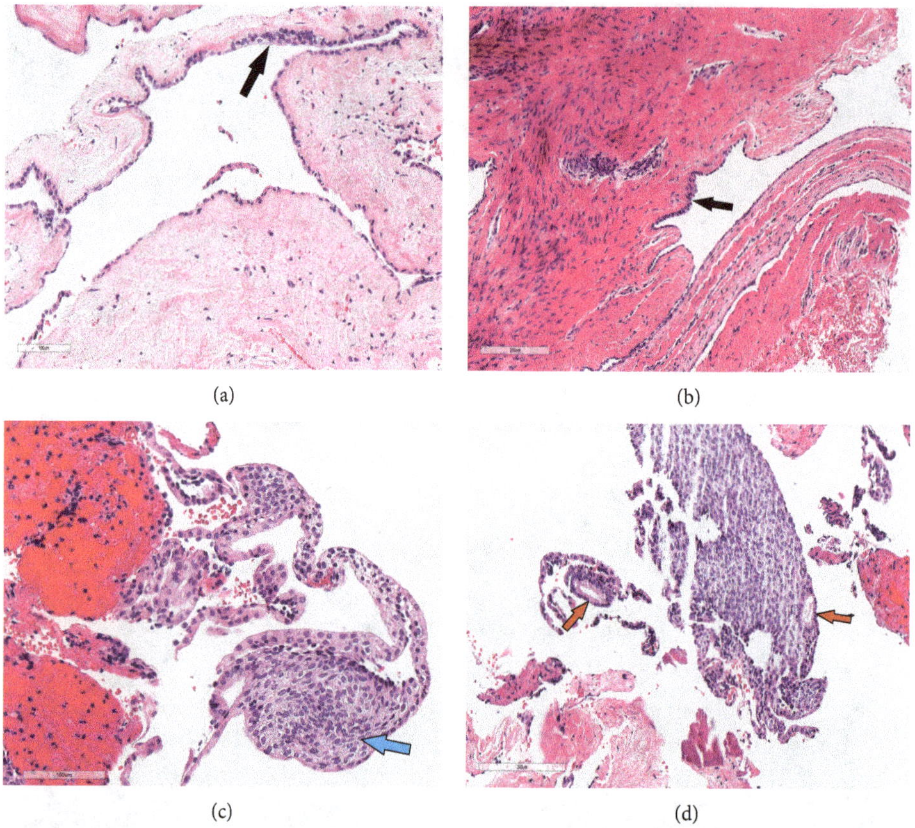

Figure 4: Histopathological examination of (a) the excised cystic lesion showing and (b) cystic lesion composed of reduced enamel epithelium-like lining comprising single or double layer(s) of flattened squamous or cuboidal cells and subtly thickened areas with more closely packed cells (arrow). The cyst wall is uninflamed throughout but demonstrates varying degrees of collagenization and cellularity. Cells with a clear cytoplasm are scattered throughout the lining (a). (c) A fragmented part of the lining showing a thickened cellular plaque with evidence of whorled (swirling) arrangement (blue arrow). Cells with a clear cytoplasm are also seen scattered in this plaque. (d) Another fragmented thickened epithelial plaque with areas showing ductal orientation (red arrow). Scale bars: 100 μm (a, c) and 200 μm (b, d).

dental lamina or cell rests of Malassez [3, 5]. It has been hypothesized that the origin of LPC could be correlated to the cell type of origin, based on histopathological findings. While the presence of nonkeratinized epithelium points to an origin from reduced enamel epithelium, evidence of glycogen-rich clear cells indicates the relationship with remnants of dental lamina [3, 18]. On the other hand, the predominantly reported location of LPC close to the root surface implies a possible origin from the cell rests of Malassez [3, 18]. Nevertheless, there is no consensus regarding a particular cell type of origin, as all the abovementioned features have been described by the majority of the cases reported in the literature [3]. In the present case, HPE revealed the presence of a thin layer of nonkeratinized odontogenic epithelium, along with clear cells and epithelial plaques in the cystic lining (Figure 4).

It must however be noted that a HPE finding similar to LPC is also reported in the botryoid odontogenic cyst (BOC) [5, 9]. In contrast to LPC which presents as circumscribed or tear-shaped radiolucency in between roots of teeth, BOC appears as a multilocular radiolucency and presents as a multicystic lesion at both the macroscopic and microscopic levels [3, 4, 9]. It derives its name from the Greek word "botryos," which means grape-like, and is considered a histopathological variant of LPC with a greater propensity for recurrence following treatment [1, 3, 9, 12]. Although a rare entity, BOC has also been reported to develop from the cystic lining of a preexisting LPC associated with aggressive intrabony expansion [9, 19]. While it is believed that BOC arises as a result of changes in LPC, it has also been reported that BOC has a multicentric origin, wherein several LPCs develop in very close proximity [4, 9, 19]. Nevertheless, there has been a unanimous agreement regarding the common odontogenic origin for both the LPC and BOC [12, 19]. Based on a hypothesis that all LPCs are capable of progressing to multicystic lesions, Altini and Shear [8] proposed a classification of LPC as unicystic, multicystic, or botryoid variants, but all of them with similar histopathological presentation [8]. Interestingly, BOC has also been classified as a "polymorphous odontogenic cyst" along with sialo-odontogenic, glandular, and median-mandibular cysts owing to their predominantly high rates of recurrence [20]. It must therefore be reiterated that HPE to identify any microcysts developing within the LPC lining and wall is required to distinguish the lesion from the aggressive multicystic or botryoid variants [12, 19, 20]. In the present case, there was no histopathological evidence of intraepithelial microcyst formation, thereby confirming the diagnosis of a unicystic LPC variant (Figure 4).

Treatment of unicystic LPC usually involves conservative surgical enucleation of the cyst and curettage of the cystic cavity to eliminate any remnants. In the majority of the cases, the associated teeth remain vital and are neither extracted nor endodontically treated [2, 5, 12]. In the present case too, a similar surgical treatment was carried out. Both the associated teeth (33 and 34) were clinically vital at the beginning of treatment and remained vital and in function after one year of follow-up. However, a primary reconstruction of the cystic cavity was carried out using guided bone regeneration (Figure 2). Similar to our case, in several reported cases of LPC in the literature, enucleation and curettage were done based on a clinical and radiographic diagnosis and confirmation through HPE was done only postoperatively [3, 10, 13, 14, 16–18]. Nevertheless, it is imperative to identify and rule out differential diagnoses of other odontogenic lesions prior to any definitive treatment. Odontogenic cysts including odontogenic keratocyst (OKC) [21], dentigerous cyst [22, 23], and glandular odontogenic cyst (GOC) [24] have mimicked LPC in their presentation. However, the abovementioned odontogenic cysts clinically and radiographically present in association with impacted teeth and are preponderant in the posterior mandibular region [3, 21, 23, 24]. On the contrary, histopathologically confirmed LPC predominantly presented in the periodontal ligament space between the lateral surfaces of teeth, either in the mandibular canine-premolar region or in the maxillary anterior region [2, 5, 12]. Considering the high rates of recurrence associated with lesions such as OKC and GOC, it is justifiable to perform an incisional biopsy of cystic lesions mimicking LPC in the mandibular posterior region.

Even though managed conservatively, enucleation of LPC leaves behind a significant bone cavity and dead space, which in the long term might affect the periodontal health of associated teeth [12]. Several modalities of tissue regenerative techniques have been reported to achieve optimum postoperative periodontal health following surgical treatment of LPC [10, 13]. GBR is routinely used for the treatment of periodontal bone defects and alveolar ridge augmentation prior to implant placement [14], wherein regeneration of an osseous defect is achieved within 6-10 months by placement of an osteoconductive bone substitute material in the defect and covering it with a barrier membrane [14]. While several osteoconductive materials including hydroxyapatite, tri-calcium phosphate, and deproteinized allograft and xenograft are reportedly used in GBR, a resorbable collagen barrier membrane (RCM) is preferred [10, 13, 14]. In addition to preventing fibrous tissue invasion into the osseous defect, RCM enables hemostasis and neovascularization and promotes attachment of osteoblasts [14]. In the present case, a bovine derived deproteinized xenograft bone was used as the osteoconductive scaffold along with RCM and at one-year follow-up, complete bone fill of the defect site was evidenced radiographically (Figure 3). Moreover, healing of periodontal tissues without any complications was also noticed clinically, in between the affected teeth.

4. Conclusion

Although LPC is an uncommon developmental odontogenic cyst, it should be considered a differential diagnosis in case of cystic lesions lateral to the surface of a tooth and without any associated inflammatory processes or symptoms. Unicystic LPC clinically and radiographically diagnosed based on the previously mentioned characteristic features can be managed with conservative surgical enucleation and GBR. However, further long-term clinical studies in larger sample sizes should be mandated to ascertain the efficacy of this treatment modality. Nevertheless, the role of HPE after surgical enucleation should not be discounted and histopathological confirmation of diagnosis serves as the benchmark for a recurrence-free follow-up period.

References

[1] M. Shear and P. Speight, *Gingival Cyst of Adults, Lateral Periodontal Cyst, Botryoid Odontogenic Cyst*, Cysts of the Oral and Maxillofacial Regions, Blackwell Munksgaard, 4th edition, 2008.

[2] R. E. Friedrich, H. A. Scheuer, and J. Zustin, "Lateral periodontal cyst," *In Vivo (Athens, Greece)*, vol. 28, no. 4, pp. 595–598, 2014.

[3] L. F. de Carvalho, C. F. Lima, L. A. Cabral, A. A. Brandao, and J. D. Almeida, "Lateral periodontal cyst: a case report and literature review," *Journal of Oral & Maxillofacial Research*, vol. 1, no. 4, p. e5, 2011.

[4] M. Siponen, B. W. Neville, D. D. Damm, and C. M. Allen, "Multifocal lateral periodontal cysts: a report of 4 cases and review of the literature," *Oral Surgery, Oral Medicine, Oral Pathology, Oral Radiology, and Endodontics*, vol. 111, no. 2, pp. 225–233, 2011.

[5] E. A. Bilodeau and B. M. Collins, "Odontogenic cysts and neoplasms," *Surgical Pathology Clinics*, vol. 10, no. 1, pp. 177–222, 2017.

[6] J. J. Sciubba, J. E. Fantasia, and L. B. Kahn, *Tumors and Cysts of the Jaw*, Atlas of Head and Neck Pathology, B. M. Wenig, Ed., Elsevier, 2008.

[7] M. Soluk-Tekkesin and J. M. Wright, "The World Health Organization Classification of odontogenic lesions: a summary of the changes of the 2017 (4th) edition," *Turk Patoloji Dergisi*, vol. 34, no. 1, 2018.

[8] M. Altini and M. Shear, "The lateral periodontal cyst: an update," *Journal of Oral Pathology & Medicine*, vol. 21, no. 6, pp. 245–250, 1992.

[9] B. Vidakovic, I. Uljanic, J. Grgurevic, B. Peric, and S. Manojlovic, "Botryoid cyst, a rare type of odontogenic cyst," *Acta Clinica Croatica*, vol. 55, no. 3, pp. 510–514, 2016.

[10] S. Sivolella, C. Perin, M. Capecchi, V. Buongiorno, and M. Valente, "Guided bone regeneration in the treatment of a lateral periodontal cyst: 2-year clinical and radiologic follow-up," *The International Journal of Periodontics & Restorative Dentistry*, vol. 38, no. 5, pp. 747–754, 2018.

[11] A. K. El-Naggar, J. K. C. Chan, J. R. Grandis, T. Takata, and P. J. Slootweg, *WHO Classification of Head and Neck Tumours*, International Agency for Research on Cancer, 2017.

[12] B. R. Chrcanovic and R. S. Gomez, "Gingival cyst of the adult, lateral periodontal cyst, and botryoid odontogenic cyst: an updated systematic review," *Oral Diseases*, vol. 25, no. 1, pp. 26–33, 2019.

[13] S. E. Meseli, O. B. Agrali, O. Peker, and L. Kuru, "Treatment of lateral periodontal cyst with guided tissue regeneration," *European Journal of Dentistry*, vol. 8, no. 3, pp. 419–423, 2014.

[14] S. Ramalingam, A. Al-Rasheed, A. ArRejaie, N. Nooh, M. Al-Kindi, and K. Al-Hezaimi, "Guided bone regeneration in standardized calvarial defects using beta-tricalcium phosphate and collagen membrane: a real-time in vivo micro-computed tomographic experiment in rats," *Odontology*, vol. 104, no. 2, pp. 199–210, 2016.

[15] S. M. Standish and W. G. Shafer, "The lateral periodontal cyst," *The Journal of Periodontology*, vol. 29, no. 1, pp. 27–33, 1958.

[16] D. A. Cohen, B. W. Neville, D. D. Damm, and D. K. White, "The lateral periodontal cyst. A report of 37 cases," *Journal of Periodontology*, vol. 55, no. 4, pp. 230–234, 1984.

[17] L. G. Rasmusson, B. C. Magnusson, and H. Borrman, "The lateral periodontal cyst. A histopathological and radiographic study of 32 cases," *The British Journal of Oral & Maxillofacial Surgery*, vol. 29, no. 1, pp. 54–57, 1991.

[18] M. de Andrade, A. P. P. Silva, F. M. de Moraes Ramos-Perez, Y. T. C. Silva-Sousa, and D. E. da Cruz Perez, "Lateral periodontal cyst: report of case and review of the literature," *Oral and Maxillofacial Surgery*, vol. 16, no. 1, pp. 83–87, 2012.

[19] P. Arora, K. A. Bishen, N. Gupta, A. Jamdade, and G. R. Kumar, "Botryoid odontogenic cyst developing from lateral periodontal cyst: a rare case and review on pathogenesis," *Contemporary Clinical Dentistry*, vol. 3, no. 3, pp. 326–329, 2012.

[20] A. S. High, D. M. G. Main, S. P. Khoo, J. Pedlar, and W. J. Hume, "The polymorphous odontogenic cyst," *Journal of Oral Pathology and Medicine*, vol. 25, no. 1, pp. 25–31, 1996.

[21] B. Manohar, D. Baidya, S. Bhuvaneswari, and A. B. Rai, "Keratocystic odontogenic tumour mimicking lateral periodontal cyst: a diagnostic dilemma," *Kathmandu University medical journal (KUMJ)*, vol. 14, no. 56, pp. 370–372, 2016.

[22] A. R. Byatnal, P. M. K, T. Rukmangada, and S. Koppal, "An unfamiliar presentation of a lateral periodontal cyst," *Case Reports*, vol. 2013, 2013.

[23] F. M. Buckley, P. Huntley, and P. M. Speight, "A lateral periodontal cyst in association with a follicular cyst," *British Dental Journal*, vol. 167, no. 1, pp. 26–28, 1989.

[24] Y. Takeda, "Glandular odontogenic cyst mimicking a lateral periodontal cyst: a case report," *International Journal of Oral and Maxillofacial Surgery*, vol. 23, no. 2, pp. 96-97, 1994.

17

The Gingival Oral Lichen Planus: A Periodontal-Oral Medicine Approach

Abdulhameed Alsarraf,[1] Kunj Mehta,[2] and Nabil Khzam[3]

[1]*Ministry of Health, Kuwait*
[2]*Private Practice, Perth 6000 Western Australia, Australia*
[3]*NK Perio & Implants, Perth 6172 Western Australia, Australia*

Correspondence should be addressed to Nabil Khzam; nokhzam@gmail.com

Academic Editor: Jose López-López

We present a case of a 77-year-old female who suffered from oral lichen planus (OLP) involving her gingiva and bilateral buccal mucosa for over 6 months. We showed that oral hygiene measures and conventional periodontal treatment and strict maintenance were sufficient to control the gingival involvement of OLP. The mechanism of OLP is complex and not yet fully understood. The focus of discussion in our case was that knowledge and understanding of gingival pathology are fundamental for a determined management approach. Our case was managed according to the suggested protocols in previous case studies. A multidisciplinary approach allowed for accurate diagnosis and treatment tailored to the presented case.

1. Introduction

Lichen planus is a chronic immune-mediated inflammatory disease that affects the skin and mucous membranes. Oral lichen planus (OLP) is the mucosal counterpart of cutaneous lichen planus and it was first described in 1866 as white papular eruptions in the oral cavity [1]. According to the American Academy of Periodontology, OLP is classified as nonplaque-induced gingival lesions [2]. Classically, OLP appears in a roughly symmetrical distribution of well-defined white striations on a background of mild erythema, commonly involving the buccal mucosa and tongue [3]. Other clinical patterns reported in the literature include atrophic, erosive, papular, plaque-like, and bullous-type lesions [4]. To ensure accurate diagnosis of OLP, key histopathological features from biopsy specimens should be reported by an oral pathologist to allow clinicopathological correlation and exclusion of oral epithelial dysplasia. The pathogenesis of the disease is characterized by cytotoxic $CD8^+$ T lymphocytes migration to the epithelium inducing apoptosis of basal keratinocytes [5]. A number of etiological factors in OLP have been proposed such as local and systemic inducers of cell-mediated hypersensitivity, drugs, dental materials, infectious agents, and stress [6]. OLP management is directed at controlling active inflammation and the reduction of associated symptoms; therefore, patient education and awareness is important [7]. In addition, maintaining good oral hygiene, absence of oral candidosis, periodontal disease, and salivary gland hypofunction are all factors to successful management outcomes [8]. Various therapeutic agents are described for controlling OLP including topical, intralesional, and systemic corticosteroids, immunosuppressive agents, retinoids, and immunomodulators. These treatment regimens may be used sequentially until effective symptomatic control is reached due to variations in patient responses [9–11]. Of note, the malignant potential of OLP is reported in the literature with an overall malignant transformation of 1%. This is due to cases of oral cancer arising from patients with OLP demonstrating absence of epithelial dysplasia [12, 13]. OLP has therefore been designated as an oral potentially malignant disorder. It must also be noted that similar clinical presentations of OLP are induced by oral lichenoid reactions; however, it is not always simple to distinguish between the two different

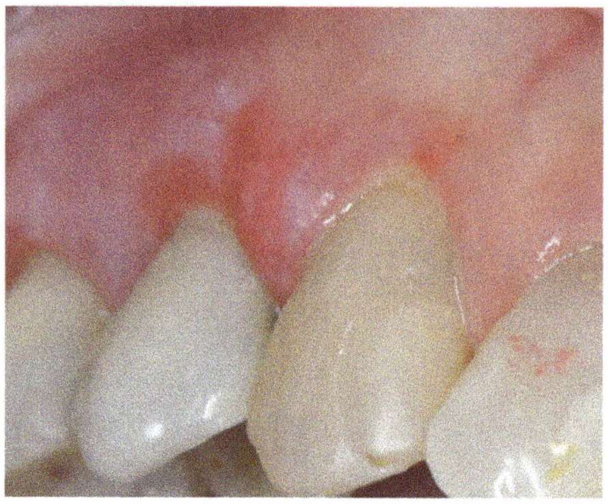

FIGURE 1: Gingival OLP: a mixed red and white lesion in the background of white striations involving the gingiva between teeth 13 and 14. No to minimal plaque is noted and the involvement of the attached gingiva distinguishes OLP from plaque-induced gingivitis.

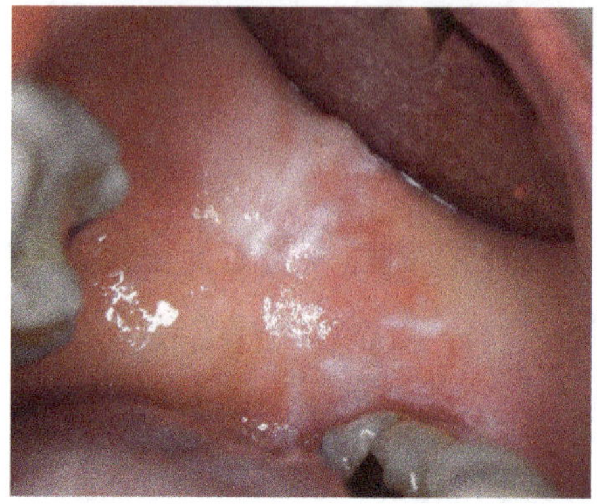

FIGURE 2: Left buccal mucosa: predominantly white plaque-type lesion and white striations noted in the background of mild erythema.

diseases clinically as well as histopathologically [9]. With that being said, most oral lichenoid lesions are directly presented adjacent to direct restorative materials such as amalgam and composite [9]. Further understanding and clinical experience aids in implementing a long-term management plan for OLP cases.

2. Case Report

A 77-year-old female patient presented to her general dentist due to bleeding gums. The dentist referred the patient to a specialist periodontist for a consultation regarding the assessment and treatment of generalized chronic periodontitis. A full comprehensive periodontal and radiographic examination revealed a periodontal diagnosis of generalized moderate to advanced chronic periodontitis. Clinical signs of gingival inflammation and periodontal pockets of 5 mm and more with calculus and bleeding upon probing were present on two or more aspects of each tooth. The radiographic examination revealed a generalized horizontal bone loss of 40 to 50% around most of the dentition. The patient was then referred to the Oral Medicine Clinic for diagnosis and further management of OLP-like lesions. Incisional biopsies were performed from the left buccal mucosa and 13/14 labial gingiva (Figures 1 and 2). Histopathological assessment showed hyperkeratosis and band-like lymphocytic infiltrate in the lamina propria (Figure 3). No epithelial dysplasia was noted. These features are consistent with the diagnosis of OLP. Patient education and awareness was delivered in the context of diagnosis, potential triggering factors, and disease malignant potential. Long-term observation is necessary, and the patient will be followed up regularly to monitor disease behavior and progression.

3. Discussion

The diagnosis of OLP requires both clinical manifestations and characteristic histopathological features. The practice of good oral hygiene and achieving optimum periodontal health contribute to successful management outcomes. From

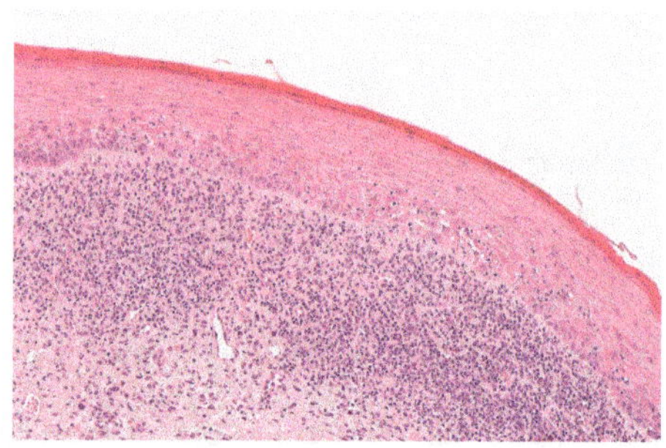

FIGURE 3: Histopathological assessment from an incisional biopsy performed from the left buccal mucosa showed hyperkeratosis and band-like lymphocytic infiltrate in the lamina propria.

a clinical standpoint, the proposed periodontal treatment plan was patient education, in the form of information on periodontitis in terms of pathogenesis, treatment, and prevention. Detailed oral hygiene instructions include recommendations for the use of electric ultrasoft tooth brush, spongy dental floss, and soft interdental brushes. The patient was encouraged to maintain high level of oral hygiene and attend regular periodontal review appointments in order to maintain periodontal stability. The patient underwent two sessions of nonsurgical periodontal therapy on the same month, followed by reevaluation of periodontal tissue conditions 12 weeks after completion of debridement. This was followed by supportive periodontal treatment (3 monthly intervals). Overall, the patient had an excellent response to the nonsurgical periodontal therapy with good oral hygiene. In view of the involved OLP, additional attention is required in the overall management of the case. OLP is frequently asymptomatic or associated with minor discomfort only. This is especially true for papular, reticular, and plaque-type lesions which are often unnoticed by the patient and the general dentist. In contrast, atrophic and ulcerative lesions may give rise to severe pain, particularly related to food intake and aggressive oral hygiene procedures. In the presented case, the OLP lesion involving the gingiva of teeth 13 and 14 was symptomatic; therefore, the patient was instructed to use a

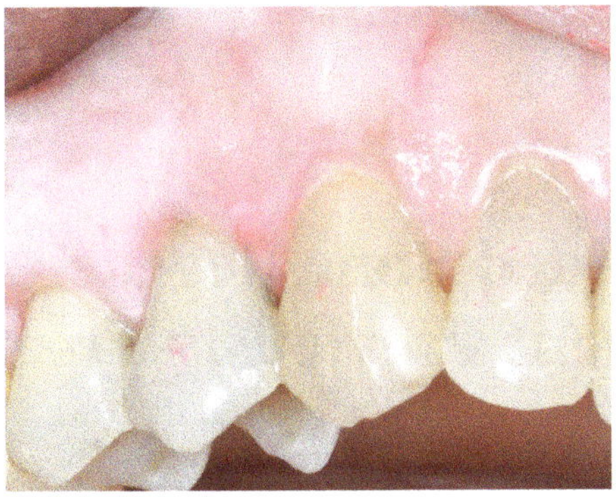

FIGURE 4: Resolution of erythema and active gingival inflammation due to OLP lesion involving the gingiva between teeth 13 and 14 following use of topical corticosteroid ointment.

topical corticosteroid ointment three times daily for two weeks applied directly to the lesion. Specifically, betamethasone valerate 0.05% was used as a topical application to the affected areas. Successful resolution of background erythema and active gingival inflammation was noted in the review appointment (Figure 4). Other areas involving the oral cavity such as the left buccal mucosa improved significantly. From a periodontal perspective, the most important part of the therapeutic regimen is treatment of periodontal disease (conservative nonsurgical approach), an atraumatic oral hygiene in terms of gentle tooth brushing and flossing using spongy type floss. Evidence of the literature supports this statement in the context of personalized plaque control for OLP gingival manifestations [14]. This will in turn result in significant improvement in a large number of patients. Effective plaque removal without traumatic influence on the gingival tissues must be established. In case of persistent pain typically associated with ulcerative and atrophic types, antifungal treatment may be necessary if the lesion contains candida species [8]. In chronic and symptomatic OLP cases, the response to the above treatment regimens is usually poor; therefore, topical corticosteroids are considered the first-line medications to control patients' symptoms. However, relapse in such cases is very common and intermittent episodes of treatment may be required over an extended period of time.

4. Conclusion

This case has demonstrated the periodontal management of a patient with oral lichen planus. While oral hygiene measures and conventional periodontal treatment were sufficient to control the gingival involvement of OLP, patient education and awareness of triggering factors were important to control OLP activity with the aid of topical corticosteroids. It is however important to consider the side effects related to long-term use of topical corticosteroids in the oral cavity. It is therefore important that both knowledge and understanding of gingival pathology are fundamental for a determined management approach in such cases.

References

[1] E. Wilson, "On lichen planus: the lichen ruber of Hebra," *BMJ*, vol. 2, no. 302, pp. 399–402, 1866.

[2] G. C. Armitage, "Development of a classification system for periodontal diseases and conditions," *Annals of Periodontology*, vol. 4, no. 1, pp. 1–6, 1999.

[3] F. Gorouhi, P. Davari, and N. Fazel, "Cutaneous and mucosal lichen planus: a comprehensive review of clinical subtypes, risk factors, diagnosis, and prognosis," *The Scientific World Journal*, vol. 2014, Article ID 742826, 22 pages, 2014.

[4] Y.-S. L. Cheng, A. Gould, Z. Kurago, J. Fantasia, and S. Muller, "Diagnosis of oral lichen planus: a position paper of the American Academy of Oral and Maxillofacial Pathology," *Oral Surgery, Oral Medicine, Oral Pathology and Oral Radiology*, vol. 122, no. 3, pp. 332–354, 2016.

[5] Z. B. Kurago, "Etiology and pathogenesis of oral lichen planus: an overview," *Oral Surgery, Oral Medicine, Oral Pathology and Oral Radiology*, vol. 122, no. 1, pp. 72–80, 2016.

[6] D. Farhi and N. Dupin, "Pathophysiology, etiologic factors, and clinical management of oral lichen planus, part I: facts and controversies," *Clinics in Dermatology*, vol. 28, no. 1, pp. 100–108, 2010.

[7] V. Crincoli, M. B. Di Bisceglie, M. Scivetti, A. Lucchese, S. Tecco, and F. Festa, "Oral lichen planus: update on etiopathogenesis, diagnosis and treatment," *Immunopharmacology and Immunotoxicology*, vol. 33, no. 1, pp. 11–20, 2011.

[8] I. M. C. Lundström, G. B. Anneroth, and K. Holmberg, "Candida in patients with oral lichen planus," *International Journal of Oral Surgery*, vol. 13, no. 3, pp. 226–238, 1984.

[9] I. Al-Hashimi, M. Schifter, P. B. Lockhart et al., "Oral lichen planus and oral lichenoid lesions: diagnostic and therapeutic considerations," *Oral Surgery, Oral Medicine, Oral Pathology, Oral Radiology, and Endodontology*, vol. 103, pp. S25.e1–S25.e12, 2007.

[10] F. Agha-Hosseini, N. Sheykhbahaei, and M.-S. SadrZadeh-Afshar, "Evaluation of potential risk factors that contribute to malignant transformation of oral lichen planus: a literature review," *The Journal of Contemporary Dental Practice*, vol. 17, no. 8, pp. 692–701, 2016.

[11] E. M. Otero-Rey, F. Suarez-Alen, M. Penamaria-Mallon, J. Lopez-Lopez, and A. Blanco-Carrion, "Malignant transformation of oral lichen planus by a chronic inflammatory process. Use of topical corticosteroids to prevent this progression?," *Acta Odontologica Scandinavica*, vol. 72, no. 8, pp. 570–577, 2014.

[12] G. Lodi, C. Scully, M. Carrozzo, M. Griffiths, P. B. Sugerman, and K. Thongprasom, "Current controversies in oral lichen planus: report of an international consensus meeting. Part 1. Viral infections and etiopathogenesis," *Oral Surgery, Oral Medicine, Oral Pathology, Oral Radiology, and Endodontology*, vol. 100, no. 1, pp. 40–51, 2005.

[13] S. Warnakulasuriya, N. W. Johnson, and I. van der Waal, "Nomenclature and classification of potentially malignant disorders of the oral mucosa," *Journal of Oral Pathology & Medicine*, vol. 36, no. 10, pp. 575–580, 2007.

[14] S. J. Stone, G. I. McCracken, P. A. Heasman, K. S. Staines, and M. Pennington, "Cost-effectiveness of personalized plaque control for managing the gingival manifestations of oral lichen planus: a randomized controlled study," *Journal of Clinical Periodontology*, vol. 40, no. 9, pp. 859–867, 2013.

18

Customized Titanium Mesh for Guided Bone Regeneration in the Posterior Mandible in a Patient Previously Treated with Bisphosphonates

Johannes Müller[1,2] **and Rüdiger Junker**[1]

[1]*Department of Prosthodontics and Biomaterials, Danube Private University, Krems, Austria*
[2]*Deputy Medical Director, Danube Private University, Krems, Austria*

Correspondence should be addressed to Rüdiger Junker; ruediger.junker@dp-uni.ac.at

Academic Editor: Asja Celebic

We describe the restorative treatment of an 86-year-old female patient who was referred to our specialist prosthodontics clinic. Due to secondary osteoporosis, she underwent oral antiresorptive therapy with ibandronic acid for 10 years. Although she was classified as a patient at increased risk of drug-induced osteonecrosis of the jaw, she eventually signed a consent form for fixed implant-supported prosthetic rehabilitation in her 4th sextant. However, after tooth extraction, the bone ridge was too small at the intended implant positions. Therefore, guided bone regeneration was performed with a computer-aided design/computer-aided manufacturing three-dimensional printed titanium mesh. Finally, a continuous augmented hard tissue ridge above 7 mm was found, and three implants were inserted. Eventually, after four months of submerged healing, the implants were loaded with single crowns. Now, the patient is seen regularly for supportive peri-implant therapy.

1. Introduction

In our time, prosthetic rehabilitation of missing teeth with dental implants has become a predictable treatment option [1, 2]. However, a common clinical problem in implant dentistry is the lack of sufficient bone width and bone height to allow for prosthetically driven implant position and placement [3]. In view of this, scientific evidence supports lateral [3, 4] and vertical [3, 5] bone augmentation prior to implant placement as effective procedures to achieve sufficient ridge width and height for implant placement. In this context, guided bone regeneration (GBR)—in principle, the application of a barrier membrane to exclude cells from the soft tissue to allow protected migration of osteoblasts and eventually bone formation [6]—with resorbable, collagenous barrier membranes in combination with space maintaining xenografts is considered useful and predictable [3–5, 7]. However, such a combination might lack mechanical stability, which ultimately leads to a smaller increase in bone volume [4, 9]. To overcome this, individualized computer-aided design/computer-aided manufacturing (CAD/CAM) three-dimensional printed titanium meshes have been successfully introduced into GBR [10].

Here, we present the rehabilitation of the posterior mandible—in an elderly patient previously under bone resorptive therapy—with implants and implant-supported single crowns after guided bone augmentation supported by a printed titanium mesh.

2. Patient Information

An 86-year-old female patient was referred to our specialist prosthodontic clinic in August 2018 for comprehensive therapy due to a vertical root fracture on tooth 35 (Figure 1) and the patient's desire for fixed rehabilitation. She presented with fixed, tooth- and implant-supported prosthetic restorations that were fitted about 17 years ago. But in recent years, she has not seen a dental hygienist or a general dentist regularly. She has also never smoked and is mentally and physically fit. However, due to secondary osteoporosis, she underwent oral antiresorptive therapy with ibandronic acid (i.e., one

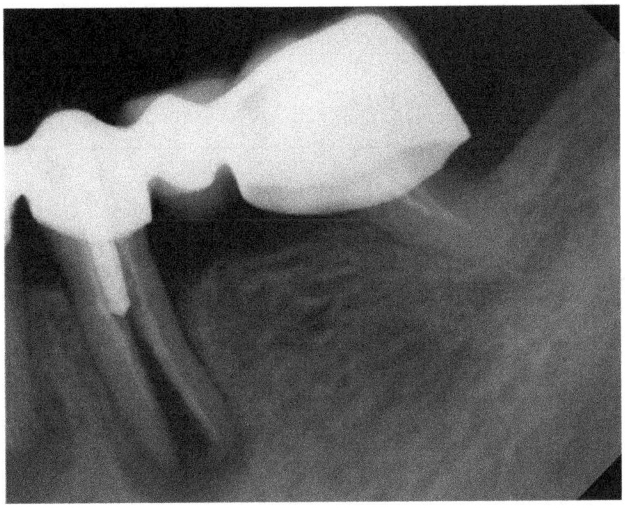

FIGURE 1: Radiograph tooth 35 at intake August 2018.

150 mg tablet once a month; Bonviva®, Future Health Pharma GmbH, Wetzikon, Switzerland) from 2005 to 2015. For the treatment of osteoporosis, she continues to take Calciduran® vitamin D3 tablets (calcium carbonate; Recipharm Stockholm AB, Jordbro, Sweden) once a day and Oleovit® D3 drops (colecalciferol; Fresenius Kabi Austria GmbH, Graz, Austria) once a week. The patient is otherwise healthy. Her chief complaint was bite pain in the lower left posterior mandible. In addition, she insisted on fixed prosthodontic rehabilitation.

3. Clinical and Radiographic Findings

In brief, at intake, teeth 13, 12, 11, 21, 22, 23, 24, 25, and 27 as well as implants in regions 15 and 16 were present with corresponding fixed prostheses (Figure 2). Due to insufficient crown margins, caries, tooth mobility, and peri-implant bone loss, it was decided to extract all teeth in the maxilla and rehabilitate it with a one-piece fixed dental prosthesis (FDP) on seven implants (Table 1 and Figure 3). This treatment will not be presented and discussed in detail in this case report. In the mandible, teeth 37, 35, 34, 33, 32, 31, 41, 42, 43, 44, and 48 were present with corresponding fixed prostheses (Figure 2). Here, extractions of 37 (insufficient root canal treatment), 35 (vertical root fracture), and 34 (insufficient root canal treatment associated with peri-apical radiolucency), and replacement with three implant-borne single crowns were planned. No intervention was planned for the 6th sextant (Table 1). In addition, the patient had acceptable oral hygiene (Approximal Plaque Index 28%) but is prone to periodontitis (could be classified as stage III, grade B [11]).

4. Timeline

The timeline for the treatment of the left posterior mandible is shown in Table 2.

5. Therapeutic Intervention

As mentioned above, in the 4th sextant, the extractions of teeth 34 due to insufficient root canal treatment associated with peri-apical radiolucency, 35 due to a vertical root fracture, and 37 due to insufficient root canal treatment (as well as assuming that it would be unreasonable to treat and retain this tooth under the concept of prosthetic rehabilitation with implant-supported single crowns), and subsequent rehabilitation with three implant-supported single crowns were planned.

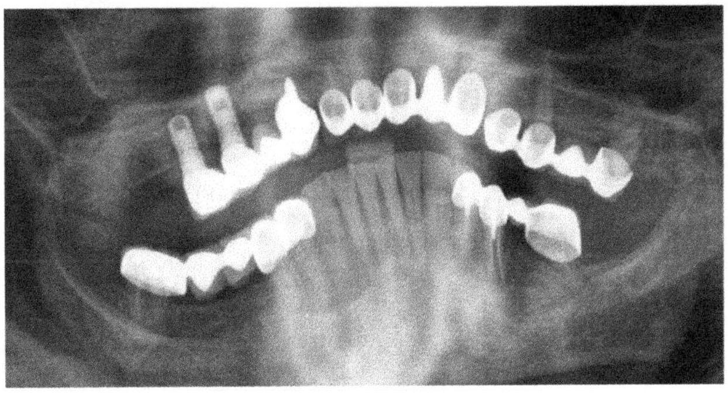

FIGURE 2: DPT section at intake August 2018.

6. Risk Assessment for Medication-Related Osteonecrosis of the Jaw

Due to secondary osteoporosis, the patient had been taking oral antiresorptive medication (i.e., the bisphosphonate ibandronic acid, one 150 mg tablet once per month; Bonviva®, Future Health Pharma GmbH) from 2005 to 2015. Unfortunately, drug-induced osteonecrosis of the jaw (medication-related osteonecrosis of the jaw [MRONJ]) has been reported as a rare side effect of bisphosphonates. It is defined as exposed bone or bone that can be probed through an intraoral or extraoral fistula in the jaw region that has been present for more than eight weeks in patients who have been treated with anti-resorptive drugs in the past, without radiotherapy to the jaw or obvious metastatic disease of the jaw [12]. In this context, it should be understood that dentoalveolar surgery (e.g., GBR or placement of dental implants) is considered a risk factor for MRONJ [13]. However, the risk of MRONJ, for example, after the placement of dental implants, is unknown [14, 15]. However, as bisphosphonates are known to remain in the body for a considerable time after cessation of use, it is recommended that patients who have taken the drug for more than five years should be assigned to a risk group as if they were still taking the drug. [13]. Therefore, the patient was classified as a higher risk patient [13]. This risk assessment was discussed between the treating dentists and, of course, with the patient. Finally, the patient gave informed consent to the treatment (i.e., GBR and dental implants).

7. GBR—Planning

After the extraction of teeth 34, 35, and 37 and thirteen months of bone healing, a digital volume tomography (DVT) of the jaws was made in June 2020 for final treatment planning. Tapered Screw Vent TSVT MTX Zimmer Biomet™ implants (Zimmer Biomet Holdings Inc., Warsaw, IN, USA) were considered. The minimum diameter of this type of

Table 1: DPT, dental status at intake, and treatment planning.

Treatment plan								FDP								
			I		I	I		I		I	I			I		
			X	X		X	X	X	X	X	X	X	X		X	
				FDP					FDP				FDP			
Dental status	M	M	I	I	M									M		M
	8	7	6	5	4	3	2	1	1	2	3	4	5	6	7	8

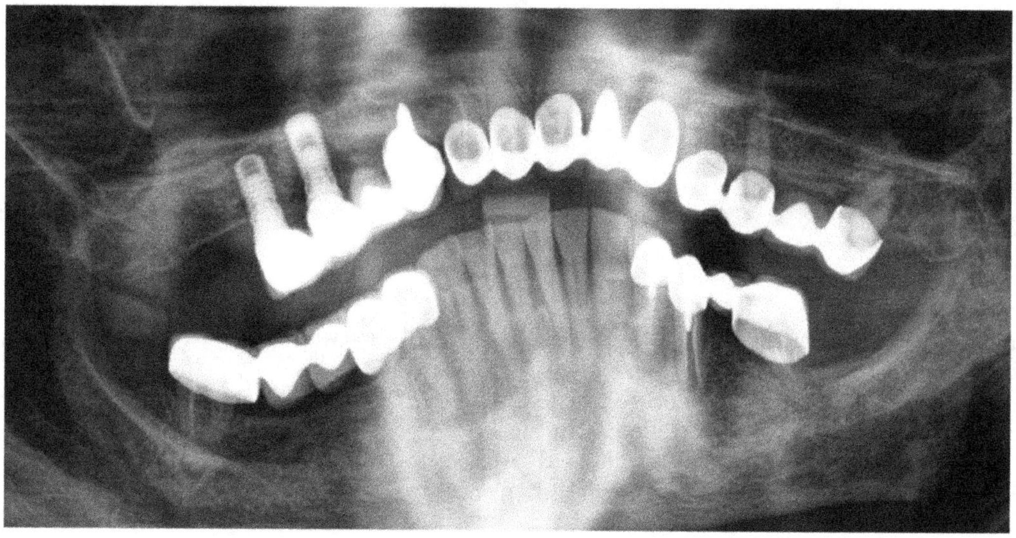

	8	7	6	5	4	3	2	1	1	2	3	4	5	6	7	8
Dental status		M	M											M		M
			FDP										FDP			
Treatment plan												I	I	I		
												SC	SC	SC		

M: Missing tooth. I: Implant. X: To be extracted or explanted. SC: Single crown. FDP: Fixed dental prosthesis.

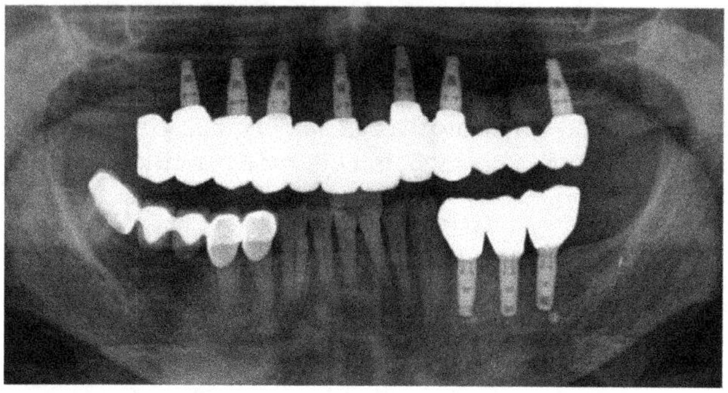

Figure 3: Section of a DPT immediately after cementation of the single crowns.

implants used for the replacement of premolars and molars is 3.7 mm, and the minimum length is 8 mm. When measuring the intended implant positions in regions 34, 35, and 36, the bone crest was found to be too narrow (<5 mm; Figures 4–6). Therefore, a GBR with a CAD/CAM-printed three-dimensional titanium mesh (YxOss CBR®; ReOss®, Filderstadt, Germany) in combination with autogenous bone (AB) and xenografts (Bio-Oss®/Bio-Gide®; Geistlich, Baden-Baden, Germany) was planned and prepared.

To create the conditions for successful implant placement and osteointegration, the first step was to simulate a primary horizontal augmentation to 8 mm in the 34–37 regions on the patient's DVT (Orthophos SL 3D, Dentsply Sirona Deutschland GmbH, Bensheim, Germany) from June 2020. The data were uploaded to and discussed with experienced clinical consultants (ReOss®, Filderstadt, Germany). Based on this, an individual YxOss CBR® titanium mesh was designed and visualized by ReOss® (Figure 7). After evaluation of the three-dimensional design and position by the treating specialist dentist, it was manufactured and delivered.

7.1. GBR—First Surgical Intervention. On July 9, 2020, the corresponding surgical procedure was performed. As premedication, the patient received 40 mg Urbason® (methylprednisolone; Sanofi-Aventis Deutschland GmbH, Frankfurt, Germany), 1 g Augmentin® (amoxicillin + clavulanic acid; GlaxoSmithKline Pharma GmbH, Vienna, Austria), and 600 mg Ibuprofen® (nonsteroidal anti-inflammatory painkiller; BASF, Ludwigshafen, Germany) one hour before the surgery. Furthermore, regions 38–33 were anaesthetized with a total of 5.1 ml Ultracain® D-S forte (Sanofi-Aventis Deutschland GmbH, Frankfurt am Main, Germany). Then, after a mid-crestal incision form region 38 into the gingival sulcus of 33 and a realising incision into the vestibulum distal to 33, a muco-periosteal flap was prepared (Figure 8).

Table 2: Chronological order of the treatment.

Timeline—left posterior mandible	
Intake	August 2018
Clinical examination	
DPT	
Articulated models of maxilla and mandible	
Preliminary treatment plan and initial treatment	Up to June 2020
Oral hygiene improvement	
Non-surgical periodontal therapy	
Extraction of teeth 34, 35, and 37	
Supportive therapy 4 times per year	
DVT	June 2020
Definitive treatment plan	
Implant positions	
CAD-titanium mesh for guided bone regeneration	
First surgical approach (i.e., GBR)	July 2020
CAM-printed titanium mesh (YxOss®; ReOss, Filderstadt, Germany)	
Xenografts (Bio-Oss®/Bio-Gide®; Geistlich, Baden-Baden, Germany)	
Submerged healing	
Second surgical approach	May 2021
Removal of the titanium mesh	
Implant placement (Tapered Screw Vent Zimmer Biomet™; Zimmer Biomet Holdings Inc., IN, USA)	
Submerged healing	
Third surgical approach	August 2021
Uncovering of the implants	
Healing abutments	
Prosthodontics (i.e., loading the implants)	
Individualized titanium abutments	
Monolithic, coloured SCs (Zirkon GEN-X®; Amman Girrbach™, Koblach, Austria)	
Cemented (KetacCem®; 3M; Vienna, Austria)	

DPT: digital panoramic tomography. DVT: digital volume tomography. GBR: guided bone regeneration. CAD: computer assisted design. CAM: computer assisted manufacturing. SC: single crown.

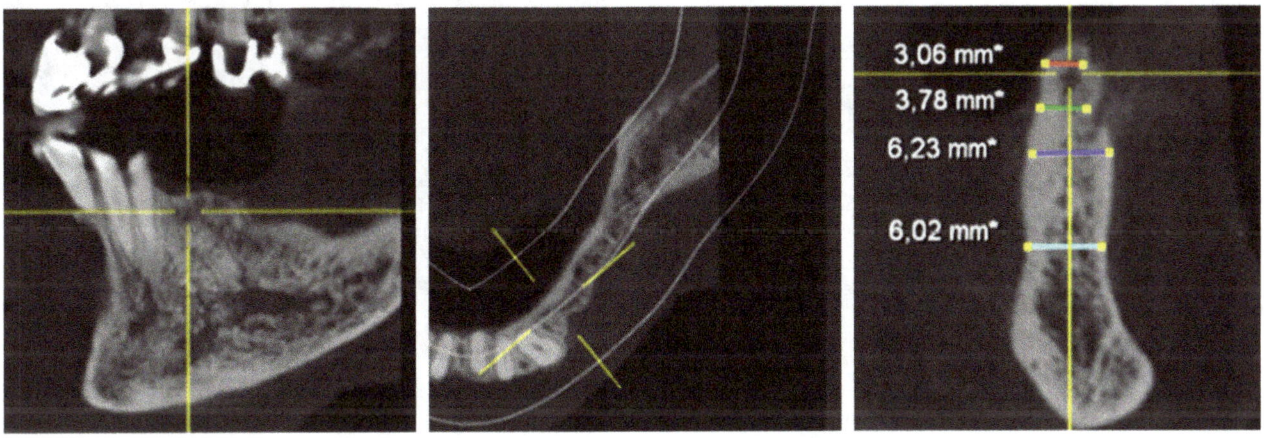

Figure 4: DVT—section region 34.

Next, the sterilized YxOss CBR® titanium mesh was tried on and checked for accuracy of fit. Buccal cortical bone was then harvested apically and distally to the final mesh position for mixing with a xenograft (Safescraper™ Twist Cortical Bone Collector; Zimmer Biomet Austria GmbH, Vienna, Austria). Subsequently, to support adequate healing of the bone graft, the crestal and buccal cortical bone of the bed to be augmented was perforated with a drill (alveolar process

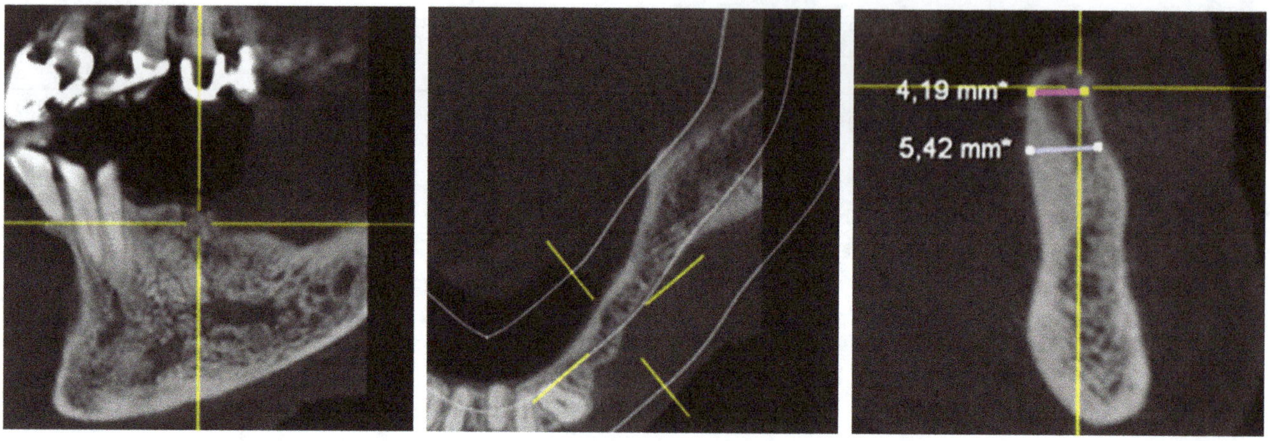

Figure 5: DVT—section region 35.

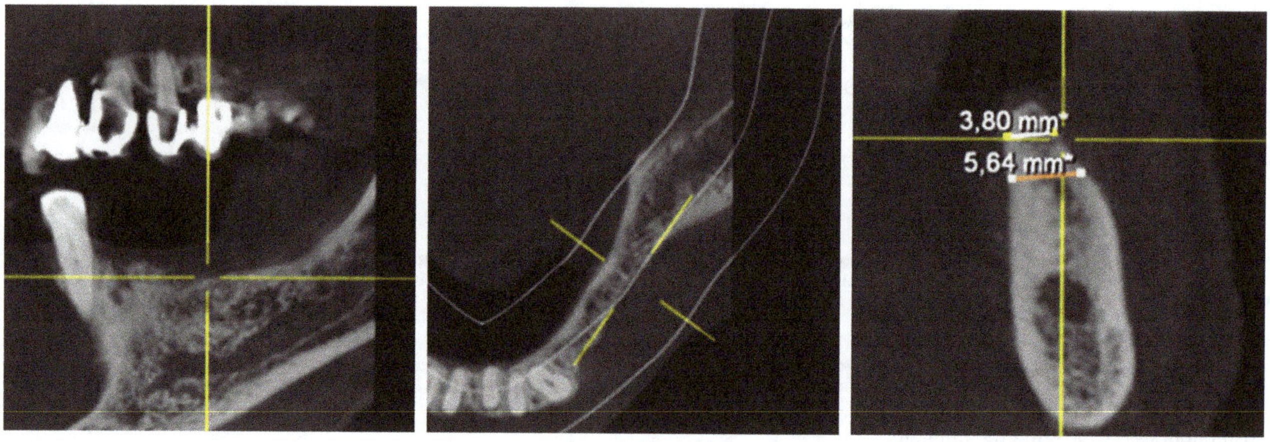

Figure 6: DVT—section region 36.

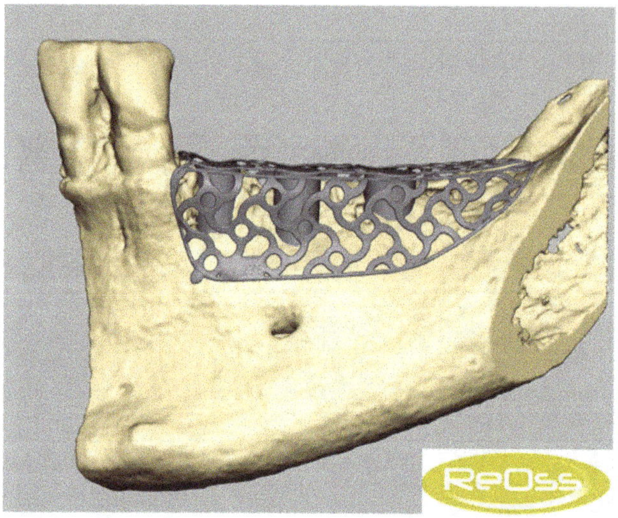

Figure 7: Individualized YxOss CBR® titanium mesh designed and visualized by ReOss®.

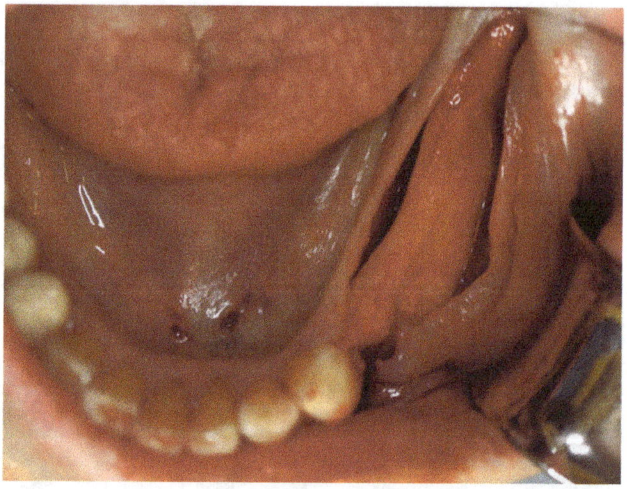

Figure 8: Muco-periosteal flap in the 4th sextant.

drill: diameter 1.2 mm and length 8 mm; Straumann Holding AG, Basel, Switzerland). After repositioning the YxOss CBR® titanium mesh, holes were drilled through the corresponding mesh openings (alveolar process drill; Straumann Holding AG), and the mesh was screwed onto the bone with four titanium screws (titanium osteosynthesis screws: diameter 1.5 mm and length 8 mm; Straumann Holding AG; Figure 9). Then, 0.5 g Bio-Oss® small granules (0.25–1 mm) and 2 g Bio-Oss® large granules (1–2 mm) were mixed with autologous bone and blood from the surgical site and placed

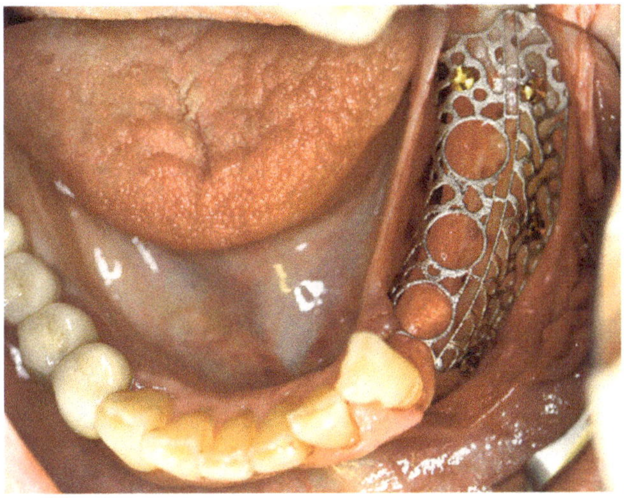

FIGURE 9: YxOss CBR® titanium mesh screwed onto the bone.

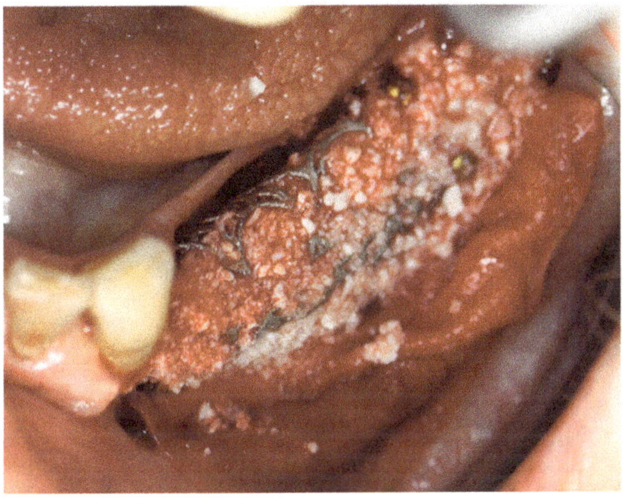

FIGURE 10: YxOss CBR® titanium mesh filled with the bone replacement graft.

in the titanium mesh (Figure 10). Thereafter, a Bio-Gide® membrane (30mm × 40mm) was cut to cover the YxOss CBR® titanium mesh and about 3 mm of the surrounding bone in a single layer. The membrane was stabilized in position with three titanium pins (Straumann Holding AG; Figure 11). To ensure tension-free wound closure, underlying vertical mattress sutures with absorbable suture material (Vicryl 4-0; Ethicon, Johnson & Johnson Medical GmbH, Norderstedt, Germany) were placed. Primary wound closure was achieved with a continuous suture (GORE-TEX® Suture CV5; W.L Gore & Associates, Phoenix, AZ, USA). In addition, a sling suture was applied to 33 for coronal positioning and stabilisation of the mucoperiosteal flap (Figure 12). A digital pantomogram (DPT) was obtained immediately after suturing (Figure 13). Augmentin® (2 g × 1 g daily, for 7 days) and Ibuprofen® (3 mg × 600 mg daily, for 3 days, then as needed) were prescribed, and the patient was again informed about postoperative behaviour (e.g., cooling). An absence of at least three weeks from her interim prosthesis was agreed with the patient. In addition, the patient was asked not to

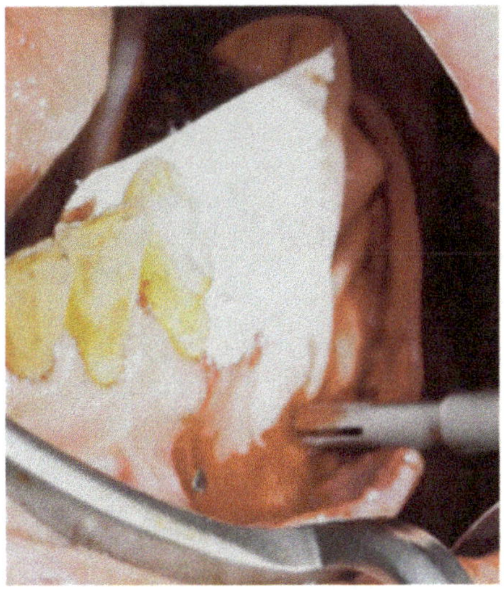

FIGURE 11: Bio-Gide® membrane stabilized in its position with titanium pins.

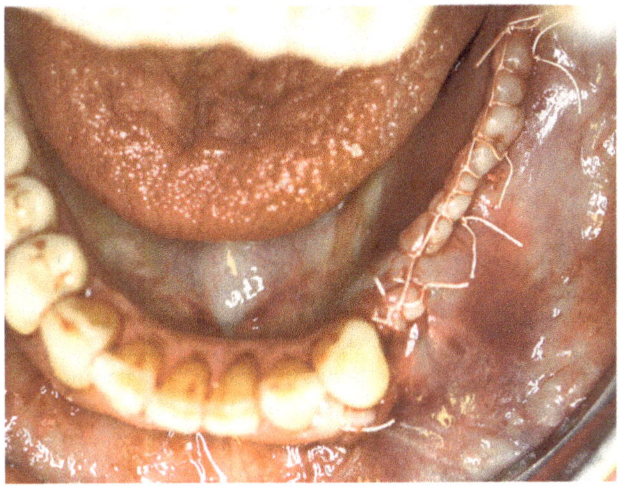

FIGURE 12: GORE-TEX® suture in place.

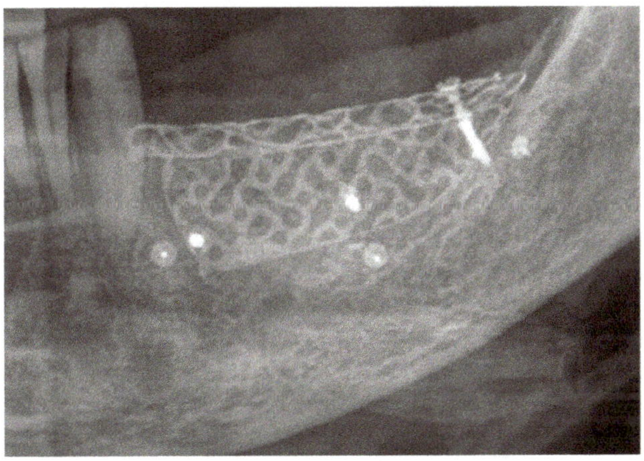

FIGURE 13: DPT section after GBR surgery was completed.

brush the surgical area until the suture was removed, but to rinse regularly (at least twice a day) with Chlorhexamed® (0.1%; GlaxoSmithKline Consumer Healthcare GmbH,

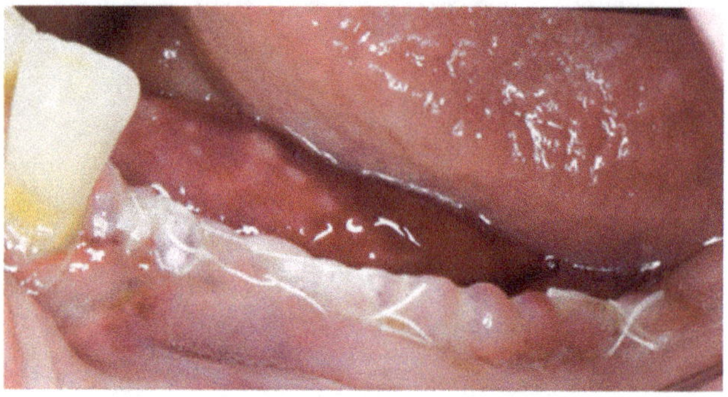

FIGURE 14: Day 1 after surgery.

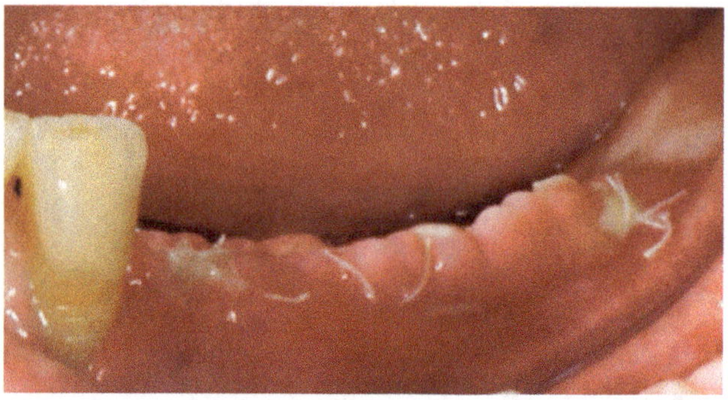

FIGURE 15: Day 7 after surgery.

Munich, Germany) according to the instructions for use. From the first postoperative day until the removal of the sutures, the surgical area was checked and cleaned (cotton swabs soaked with Chlorhexamed® 0.1%) every other day (Figures 14 and 15). In addition, plaque on adjacent teeth was removed with curettes (Hu-Friedy Mfg. Co., LLC., Frankfurt, Germany). Until suture removal, twelve days after surgery, the wound healing was uneventful.

7.2. GBR—YxOss CBR® Titanium Mesh Removal. After an uneventful—completely submerged—healing period of ten months, the titanium mesh was surgically removed on April 20, 2021 (delay due to COVID-19; usually 6 months according to Geistlich for BioOss®). As premedication, the patient received 1 g Augmentin® and 600 mg Ibuprofen® one hour before the surgery. In addition, regions 38–33 were anaesthetized with a total of 6.8 ml Ultracain® D-S forte. Then, after a mid-crestal incision from region 38 into the gingival sulcus of 33 (to keep the surgical area as small as possible without releasing incision), a muco-periosteal flap was prepared (Figure 16), and the YxOss CBR® titanium mesh, the four associated titanium screws, and one titanium pin were removed. Due to the decision to keep the surgical area as small as possible, the disto-apical and distal titanium pins were left in situ. Obviously, the graft was ossified (Figure 17).

7.3. Implant Placement. To plan the implant position, the bone edges were smoothed, and a DVT was taken immediately after removal of the YxOss CBR® titanium mesh. A continuous augmented hard tissue ridge, at the coronal margin above 7 mm, was found. Furthermore, the augmented

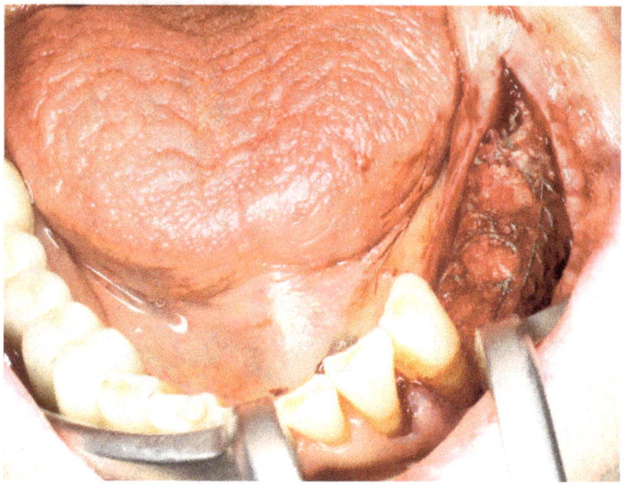

FIGURE 16: Exposed YxOss CBR® titanium mesh.

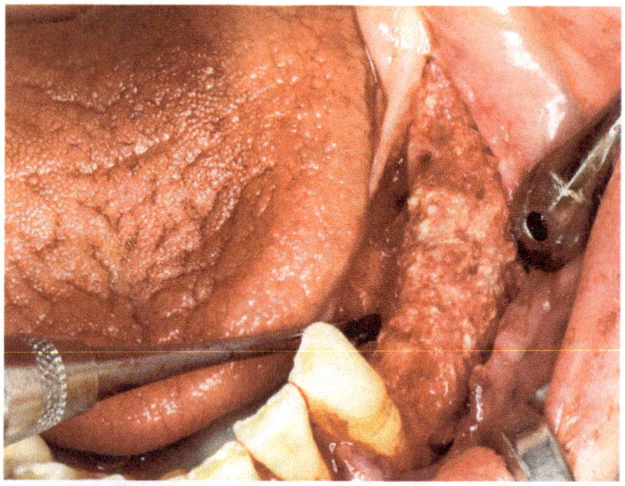

FIGURE 17: Ossified graft after YxOss CBR® titanium mesh removal.

hard tissue volume could be clearly distinguished from the native bone. As mentioned above, Tapered Screw Vent TSVT MTX Zimmer Biomet™ implants with a minimum coronal diameter of 3.7 mm and a minimum length of 8 mm had to be considered for the replacement of premolars and molars. When measuring the intended implant positions in regions 34, 35, and 36, the bone ridge was found to be sufficient in width and height (width: >7 mm, height (distance from coronal edge to upper edge of mandibular canal: >14 mm; Figures 18–20). Figures 21–23 show the approximate comparison of the hard tissue volume in the different regions where the implants were to be placed before and after GBR.

Immediately after planning the implant position, three Tapered Screw Vent TSVT MTX Zimmer Biomet™ implants (region 34: diameter 3.7 mm and length 10 mm; region 35: diameter 3.7 mm and length 10 mm; region 36: diameter 4.1 mm and length 10 mm) were implanted slightly subcrestal with an insertion torque of 35 Ncm each (Figure 24). Primary wound closure for healing of the submerged implants

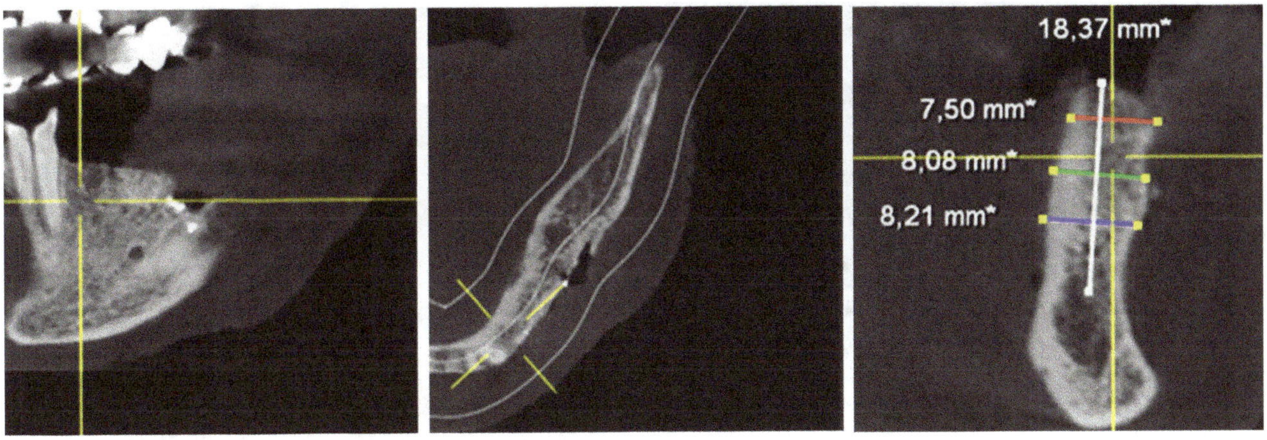

Figure 18: DVT—section; implant position region 34.

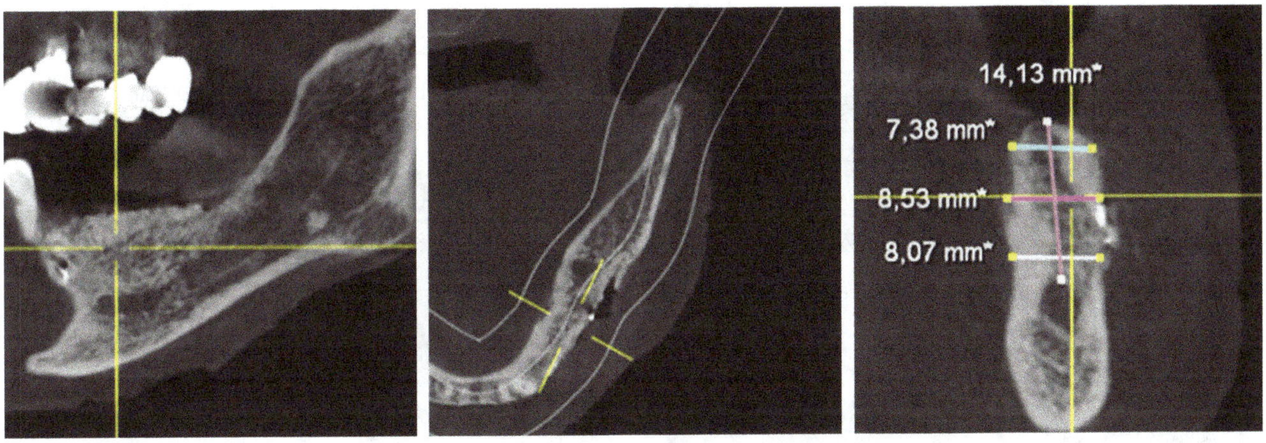

Figure 19: DVT—section; implant position region 35.

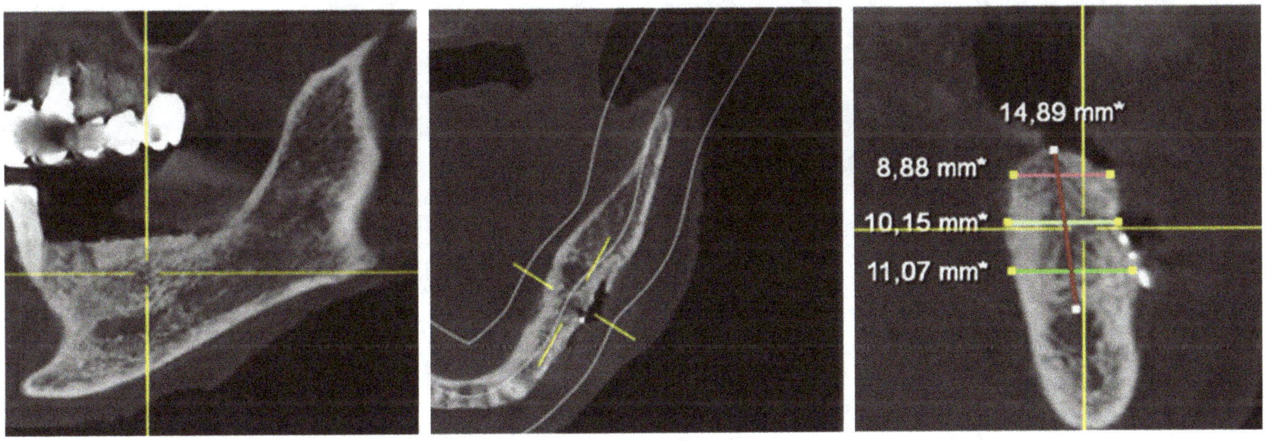

Figure 20: DVT—section; implant position region 36.

was achieved with interrupted single sutures (GORE-TEX® suture CV5). A DPT was taken immediately after suturing (Figure 25). Again, Augmentin® (2 g × 1 g daily, for 7 days) and Ibuprofen® (3 g × 600 mg daily, for 3 days, then as required) were prescribed, and the patient was asked not to brush the surgical area until the suture was removed, but to rinse regularly (at least twice a day) with 0.1% Chlorhexamed®. From the first postoperative day until the removal of the suture, the surgical area was checked and cleaned (cotton swabs soaked with Chlorhexamed® 0.1%) every fourth day. Plaque on the adjacent teeth was also removed with curettes. Until the suture was removed, thirteen days after surgery, wound healing was uneventful.

7.4. Prosthodontics and Supportive Therapy. In August 2021, after four months of submerged healing, the prosthetic

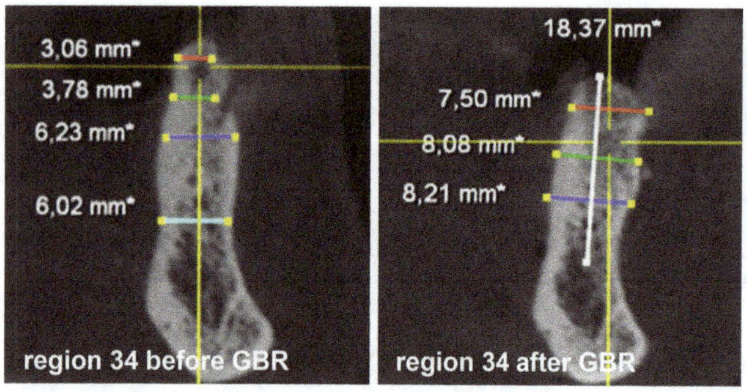

Figure 21: DVT—sections; implant position region 34 before and after GBR.

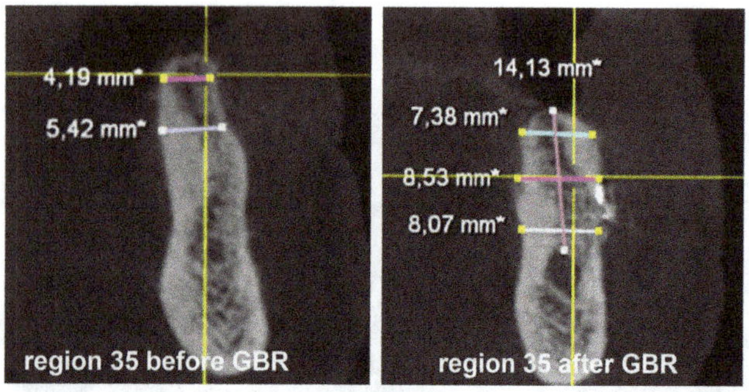

Figure 22: DVT—sections; implant position region 35 before and after GBR.

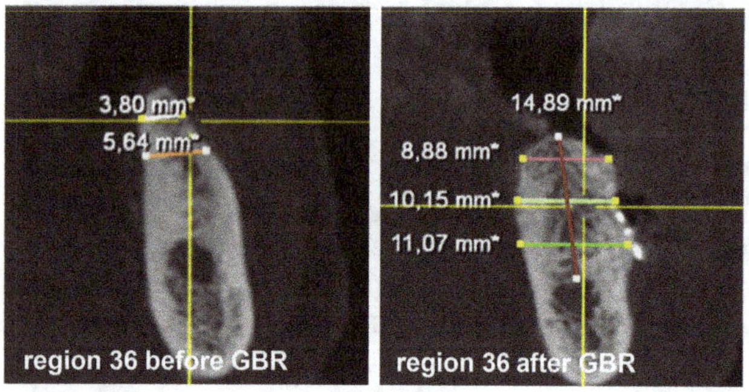

Figure 23: DVT—sections; implant position region 36 before and after GBR.

phase was initiated. In detail, after surgical exposure of the implants and open impression technique (ImpregumTM PentaTM; 3 M Deutschland GmbH, Neuss, Germany), individual single crowns and corresponding abutments were finally designed (ExocadTM GmbH, Darmstadt, Germany). The individual abutments were milled from Zimmer Biomet™ pre-milled abutment blanks (Zfx™ GenTek™ Titanium Pre-milled Abutment Blank, 4.5 mm diameter). In addition, the matching single crowns were monolithically milled from a zirconia oxide blank (zircon GEN-X®; Amman Girrbach™, Koblach, Austria) and shaded according to the patient needs. Finally, the crowns were cemented onto the titanium abutments with KetacCem® (3MTM; Vienna, Austria). Immediately after cementation, a DPT

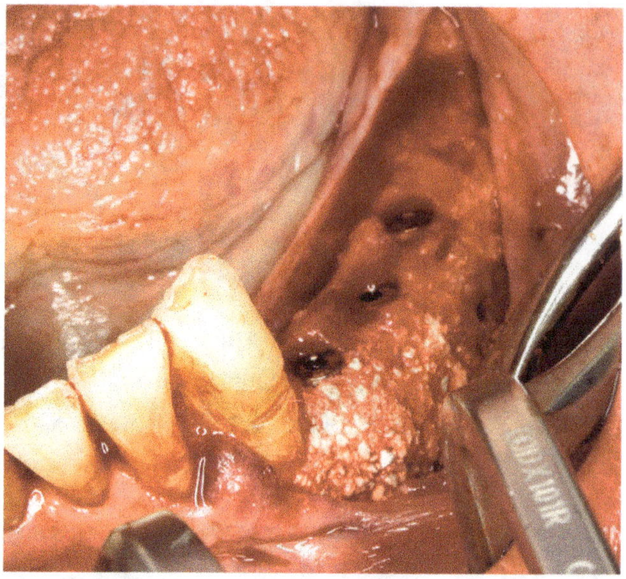

Figure 24: Tapered Screw Vent TSVT MTX Zimmer Biomet™ implants inserted in region 34, 35, and 36.

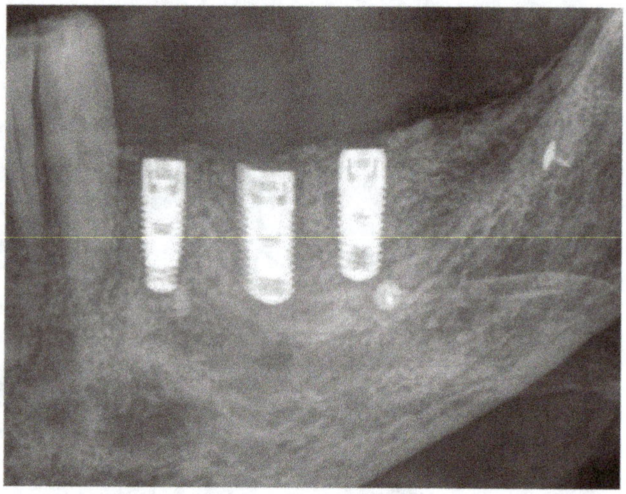

Figure 25: DPT—section; Tapered Screw Vent TSVT MTX Zimmer Biomet™ implants inserted in region 34, 35, and 36.

was taken to check the exact fit and to exclude cement residues (Figure 3).

Thereafter, the patient received two further appointments, each two weeks apart, to (1) check and, if necessary, correct static and dynamic occlusion and (2) check and, if necessary, support oral hygiene. In the further course, the patient was enrolled in a supportive therapy programme, and visits were arranged every three months.

7.5. GBR—Calculated Hard Tissue Gain. Figure 26 shows an overlay of DVTs before (2019) and after guided bone augmentation (2021). For this purpose, the corresponding 3D data sets were converted into 3D STL files using CoDiagnostiX® software (Dental Wings™, Montreal, QC, Canada) and then overlaid using Autodesk Netfabb 2020.0® software (Autodesk™, San Rafael, CA, USA). Furthermore, a

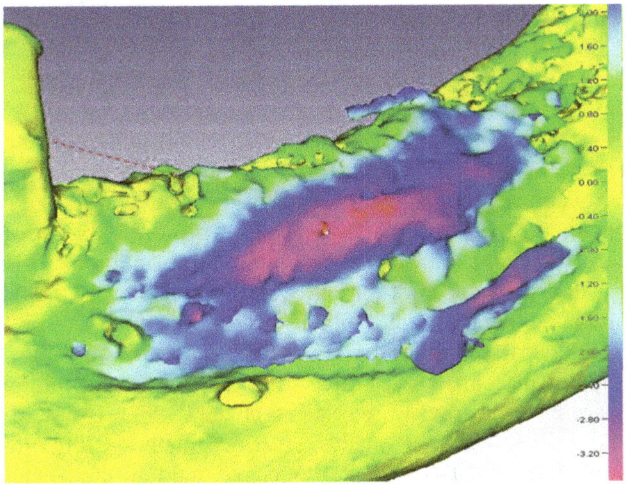

FIGURE 26: Graphical representation of the volume gain. The colour coding divides the gain from 0.0 mm (yellow) to 4.0 mm (red) at the respective positions of the third quadrant.

matching was performed with the software Final Surface® (Gesellschaft zur Förderung angewandter Informatik e.V., GFaI, Berlin, Germany; modified best-fit method), and a volume gain of 1.3–1.4 cm^3 was calculated. However, it should be clearly stated that this calculation method is not validated and that some referencing error (i.e., inaccuracies due to, e.g., artefact reduction during digital processing of the datasets used or conversion into STL files) remains in the 3D composite image.

8. Discussion

Here, we describe the restorative treatment of an 86-year-old patient who was referred to our specialist prosthodontics clinic in August 2018. Due to secondary osteoporosis, she received oral antiresorptive therapy with ibandronic acid from 2005 to 2015. Despite being classified as a patient at higher risk of MRONJ [13], she insisted on fixed implant-supported prosthetic rehabilitation in her 4th sextant and eventually signed the informed consent form. However, after extraction of teeth 34, 35, and 37 and thirteen months of bone healing, it was found that the coronal aspect of the bone ridge was too small (<5 mm horizontally) at the planned implant sites in regions 34, 35, and 36. Therefore, GBR was performed with a CAD/CAM-printed three-dimensional titanium mesh in combination with AB and a xenographic bone replacement graft. To create the conditions for successful implant placement and osseointegration, a horizontal augmentation of 8 mm ridge width in regions 34–37 was planned and performed. After ten months of submerged healing, a new DVT was taken, and a hard tissue ridge was found at the coronal margin, which was consistently above 7 mm. This allowed three implants (region 34: diameter 3.7 mm and length 10 mm; region 35: diameter 3.7 mm and length 10 mm; region 36: diameter 4.1 mm and length 10 mm) to be placed slightly subcrestal with an insertion torque of 35 Ncm each. After a four-month healing phase, the implants were finally restored with single crowns. Now the patient is seen regularly—every three months—for supportive peri-implant therapy.

During treatment planning, the previous antiresorptive therapy with Bonviva® (i.e., orally administered, 150 mg tablets once monthly; therapeutic indication: treatment of osteoporosis in postmenopausal women [16]) was critically reviewed. Each tablet of Bonviva® contains 150 mg ibandronic acid (molecular formula: $C_9H_{23}NO_7P_2$; structural formula: [1-hydroxy-3-(methylpentylamino)propylidene]diphosphonic acid), a medicine from the group of bisphosphonates for the treatment of, for example, osteoporosis. Hence, Bonviva® belongs to the pharmacological group of medicinal products for the treatment of bone diseases, bisphosphonates, and its Anatomical Therapeutic Chemical Classification System code is M05-BA06. Thereby, ibandronic acid is a highly effective bisphosphonate that belongs to the group of nitrogen-containing bisphosphonates (N-BPs; group of so called powerful antiresorptives [pARs]) that act selectively on bone tissue and specifically inhibit osteoclast activity without directly affecting bone formation. It does not interfere with osteoclast recruitment. Consequently, it leads to a progressive net increase in bone mass due to the reduction in increased bone turnover to premenopausal levels in postmenopausal women [16]. The principle molecular mechanisms underlying the inhibition of bone resorption by osteoclasts mediated by ibandronic acid are known. In brief, since bisphosphonates target bone mineral and osteoclasts are capable of releasing bone-bound bisphosphonate, a direct effect on mature osteoclasts appears to be the most important route of action. Ibandronic acid seems to act as analogues of isoprenoid diphosphate lipids, thereby inhibiting farnesyl diphosphate synthase. Inhibition of this enzyme in osteoclasts prevents the biosynthesis of isoprenoid lipids (farnesyl pyrophosphate and geranylgeranyl pyrophosphate), which are essential for posttranslational farnesylation and geranylgeranylation of small GTPase signalling proteins. Then, the loss of bone resorptive activity and osteoclast apoptosis is primarily a consequence of the loss of these geranylgeranylated small GTPases [17].

Unfavourably, MRONJ is a potentially severe adverse event affecting patients with osteoporosis (this applies also to patients with cancer, of course) who have been treated with, for example, N-BPs, pARs [18] as ibandronic acid. Thus, the European Public Assessment Report of the European Medicines Agency for Bonviva® lists osteonecrosis of the jaw (ONJ; i.e., MRNOJ) as a very rare adverse reaction (<1/10,000) reported in post-marketing settings in postmenopausal women receiving Bonviva 150 mg once monthly [16]. However, it should not be left unmentioned that this is generalized in a footnote to "Cases of osteonecrosis of the jaw have been reported, predominantly in cancer patients treated with medicinal products that inhibit bone resorption, such as ibandronic acid. Cases of ONJ have been reported in the post-marketing setting for ibandronic acid." [16] And thus, also for Bonviva®, indicating, and consistent with published data, that pAR-related MRONJ has similar general MRONJ pathophysiology in cancer and osteoporosis patients [12, 19, 20], but that pAR-related MRONJ occurs less frequently in patients treated for osteoporosis (incidence of 0.01–0.03%) than in cancer patients (incidence of 1.8–5%)

[12, 19, 21, 22]. Accordingly, that pAR-treated patients are at risk for MRONJ is reflected in guidelines [13, 23]. On this basis, we primarily classified our patient as being at higher risk of developing MRONJ. However, preclinical and clinical data suggest that most MRONJ cases require systemic risk factors (e.g., pARs) in combination with local oral risk factors, including inflammatory dental disease (e.g., periodontitis), tooth extractions, trauma from removable dentures, and possibly placement of dental implants [12, 19, 20, 24–39]. Be that as it may, even when looking very cautiously at scientific papers published to date, there seems to be convincing evidence that placing dental implants in patients receiving oral bisphosphonate therapy (as opposed to intravenous bisphosphonate therapy) has no significant negative impact on the development of MRONJ, implant survival, and implant success rate alone [15, 39–44]. Furthermore, since the teeth 34–37 would have had to be extracted anyway and periodontitis was successfully treated in advance and, moreover, as the general pathophysiology of MRONJ associated with pAR is at least similar in cancer and osteoporosis patients, and therefore trauma from removable dentures could be a theoretical risk factor for the development of MRONJ in patients with oral pAR therapy [35, 38], and since the patient presented here was otherwise healthy (i.e., beside an age of more than 60 years and female sex, no other non-dental risk factors for developing MRONJ; for review see Wan et al. [24]), we finally categorised her as a patient at lower risk for the development of MRONJ and were willing to realize the patient's request for a fixed—implant-supported—prosthetic restoration. However, the actual statistical or even individual risk of developing MRONJ (during or) after oral therapy for postmenopausal osteoporosis with Bonviva® following GBR and dental implantation remains unknown. All this was discussed with the patient in detail. Finally, the patient agreed to the therapy and signed the corresponding consent form. It should not go unmentioned that the treatment outcome confirms our assessment regarding not developing MRONJ.

Since oral surgical procedures should generally be considered risk factors for the development of MRONJ also in patients on oral pAR therapy (e.g., tooth extraction, bone augmentation, and implant placement), we chose a multistage approach. First, although the evidence especially for oral pAR therapy should be regarded as low, the teeth 34, 35, and 37 were extracted under a preventive protocol [28, 45–48]. In brief, before extraction, care was taken (especially in the 3rd quadrant) to ensure that plaque was reduced as much as possible and that there were no clinical signs of gingivitis [28]. As premedication, the patient received 1 g Augmentin® and 600 mg Ibuprofen® one hour before the intervention. In addition, immediately before tooth extraction, the oral cavity was thoroughly rinsed with Chlorhexamed® FORTE 0.2% for one minute. Furthermore, tension-relieving incisions were made for tooth extraction, bone edges were removed after the extraction, and the entire wound was completely closed in a passive manner (i.e., tension-free) [28, 46, 47]. In addition, Augmentin® (2 g × 1 g daily, for 7 days) and Ibuprofen® (3 mg × 600 mg daily, for 3 days, then as required) were prescribed. Furthermore, the patient was asked not to brush the surgical area until suture removal, but to rinse regularly (at least twice a day) with Chlorhexamed® 0.1%. Starting on the first post-surgical day until suture removal, the surgical area was checked and cleaned (cotton swabs soaked in Chlorhexamed® 0.1%) every second day. In addition, plaque on adjacent teeth was removed with curettes (Hu-Friedy Mfg. Co., LLC.). Until suture removal, wound healing was uneventful. Based on this experience, this prevention protocol was used accordingly for bone augmentation and implantation.

In general (i.e., not for patients with previous or current oral pAR therapy), the available evidence suggests that predictable correction of horizontal bone deficits that allow implant placement is possible through bone augmentation procedures (for review, see Naenni et al. [4]). In this systematic review and meta-analysis, various methods (but not graft-stabilising techniques with, e.g., a titanium mesh) and materials for lateral bone augmentation were analysed. The mean horizontal hard tissue gain was calculated to be 3.30 mm (95% confidence interval (CI): 2.81–3.79 mm; prediction interval (PI): 0.96–5.65 mm) for all available studies (i.e., twenty studies) and to 3.43 mm (95% CI: 2.83–4.03 mm; PI: 1.31–5.55 mm) for only seven studies that presented data for all three time points investigated (pre-augmentation, post-augmentation, and re-entry). Furthermore, the mean decrease of the augmented horizontal hard tissue was calculated as −1.33 mm (95% CI: −1.78 to −0.88 mm; PI: −2.98 to 0.32 mm (all studies) and −1.54 mm (95% CI: −2.17 to −0.91 mm; PI: −3.77 to 0.69 mm (seven studies with data for all three time points). This means, however, that due to the high variability of hard tissue augmentation achieved, predictability for actual treatment (for not graft-stabilising techniques with, e.g., a titanium mesh) is certainly difficult.

Moreover, for Bonviva® in particular, there was (and still is to our knowledge) no published evidence regarding bone augmentation procedures. For that reason, during treatment planning, it was assumed that since Bonviva® does not interfere with osteoclast recruitment and leads to an increase in bone mass [16], new bone formation should not be compromised during bone augmentation (i.e., GBR), and therefore, correction of the horizontal bone deficit should be predictably possible in the current patient to allow implant placement. Since, as mentioned above, any oral surgery should be considered a risk factor for the development of MRONJ, even in patients receiving oral pAR therapy, defect augmentation was not performed with bone harvested intraorally from a second surgical site (chin, ramus mandibulae), but for mixing with a xenograft, buccal cortical bone was collected apical and distal to the final mesh position with a Safescraper™.

For the augmentation method in the present case (i.e., Bio-Oss® mixed with AB, and Bio-Gide®; but not stabilized with a titanium mesh), there is some evidence regarding lateral hard tissue gain, graft reduction during wound healing, and predictability of implant placement [49]. In brief, in a randomized clinical trial (RCT) Bio-Oss®, particles were mixed by weight with AB particles either in a ratio of 90 : 10 (mean; 1.2 g Bio-Oss® : 0.14 g AB) or in a ratio of 60 : 40 (mean; 1.1 g Bio-Oss® : 0.7 g AB) together with autogenous blood from the surgical site. However, in contrast to the present case, 0.25 ml of fibrin glue was added to each of the graft mixtures to make the graft moldable and prevent the particles from migrating from the augmented area. Finally, all grafts were covered by Bio-Gide® membranes without further fixation. The width of the alveolar ridge ranged preoperatively from 1.6 to 6.1 mm and 1.4 to 6.5 mm, 3 and 6 mm from the top of the alveolar ridge, respectively. After a submerged healing period of approximately 7.5 months, the hard tissue gain was 0.4–6.3 mm (graft reduction: 0–94.9%) and 0.4–6.3 mm (graft reduction: −8.6% to 89.7%), 3 and 6 mm from the upper edge of the alveolar ridge, respectively. Finally, all the implants could be placed in all the planned locations, except for one, where the ridge was still too narrow, and the graft was very soft at this point. As noted for the review and meta-analysis by Naenni et al. [4], this again means that due to the high variability of hard tissue gain and graft reduction, predictable treatment planning (i.e., predictable implant placement) with the method and material used may indeed be difficult. In addition, Meijndert et al. [50–52] studied Bio-Oss® in combination with Bio-Gide® in one group (five patients) of a parallel-group RCT. In brief, all patients had a single-tooth diastema in the anterior region of the maxilla. Bio-Oss® was mixed with blood from the surgical site (but, unlike the present case, not mixed with AB, and no graft stabilising titanium mesh was used) and covered with a Bio-Gide® membrane. After six months of submerged healing, ridge enlargement of 2–3 mm was reported [50]. Two implants inserted in a Bio-Oss®/Bio-Gide® graft failed to osseointegrate and were lost within six months of placement [52]. In addition, the marginal peri-implant bone loss between 1 and 120 months after prosthetic loading (i.e., crown placement) was calculated to be −0.64 mm (SD: 1.46 mm) at mesial and −0.37 mm (SD: 1.47 mm) at distal sites in the Bio-Oss®/Bio-Gide® group. During this 10-year period, no further implant in the Bio-Oss®/Bio-Gide® group was lost [52]. But again, predictable treatment planning for long-term implant success may be difficult with the method and material used.

Therefore, to augment the region 34–37 predictably for successful implantation and osseointegration, a graft-stabilising three-dimensional printed titanium mesh for horizontal bone augmentation of up to 8 mm was planned and used in the present case. The graft biomaterials used were Bio-Oss® (mixed with AB and blood from the surgical site) and a Bio-Gide® membrane (to prevent ingrowth of connective tissue and to ensure osteogenic potential in the marginal area of the graft), stabilized with titanium pins. After a submerged healing period of ten months, a continuous augmented hard tissue ridge, at the coronal margin above 7 mm, was found, and all three implants could be placed in a prosthodontically driven position with an insertion torque of 35 Ncm each. Furthermore, after four months of submerged implant healing, the implants were clinically stable (i.e., osseointegrated) and restored with single crowns. Thus, the lateral bone width gain in the entire augmentation area in the 4th sextant was approximately between more than 3 mm and more than 5 mm. This is within the 95% prediction interval of bone width gain of the systematic review and meta-analysis on lateral bone augmentation before implant placement without graft stabilising techniques (e.g., a titanium mesh) published by Naenni et al. [4] and within the range of bone width gain (without graft stabilising technique) in the study by Mordenfeld et al. [49]. Moreover, such a continuous increase in hard tissue was never observed in our hands in similar GBRs without titanium mesh and might be attributed to the positional stability of the augmentation, which allows undisturbed bone healing free from compressive loads and other physical influences. Furthermore, compared to the data of Naenni et al. [4] and Mordenfeld et al. [49], the associated graft reduction was minimal in the current case.

Besides, there is a limited evidence for lateral bone augmentation with a graft-stabilising titanium mesh in general (for review see [53, 54]) and for the YxOss titanium mesh in combination with Bio-Oss® mixed with AB and Bio-Gide® in particular [55, 56] for lateral hard tissue gain, wound healing, and predictability of implant placement. In brief, Sagheb et al. [55] retrospectively analysed GBR (i.e., Bio-Oss® mixed with AB (AB form different intraoral donor sites and from the iliac crest or AB alone/YxOss titanium mesh/Bio-Gide® plus platelet-rich fibrin (PRF) membrane or Bio-Gide® alone) in 17 patients with 21 principally three-dimensional bone defects (i.e., vertical and horizontal bone augmentation). The postoperative healing was uneventful in 14 GBR sites (67%) during the follow-up time of six months until re-entry. However, at seven GBR sites (33%), exposure of the YxOss titanium mesh was observed after periods of five to twelve weeks after the first-stage surgery. Re-entry with explantation of the YxOss titanium mesh and simultaneous implantation of 44 implants was performed after six months. Cone beam computed tomography was performed preoperatively and six months postoperatively to measure bone height and width. A mean vertical bone gain of 6.5 mm (SD: 1.7 mm) and a mean horizontal bone gain of 5.5 mm (SD: 1.9 mm) were observed. Furthermore, after a mean follow-up time of 12 months (SD: 6 months) after second-stage surgery, none of the 44 inserted implants were lost, which corresponds to a survival rate of 100%. In the end, the authors only very generally concluded that individualized CAD-CAM fabricated titanium meshes are a safe and predictable procedure for large vertical and horizontal ridge augmentations. Similar results are reported by Hartmann and Seiler [56]. They also retrospectively analysed GBR (i.e., Bio-Oss® mixed with AB (in one patient, only Bio-Oss®; AB from different intraoral donor sites and from the iliac crest; ratio 1:1/YxOss titanium mesh/Bio-Gide® or Bio-Gide® plus an Advanced- (A-PRF®) membrane) in 55 patients with 68 three-dimensional bone defects (i.e., vertical and horizontal bone augmentation). Overall (i.e., Bio-Gide® or Bio-Gide® plus A-PRF® membrane), exposure of the YxOss titanium mesh was observed in 25% of treated defect sites ($n = 17$) in association with partial (11.8%, $n = 8$) and complete (15%, $n = 1$) loss of graft material. The YxOss titanium meshes were removed after a mean healing time of 6.5 months (SD: 2.7 months). A total of 98 implants were placed as planned. These authors also very generally concluded that the surgical protocol of individual bone regeneration has proven to be a promising technique for complex bone reconstructions. But the variability of GBR treatment performed in the studies of Sagheb et al. [55] and Hartmann and Seiler [56] (vertical and horizontal bone augmentation/different biomaterials) makes an actual evidence-based, meaningful comparison with the case presented here difficult.

Nevertheless, this case shows that GBR with a CAD/CAM-printed three-dimensional titanium mesh can predictably fulfil the desire for fixed, implant-supported single crowns, and a corresponding quality of life even in an older, medically compromised patient.

However, this result should not be generalized (predictable horizontal bone augmentation width, minimum reduction of the graft) as such a statement would require clinical trials with appropriate patient numbers.

9. Patient Perspective

To be able to describe an objective assessment of patient satisfaction, the Oral Health Quality questionnaire with 53 questions was used for the evaluation. There was a clear increase in the quality of life, and in particular, the patient did not describe any problems or complaints with chewing functionality or phonetics.

Consent

The patient gave informed consent on 20th July 2020.

Acknowledgments

This case report was not funded by third parties and was performed as a part of the employment of the authors (Danube Private University).

References

[1] D. Buser, L. LSennerby, and H. De Bruyn, "Modern implant dentistry based on osseointegration: 50 years of progress, current trends and open questions," *Periodontology 2000*, vol. 73, no. 1, pp. 7–21, 2017.

[2] N. P. Lang, "Oral implants: the paradigm shift in restorative dentistry," *Journal of Dental Research*, vol. 98, no. 12, pp. 1287–1293, 2019.

[3] S. Jepsen et al., "Regeneration of alveolar ridge defects. Consensus report of group 4 of the 15th European workshop on periodontology on bone regeneration," *Journal of Clinical Periodontology*, vol. 46, no. S21, pp. 277–286, 2019.

[4] N. Naenni, H. C. Lim, S. N. Papageorgiou, and C. H. F. Hämmerle, "Efficacy of lateral bone augmentation prior to implant placement: a systematic review and meta-analysis," *Journal of Clinical Periodontology*, vol. 46, Suppl 21, pp. 287–306, 2019.

[5] I. A. Urban, E. Montero, A. Monje, and I. Sanz-Sánchez, "Effectiveness of vertical ridge augmentation interventions: a systematic review and meta-analysis," *Journal of Clinical Periodontology*, vol. 46, Suppl 21, pp. 319–339, 2019.

[6] A. H. Melcher, "On the repair potential of periodontal tissues," *Journal of Periodontology*, vol. 47, no. 5, pp. 256–260, 1976.

[7] M. Sanz, C. Dahlin, D. Apatzidou et al., "Biomaterials and regenerative technologies used in bone regeneration in the craniomaxillofacial region: consensus report of group 2 of the 15th European workshop on periodontology on bone regeneration," *Journal of Clinical Periodontology*, vol. 46, Suppl 21, pp. 82–91, 2019.

[8] H. J. Haugen, S. P. Lyngstadaas, F. Rossi, and G. Perale, "Bone grafts: which is the ideal biomaterial?," *Journal of Clinical Periodontology*, vol. 46, Suppl 21, pp. 92–102, 2019.

[9] C. H. F. Hämmerle and R. E. Jung, "Bone augmentation by means of barrier membranes," *Periodontology*, vol. 2003, no. 33, pp. 36–53, 2000.

[10] A. Hartmann, M. Peetz, B. al-Nawas, and M. Seiler, "Patient-specific titanium meshes: future trend or current technology?," *Clinical Implant Dentistry and Related Research*, vol. 23, no. 1, pp. 3–4, 2021.

[11] P. N. Papapanou, M. Sanz, N. Buduneli et al., "Periodontitis: consensus report of workgroup 2 of the 2017 world workshop on the classification of periodontal and peri-implant diseases and conditions," *Journal of Clinical Periodontology*, vol. 45, Suppl 20, pp. S162–S170, 2018.

[12] S. L. Ruggiero, T. B. Dodson, J. Fantasia et al., "American Association of Oral and Maxillofacial Surgeons position paper on medication-related osteonecrosis of the jaw–2014 update," *Journal of Oral and Maxillofacial Surgery*, vol. 72, no. 10, pp. 1938–1956, 2014.

[13] (SDCEP), S.D.C.E.P. Oral Health Management of Patients at Risk of Medication-related Osteonecrosis of the Jaw—Dental Clinical Guidance, 2017, http://www.sdcep.org.uk.

[14] B. Owen and H. Bradley, "Is it safe to place implants in patients at risk of MRONJ?," *Evidence-Based Dentistry*, vol. 22, no. 3, pp. 108–109, 2021.

[15] V. Mendes, G. O. dos Santos, M. D. Calasans-Maia, J. M. Granjeiro, and V. Moraschini, "Impact of bisphosphonate therapy on dental implant outcomes: an overview of systematic review evidence," *International Journal of Oral and Maxillofacial Surgery*, vol. 48, no. 3, pp. 373–381, 2019.

[16] EMAEPAR-BONOVIA-INFORMATION_EN. Annex I Summary of Product characteristics, 2022.

[17] M. J. Rogers, "New insights into the molecular mechanisms of action of bisphosphonates," *Current Pharmaceutical Design*, vol. 9, no. 32, pp. 2643–2658, 2003.

[18] J. I. Aguirre, E. J. Castillo, and D. B. Kimmel, "Preclinical models of medication-related osteonecrosis of the jaw (MRONJ)," *Bone*, vol. 153, pp. 116184–116184, 2021.

[19] A. A. Khan, A. Morrison, D. A. Hanley et al., "Diagnosis and management of osteonecrosis of the jaw: a systematic review and international consensus," *Journal of Bone and Mineral Research*, vol. 30, no. 1, pp. 3–23, 2015.

[20] T. Kikuiri, I. Kim, T. Yamaza et al., "Cell-based immunotherapy with mesenchymal stem cells cures bisphosphonate-

related osteonecrosis of the jaw-like disease in mice," *Journal of Bone and Mineral Research*, vol. 25, no. 7, pp. 1668–1679, 2010.

[21] P. Rugani et al., "Prevalence of medication-related osteonecrosis of the jaw in patients with breast cancer, prostate cancer, and multiple myeloma," *Dentistry Journal*, vol. 4, no. 4, p. 32, 2016.

[22] R. E. Coleman, M. Collinson, W. Gregory et al., "Benefits and risks of adjuvant treatment with zoledronic acid in stage II/III breast cancer. 10 years follow-up of the AZURE randomized clinical trial (BIG 01/04)," *Journal of Bone Oncology*, vol. 13, pp. 123–135, 2018.

[23] S. Ruggiero, E. R. Carlson, and L. A. Assael, "Comprehensive review of bisphosphonate therapy: implications for the oral and maxillofacial surgery patient," *Journal of Oral and Maxillofacial Surgery*, vol. 67, no. s1, pp. 1–12, 2009.

[24] J. T. Wan, D. M. Sheeley, M. J. Somerman, and J. S. Lee, "Mitigating osteonecrosis of the jaw (ONJ) through preventive dental care and understanding of risk factors," *Bone Research*, vol. 8, no. 1, p. 14, 2020.

[25] A. Soundia, D. Hadaya, N. Esfandi et al., "Osteonecrosis of the jaws (ONJ) in mice after extraction of teeth with periradicular disease," *Bone*, vol. 90, pp. 133–141, 2016.

[26] M. Song, A. Alshaikh, T. Kim et al., "Preexisting periapical inflammatory condition exacerbates tooth extraction-induced bisphosphonate-related osteonecrosis of the jaw lesions in mice," *Journal of Endodontia*, vol. 42, no. 11, pp. 1641–1646, 2016.

[27] H. Katsarelis, N. P. Shah, D. K. Dhariwal, and M. Pazianas, "Infection and medication-related osteonecrosis of the jaw," *Journal of Dental Research*, vol. 94, no. 4, pp. 534–539, 2015.

[28] T. Hasegawa, S. Hayashida, E. Kondo et al., "Medication-related osteonecrosis of the jaw after tooth extraction in cancer patients: a multicenter retrospective study," *Osteoporosis International*, vol. 30, no. 1, pp. 231–239, 2019.

[29] T. L. Aghaloo, B. Kang, E. C. Sung et al., "Periodontal disease and bisphosphonates induce osteonecrosis of the jaws in the rat," *Journal of Bone and Mineral Research*, vol. 26, no. 8, pp. 1871–1882, 2011.

[30] J. I. Aguirre, M. P. Akhter, D. B. Kimmel et al., "Oncologic doses of zoledronic acid induce osteonecrosis of the jaw-like lesions in rice rats (Oryzomys palustris) with periodontitis," *Journal of Bone and Mineral Research*, vol. 27, no. 10, pp. 2130–2143, 2012.

[31] R. S. de Molon, S. Cheong, O. Bezouglaia et al., "Spontaneous osteonecrosis of the jaws in the maxilla of mice on antiresorptive treatment: a novel ONJ mouse model," *Bone*, vol. 68, pp. 11–19, 2014.

[32] J. G. Messer, J. M. Jiron, J. L. Mendieta Calle et al., "Zoledronate treatment duration is linked to bisphosphonate-related osteonecrosis of the jaw prevalence in rice rats with generalized periodontitis," *Oral Diseases*, vol. 25, no. 4, pp. 1116–1135, 2019.

[33] J. G. Messer, J. L. Mendieta Calle, J. M. Jiron et al., "Zoledronic acid increases the prevalence of medication-related osteonecrosis of the jaw in a dose dependent manner in rice rats (Oryzomys palustris) with localized periodontitis," *Bone*, vol. 108, pp. 79–88, 2018.

[34] B. Kang, S. Cheong, T. Chaichanasakul et al., "Periapical disease and bisphosphonates induce osteonecrosis of the jaws in mice," *Journal of Bone and Mineral Research*, vol. 28, no. 7, pp. 1631–1640, 2013.

[35] K. Vahtsevanos, A. Kyrgidis, E. Verrou et al., "Longitudinal cohort study of risk factors in cancer patients of bisphosphonate-related osteonecrosis of the jaw," *Journal of Clinical Oncology*, vol. 27, no. 32, pp. 5356–5362, 2009.

[36] L. Levin, A. Laviv, and D. Schwartz-Arad, "Denture-related osteonecrosis of the maxilla associated with oral bisphosphonate treatment," *Journal of the American Dental Association (1939)*, vol. 138, no. 9, pp. 1218–1220, 2007.

[37] L. M. Hess, J. M. Jeter, M. Benham-Hutchins, and D. S. Alberts, "Factors associated with osteonecrosis of the jaw among bisphosphonate users," *The American Journal of Medicine*, vol. 121, no. 6, pp. 475–483.e3, 2008.

[38] A. Kyrgidis, K. Vahtsevanos, G. Koloutsos et al., "Bisphosphonate-related osteonecrosis of the jaws: a case-control study of risk factors in breast cancer patients," *Journal of Clinical Oncology*, vol. 26, no. 28, pp. 4634–4638, 2008.

[39] C. Walter, B. al-Nawas, T. Wolff, E. Schiegnitz, and K. A. Grötz, "Dental implants in patients treated with antiresorptive medication – a systematic literature review," *International Journal of Implant Dentistry*, vol. 2, no. 1, p. 9, 2016.

[40] R. Gelazius, L. Poskevicius, D. Sakavicius, V. Grimuta, and G. Juodzbalys, "Dental implant placement in patients on bisphosphonate therapy: a systematic review," *Journal of Oral & Maxillofacial Research*, vol. 9, no. 3, article e2, 2018.

[41] A. Stavropoulos, K. Bertl, P. Pietschmann, N. Pandis, M. Schiødt, and B. Klinge, "The effect of antiresorptive drugs on implant therapy: systematic review and meta-analysis," *Clinical Oral Implants Research*, vol. 29, Suppl 18, pp. 54–92, 2018.

[42] M. Nisi, F. la Ferla, D. Karapetsa et al., "Risk factors influencing BRONJ staging in patients receiving intravenous bisphosphonates: a multivariate analysis," *International Journal of Oral and Maxillofacial Surgery*, vol. 44, no. 5, pp. 586–591, 2015.

[43] M. Tallarico, L. Canullo, E. Xhanari, and S. M. Meloni, "Dental implants treatment outcomes in patient under active therapy with alendronate: 3-year follow-up results of a multicenter prospective observational study," *Clinical Oral Implants Research*, vol. 27, no. 8, pp. 943–949, 2016.

[44] V. Chappuis, G. Avila-Ortiz, M. G. Araújo, and A. Monje, "Medication-related dental implant failure: systematic review and meta-analysis," *Clinical Oral Implants Research*, vol. 29, Suppl 16, pp. 55–68, 2018.

[45] S. Ferlito, C. Liardo, and S. Puzzo, "Dental extractions in patient treated with intravenous bisphosphonates and risk of osteonecrosis of jaws: presentation of a preventive protocol and case series," *Minerva Stomatologica*, vol. 59, no. 11–12, pp. 593–601, 2010.

[46] S. Ferlito, S. Puzzo, and C. Liardo, "Preventive protocol for tooth extractions in patients treated with zoledronate: a case series," *Journal of Oral and Maxillofacial Surgery*, vol. 69, no. 6, pp. e1–e4, 2011.

[47] M. J. Heufelder, J. Hendricks, T. Remmerbach, B. Frerich, A. Hemprich, and F. Wilde, "Principles of oral surgery for prevention of bisphosphonate-related osteonecrosis of the jaw," *Oral Surgery, Oral Medicine, Oral Pathology, Oral Radiology*, vol. 117, no. 6, pp. e429–e435, 2014.

[48] E. Gaudin, L. Seidel, M. Bacevic, E. Rompen, and F. Lambert, "Occurrence and risk indicators of medication-related

osteonecrosis of the jaw after dental extraction: a systematic review and meta-analysis," *Journal of Clinical Periodontology*, vol. 42, no. 10, pp. 922–932, 2015.

[49] A. Mordenfeld, C. B. Johansson, T. Albrektsson, and M. Hallman, "A randomized and controlled clinical trial of two different compositions of deproteinized bovine bone and autogenous bone used for lateral ridge augmentation," *Clinical Oral Implants Research*, vol. 25, no. 3, pp. 310–320, 2014.

[50] L. Meijndert, G. M. Raghoebar, P. Schüpbach, H. J. A. Meijer, and A. Vissink, "Bone quality at the implant site after reconstruction of a local defect of the maxillary anterior ridge with chin bone or deproteinised cancellous bovine bone," *International Journal of Oral and Maxillofacial Surgery*, vol. 34, no. 8, pp. 877–884, 2005.

[51] L. Meijndert, G. M. Raghoebar, H. J. A. Meijer, and A. Vissink, "Clinical and radiographic characteristics of single-tooth replacements preceded by local ridge augmentation: a prospective randomized clinical trial," *Clinical Oral Implants Research*, vol. 19, no. 12, pp. 1295–1303, 2008.

[52] C. M. Meijndert, G. M. Raghoebar, L. Meijndert, K. Stellingsma, A. Vissink, and H. J. A. Meijer, "Single implants in the aesthetic region preceded by local ridge augmentation; a 10-year randomized controlled trial," *Clinical Oral Implants Research*, vol. 28, no. 4, pp. 388–395, 2017.

[53] Y. Xie, S. Li, T. Zhang, C. Wang, and X. Cai, "Titanium mesh for bone augmentation in oral implantology: current application and progress," *International Journal of Oral Science*, vol. 12, no. 1, p. 37, 2020.

[54] F. Briguglio, D. Falcomatà, S. Marconcini, L. Fiorillo, R. Briguglio, and D. Farronato, "The use of titanium mesh in guided bone regeneration: a systematic review," *International Journal of Dentistry*, vol. 2019, 2019.

[55] K. Sagheb, E. Schiegnitz, M. Moergel, C. Walter, B. al-Nawas, and W. Wagner, "Clinical outcome of alveolar ridge augmentation with individualized CAD-CAM-produced titanium mesh," *International Journal of Implant Dentistry*, vol. 3, no. 1, p. 36, 2017.

[56] A. Hartmann and M. Seiler, "Minimizing risk of customized titanium mesh exposures – a retrospective analysis," *BMC Oral Health*, vol. 20, no. 1, p. 36, 2020.

19

Palatal Obturator after Maxillectomy following Squamous Cell Carcinoma

Karim Chebbi, Khaoula Bouaziz, Oumaima Tayari, Azza Berkaoui, Mohamed Ali Bouzidi, and Jamila Jaouadi

Complete Removable Prosthodontic Department, Research Laboratory LR12ES11, Faculty of Dental Medicine, University of Monastir, Monastir, Tunisia

Correspondence should be addressed to Karim Chebbi; karimchebbi13@gmail.com

Academic Editor: Tommaso Lombardi

After surgical excision of tumors involving the maxilla, depending on their location and size, maxillary defects can have harmful consequences, both esthetic and functional. These effects disrupt all the functions of the manducatory system, namely breathing, swallowing, and especially phonation, thus affecting negatively the patient's psychological state. Despite the evolution of reconstructive surgical techniques and the development of microsurgery, conventional obturator prostheses are still relevant. In fact, these prostheses restore the main functions of chewing, phonation, and swallowing. They also provide the patient with a satisfactory esthetic appearance. Moreover, they have an advantage in regard to oncology, making the possibility of surveying much easier. Maxillary defects are characterized by their highly polymorphic aspect, having a great impact on the nature of prosthetic rehabilitation. The aim of this work was to present the different clinical and laboratory steps of prosthetic rehabilitation of an acquired maxillary defect following excision of a mucoepidermoid carcinoma.

1. Introduction

Mucoepidermoid carcinoma is a common salivary tumor with varying potential for aggressive behavior [1].

In malignant tumors, mucoepidermoid carcinoma remains the most frequently observed tumor in the salivary glands. The average age of discovery varies between 40 and 60 years depending on the authors. The occurrence in young children and adolescents remains rare, around thirty cases have been described in the literature since 1952 [2].

The classification of mucoepidermoid carcinoma as high-grade connotes the potential for disease progression and possibly disease-related mortality. In addition to complete resection, postoperative adjuvant radiotherapy is indicated for high-grade mucoepidermoid carcinoma [1].

The grading of this tumor has evolved over time from descriptive two-tiered schemata to more objective three-tiered systems. Patients with mucoepidermoid carcinoma classified as high-grade (grade 3) are at significant risk for presenting with positive lymph nodes and developing disease progression, and possibly disease-related mortality [1].

The morphological and spatial characteristics of the tumor, its extension to the neighboring structures, the presence of metastases, the involvement of the lymph node, and the patient's general condition determine the therapeutic choices [3].

The management of mucoepidermoid carcinoma depends on the pathological diagnosis. Surgical treatment remains the therapy of choice. It consists of excision of the tumor with a mucosal and bone carcinological margin. Lymph node dissection is indicated in high-grade tumors where the risk of lymph node metastases is greater than 50% [2].

Its treatment includes surgery associated or not with radiotherapy depending on the histological grade [2].

Surgery can cause maxillary defects, eventually leading to oronasal or orosinusal communication. It must be followed by a prosthetic rehabilitation that allows the patient to regain his manducatory functions [4].

In this work, through a case report, the specificity of prosthetic rehabilitation of a patient with an acquired maxillary defect requiring the placement of an obturator prosthesis was presented.

2. Observation

A 65-year-old man, smoker, hypertensive, non-insulin-dependent diabetic, and with a history of hyperthyroidism was referred by the Cancerology department of Salah Azaiez hospital in Tunis (Tunisia) to the department of Maxillofacial Prosthodontics at the Dental Clinic of Monastir (Tunisia) for prosthetic rehabilitation.

Resection of a high-grade squamous cell carcinoma of the palate was performed two years earlier. The patient was also subjected to underwent adjuvant chemotherapy and radiotherapy on the tumor zone and the lymph node areas.

The chief complaint was functional: chewing problems, nasal leakage of fluids, and improper speech.

Extraoral examination revealed a facial symmetry, an absence of cervical lymphadenopathy, a moderately sufficient mouth opening, and a straight mouth opening/closing path.

Intraoral examination revealed the presence of the remaining natural teeth (11, 12, 13, 21, 22, and 23) in the maxilla. These teeth were vital and showed generalized physiological attrition.

The osteomucosal-bearing surface showed a moderate deep palate and a high and wide ridge on the right side, covered with a thick, adherent fibromucosa.

On the left side, an existing surgical maxillary defect with adequate healing was noticed in the hard palate. This defect was connecting the oral cavity to the left maxillary sinus and the nasal fossae (Figure 1). It also presented two moderately deep anterior and posterior undercuts.

In the mandible, all the teeth were vital and showed generalized physiological attrition (Figure 2).

The radiological examination panoramic radiography (Figure 3) and cone-beam computed tomography (CBCT) (Figure 4) confirm the existence of the maxillary defect.

Examination of occlusion showed an unpreserved Occlusal Vertical Dimension (OVD) and Maximum Intercuspid Occlusion (MIO).

The treatment plan involved an obturator prosthesis.

Mucostatic primary impressions were made with irreversible hydrocolloid (Alginate) using perforated stock trays, whose sizes were carefully determined (Figure 5). Before taking the maxillary impression, the anterior and posterior undercuts of the maxillary defect were filled with a gauze.

Some adjustments were made using wax, which has been added to the peripheral outline of the upper stock tray on the right side in order to record the vestibular depth as well as the right paratuberosity pocket.

The maxillary impression was poured with white plaster and a custom tray was made with light-curing resin, served as a support for the anatomo-functional impression.

For the mandibular impression, the cast was made with yellow plaster, and it was used for articulator mounting.

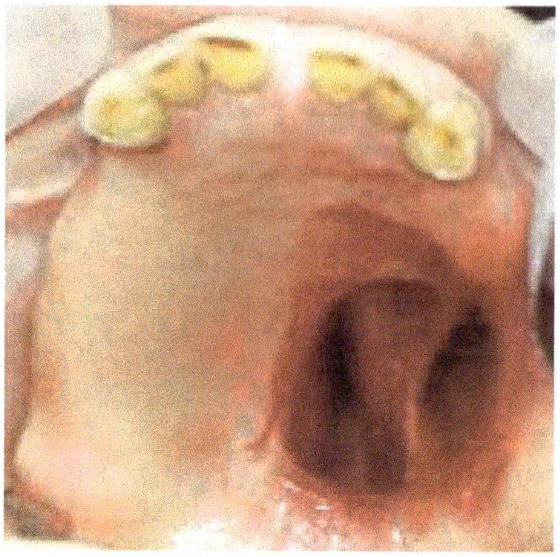

FIGURE 1: Maxillary defect was connecting the oral cavity to the left maxillary sinus and the nasal fossae.

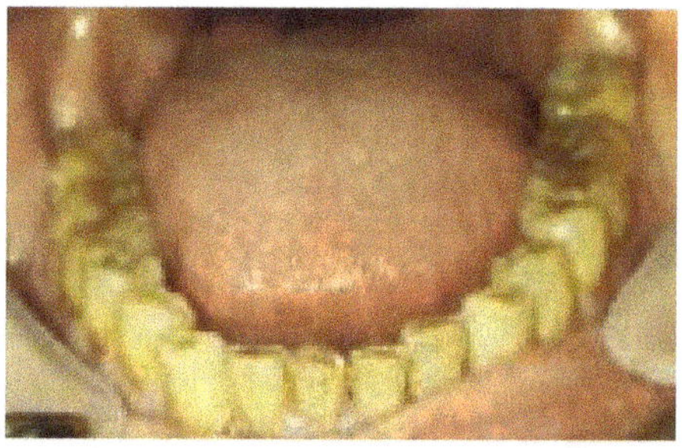

FIGURE 2: Mandibular teeth showed generalized physiological attrition.

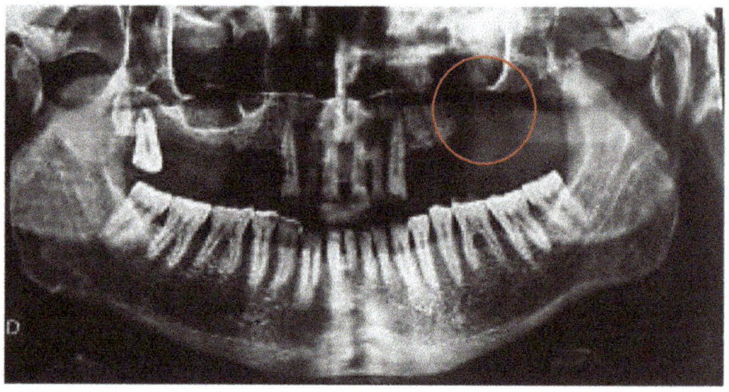

FIGURE 3: Panoramic radiography. The maxillary defect is shown with the circle above.

The maxillary custom tray was carefully adjusted in the mouth. After validation of the peripheral seal using thermoplastic paste (Kerr®) next to the edentulous ridges, perforations facing the palatal defect were made.

The upper anatomofunctional impression was taken with FITT material (Functional Impression Tissue Toner) (Kerr®) (Figures 6(a) and 6(b)) and was poured with yellow plaster (Figure 7).

Jaw relation was made in centric relation and in the correct occlusal vertical dimension. It was followed by mounting the casts on the articulator and the selection of the artificial teeth color.

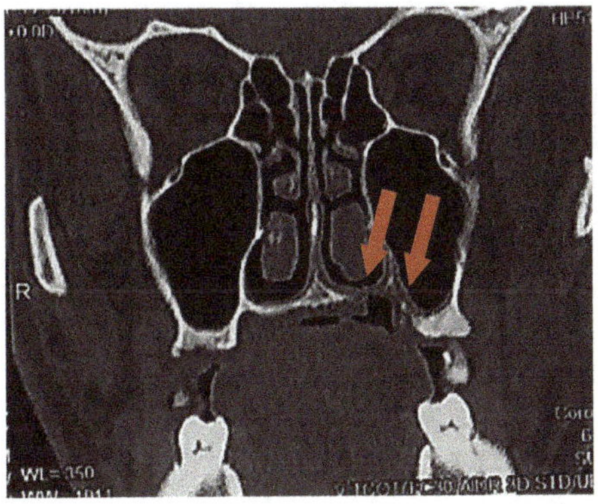

FIGURE 4: Cone-beam computed tomography (coronal cut) showing the maxillary defect, connecting the oral cavity to the left maxillary sinus and the nasal fossae.

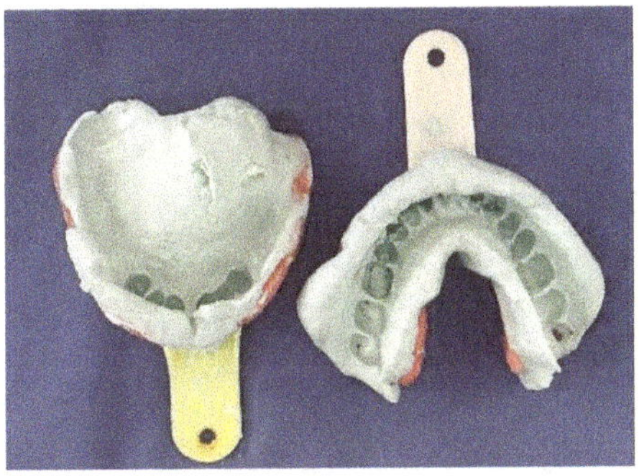

FIGURE 5: Primary impressions.

After setting up the teeth, try-in was done to evaluate both esthetics and occlusion (Figures 8(a) and 8(b)).

Once polymerized, the prosthesis was hollowed in the external surface, facing the obturator, to light it and prevent possible static instability (Figures 9(a) and 9(b)). Then, the prosthesis was polished (Figure 10) and inserted in mouth (Figures 11(a) and 11(b)).

The patient was advised to insert the prosthesis after repetitive trials in front of a mirror. Wearing and oral hygiene advice were instructed to the patient, and follow-up appointments were scheduled.

3. Discussion

Orofacial cancer therapeutics complicates prosthetic rehabilitation. Resection surgery modifies local anatomical conditions. All of these criteria, combined with complex psychological contexts, influence the prognosis of a successful prosthetic management [5].

The obturator prosthesis is a therapeutic option that is still used in many clinical cases where esthetic and functional rehabilitation cannot be achieved using another alternative [6]. It is an artificial device designed to ensure a tight closure of a bucconasal and/or buccosinusal communication. It is therefore considered as a complementary treatment to surgery and it requires some prerequisites [7].

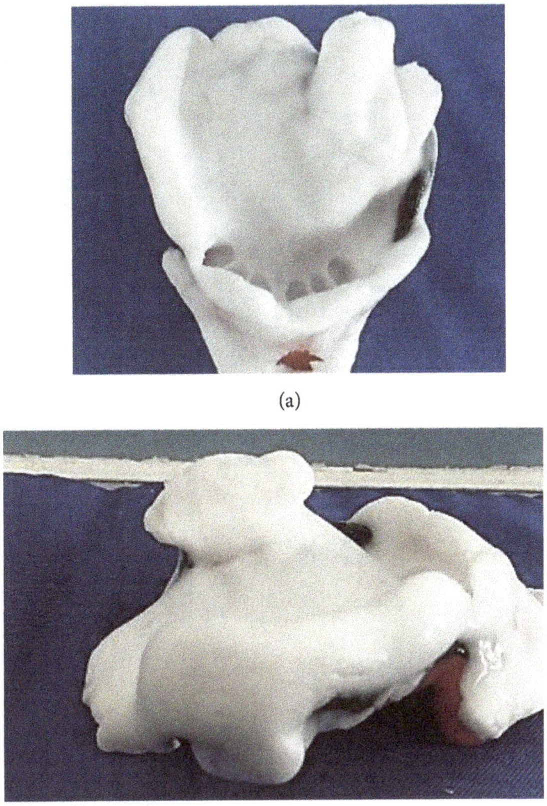

(a)

(b)

FIGURE 6: Anatomofunctional impression with FITT material: (a) upper view; (b) lateral view.

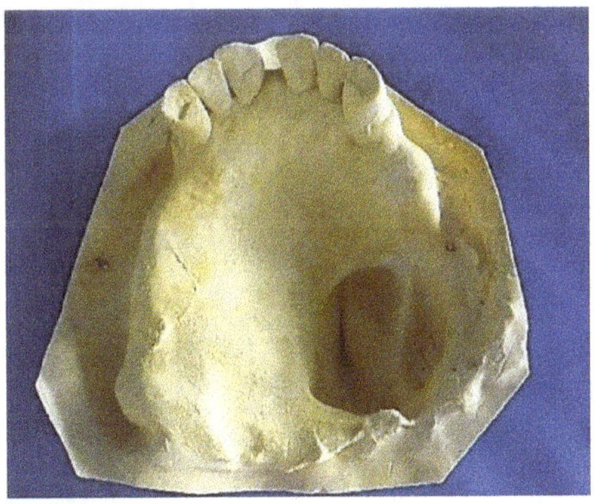

FIGURE 7: Maxillary cast.

The consequences of maxillary defects depend on their location and size [8]. In our case, the defect was of moderate size. The consequences faced with those cases are classified in Functional disorders, Infectious problems, Esthetic alterations, and Psychological and relational repercussions.

For the Functional disorders, we note speech difficulties due to nasal leakage of air, the voice is nasalized with incomprehensible words [8]; the alimentation becomes very disturbed by the reflux of food and liquids into the nasal and sinus fossae [9].

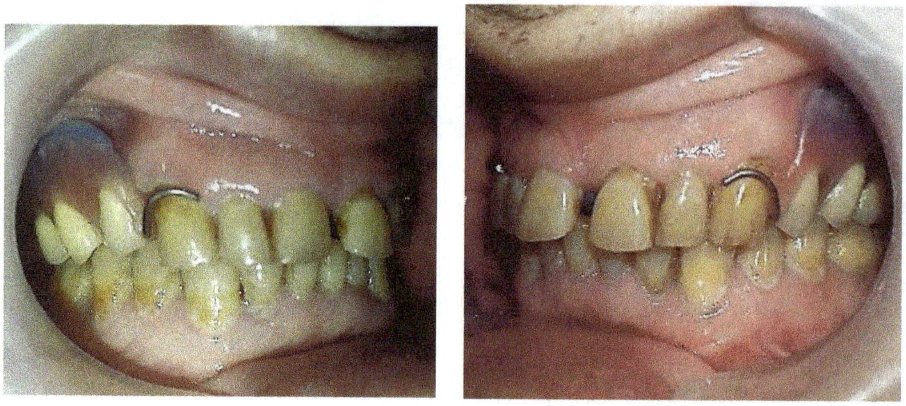

(a) (b)

Figure 8: Try-in. (a) Right side. (b) Left side.

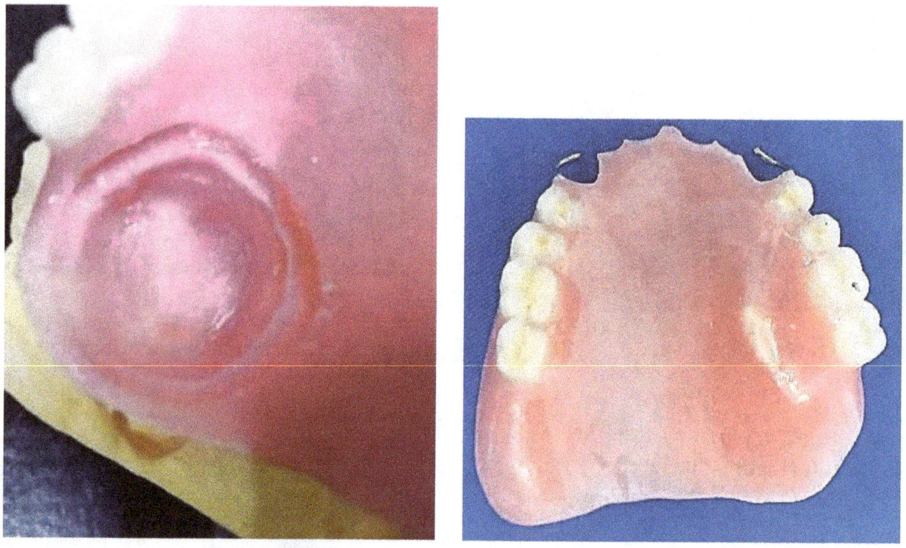

(a) (b)

Figure 9: (a) Hollowing the prosthesis. (b) Prosthetic extrados aspect.

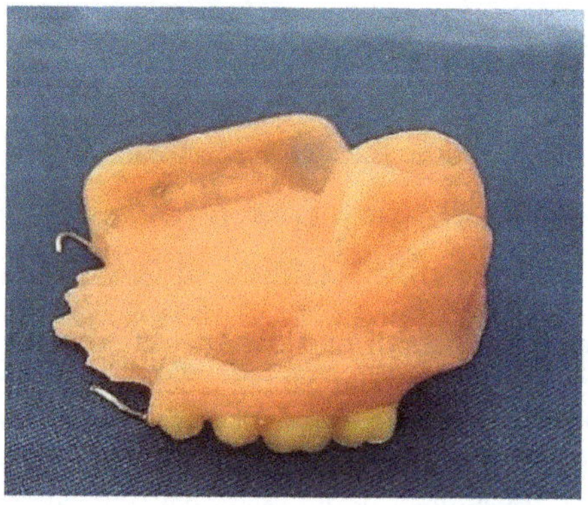

Figure 10: Obturator prosthesis.

Infectious problems consist of chronic infection of the sinus cavities that may set in [9].

Regarding esthetic alterations, resection of the underlying bone leads to sagging of the soft tissue with deterioration of the patient's esthetics [9].

Concerning psychological and relational repercussions, since the maxillofacial complex is the seat of mimics of the organs of olfaction, vision, hearing and taste, and the origin of the respiratory and digestive tracts. This gives this anatomical part a major psychological and relational importance. Any mutilation to this part profoundly affects the patients and makes them vulnerable and isolated from their social environment [8, 9].

In order to avoid these severe and handicapping consequences, it is imperative to place an obturator prosthesis. This prosthesis can only be designed within a surgical-prosthetic symbiosis plan. Thus, before starting the treatment, a multidisciplinary consultation meeting involving

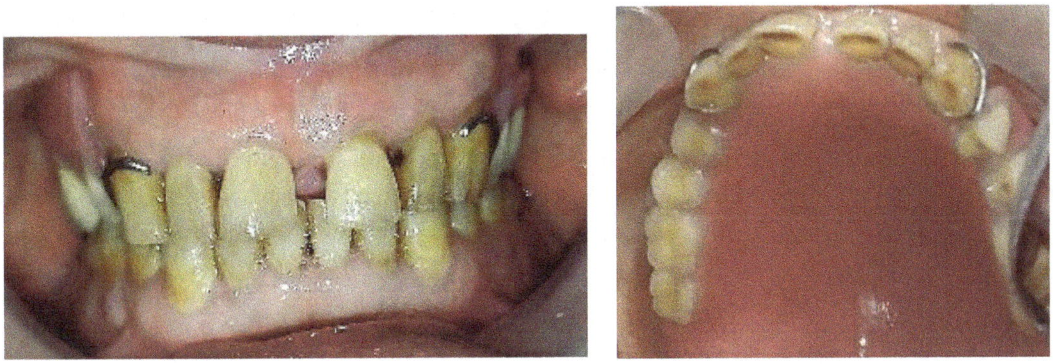

(a) (b)

FIGURE 11: Mouth insertion: (a) frontal view; (b) occlusal view.

the different specialists (maxillofacial surgeon, prosthodontist, radiologist, and social worker) must be held to outline the main lines of the treatment plan [4].

The definitive obturator prosthesis can be used for only 3 months to 1 year after the resection surgery. Dimensional changes due to remodeling and scarring of the defect's contours last approximately 1 year and are more related to soft tissue remodeling than to bone tissue remodeling. The decision for definitive rehabilitation depends on the size of the defect, the tumor prognosis, the mouth opening which must be sufficient, and the patient's edentulism. Healing is considered satisfying in the absence of sequestrum removal and in the presence of a well-reepithelialized and uninfected excision cavity [10].

In our case, a rigid obturator was indicated because the patient was partially edentulous and the maxillary defect was of moderate size (classification of M. Benoist). For the fabrication, the partial denture and the obturator were fabricated at the same time. Rigid obturator was made of methyl methacrylate. This material has the advantage of being durable in the long term, can be easily cleaned, and being perfectly polished. In addition, the weight of the denture can be reduced by hollowing the obturator [11]. For this, many materials can be used. For our case, it was the wax while salt or sand are also described for the same purpose in the literature. [12]

The impression of the maxillary defect was taken with FITT material (Kerr®) because it presented undercuts. It is a delayed-setting resin obtained by mixing powder and liquid and whose setting reaction goes through four phases: gel phase, plastic phase, elastic phase, and drying phase. Its plastic nature allowed us to mold the undercuts of the maxillary defect during the insertion of the custom tray. Its elasticity after setting allowed us to disinsert it without tearing or detachment of the impression [13].

Computer-assisted design and computer-assisted manufacturing (CAD/CAM) of obturators are also reported in the literature. Indeed, this method has many advantages, including saving time by reducing the number of steps and the possibility of avoiding some painful impressions by taking optical ones [14].

For many years, management in cancerology has been a controversial issue: should we surgically reconstruct following carcinological excision?

It is obvious that the surgical reconstruction rate is much higher. Nevertheless, we are still awaiting a scientific study on this subject to determine whether reconstruction compromises postsurgical monitoring and possibly modifies the survival time [15].

There are few comparative studies between the techniques of prosthetic rehabilitation and surgical reconstruction. Boutault et al. noted problems of food or fluid leakage in patients rehabilitated with obturators and phonatory problems in surgically reconstructed patients [16].

Based on a study involving 47 patients, Bertrand concluded that in the case of a maxillary defect with a size less than a quarter of the hard palate, the obturator prosthesis gives excellent functional results [17].

There is no doubt that prosthetic rehabilitation procedures still have an important role to play, especially in modest defects in the field of carcinology. On the other hand, there is a growing consensus that a severe defect is an indication for surgery. The choice of the best technique to be used remains rather subjective, as shown by numerous publications which are sometimes contradictory. It is sometimes possible to combine surgical and prosthetic approaches [15, 16].

Prosthetic materials can be improved and tissue engineering can be developed for the patients' benefit. There is no doubt that this subject is expected to evolve continuously and probably for quite a long time regarding its complexity [18].

4. Conclusion

Maxillofacial cancers most often require surgical excision of the developed tumors. This leads to a maxillary defect that can affect the esthetic balance of the face and have important consequences on the functional performances, especially, in case of a large bucconasal communication.

In spite of the evolution of surgical techniques, conventional obturator prostheses are still the gold standard to compensate maxillary defects.

References

[1] S. Bai, R. Clubwala, E. Adler et al., "Salivary Mucoepidermoid carcinoma: a multi-institutional review of 76 patients," *Head and Neck Pathology*, vol. 7, no. 2, pp. 105–112, 2013.

[2] T. Bridonneau, E. Quinque, S. Zink et al., "Le carcinome muco-épidermoïde du palais: présentation de deux cas et revue de la littérature," *Médecine Buccale Chirurgie Buccale*, vol. 23, no. 1, pp. 37–44, 2017.

[3] F. P. de Caxias, D. M. dos Santos, L. C. Bannwart, C. L. de Moraes Melo Neto, and M. C. Goiato, "Classification, History, and Future Prospects of Maxillofacial Prosthesis," *Journal of Dentistry*, vol. 2019, article 8657619, pp. 1-7, 2019.

[4] M. M. Ali, N. Khalifa, and M. N. Alhajj, "Quality of life and problems associated with obturators of patients with maxillectomies," *Head & Face Medicine*, vol. 14, no. 1, p. 2, 2018.

[5] B. H. Satheesh and K. S. Farhan, "Prosthetic rehabilitation of a patient with adenoid cystic carcinoma with continuous orbital-maxillary defect," *BML Case Reports*, vol. 20, no. 1, p. 3, 2013.

[6] H. Shivakumar, S. Rayannavar, D. Chougule, and S. Sharan, "Prosthetic rehabilitation of a maxillary defect caused by Ameloblastoma of rare occurrence: a clinical case report," *Contemporary Clinical Dentistry*, vol. 11, no. 1, pp. 87–90, 2020.

[7] G. Tirelli, R. Rizzo, M. Biasotto et al., "Obturator prostheses following palatal resection: clinical cases," *Acta Otorhinolaryngologica Italica*, vol. 30, no. 1, article 289509, pp. 33–39, 2010.

[8] X. Dong, C. Zhu, Y. Qian, F. Zhang, and T. Jiao, "The influence of obturators on the respiration of patients with maxillary defects: a clinical study," *PLoS One*, vol. 10, no. 5, article e0127597, 2015.

[9] M. Matsuyama, Y. Tsukiyama, M. Tomioka, and K. Koyano, "Subjective assessment of chewing function of obturator prosthesis wearers," *International Journal of Prosthodontics*, vol. 1, article e0127597, pp. 46–50, 2007.

[10] T. V. Ramasamy and J. Chandra, "An innovative sectional silicone obturator in a patient with partial maxillectomy: a case report," *The Journal of the Indian Prosthodontic Society*, vol. 20, no. 1, article 276821, pp. 115–119, 2020.

[11] P. Pomar and J. Dichamp, *Introduction à la prothèse maxillo-faciale*, EMC (Elsevier Masson SAS, Paris), Stomatologie, 2004.

[12] Y. H. Beh, T. H. Farook, N. B. Jamayet et al., "Evaluation of the differences between conventional and digitally developed models used for prosthetic rehabilitation in a case of untreated palatal cleft," *The Cleft Palate-Craniofacial Journal*, vol. 58, no. 3, pp. 386-390, 2021.

[13] M. Singh, I. K. Limbu, P. K. Parajuli, and R. K. Singh, "Definitive obturator fabrication for partial maxillectomy patient," *Case Reports in Dentistry*, vol. 2020, Article ID 6513210, 4 pages, 2020.

[14] A. Canan and Y. Suat, "Biomechanical 3-dimensional finite element analysis of obturator Protheses retained with zygomatic and dental implants in maxillary defects," *Medical Science Monitor*, vol. 21, article 892680, pp. 604–611, 2015.

[15] S. Iyer and K. Thankappan, "Maxillary reconstruction: current concepts and controversies," *Indian journal of plastic surgery: official publication of the Association of Plastic Surgeons of India*, vol. 47, no. 1, article 129618, pp. 8–19, 2014.

[16] F. Boutault, J. R. Paoli, and F. Lauwers, *Reconstruction chirurgicale des pertes de substance des maxillaires*, EMC (Elsevier Masson SAS, Paris), Stomatologie, 2005.

[17] J. C. Bertrand, "Tumeurs de l'infrastructure, reconstruction ou prothèse," in *Les tumeurs du massif facial et des cavités naso-sinusiennes*, J. P. Fontanel and J. M. Klossek, Eds., Éditions EDK, Paris, 2004.

[18] M. Arshad, G. Shirani, and X. Mahmoudi, "Rehabilitation after severe maxillectomy using a magnetic obturator (a case report)," *Clinical Case Reports*, vol. 6, no. 12, pp. 2347–2354, 2018.

20

Adenoid (Acantholytic) Squamous Cell Carcinoma of Mandibular Gingiva

T. Raut,[1] S. Keshwar,[1] M. R. Jaisani,[2] and A. Shrestha[1]

[1]*Department of Oral Pathology, College of Dental Surgery, BP Koirala Institute of Health Sciences, Dharan, Nepal*
[2]*Department of Oral and Maxillofacial Surgery, College of Dental Surgery, BP Koirala Institute of Health Sciences, Dharan, Nepal*

Correspondence should be addressed to A. Shrestha; ashish.shrestha@bpkihs.edu

Academic Editor: Mark Darling

Introduction. Adenoid (acantholytic) squamous cell carcinoma (ASCC) is a histological variant of squamous cell carcinoma which occurs mainly in the sun-exposed areas of the head and neck region. It is commonly seen among males which mainly occurs in the sixth and seventh decade of life with lip being predominately affected. Limited scientific literature is documenting the intraoral presentation of ASCC in contrast to its usual extraoral lesions associated with the skin. Characteristic pseudo glandular alveolar space formation seen in ASCC often mimics carcinoma of salivary gland origin. In-depth knowledge of histopathological features of ASCC is important to diagnose this uncommon variant. *Case Description.* An 80-year-old female presented with the chief complaint of the nonhealing lesion in the right lower back region of the jaw for 2 months, associated with pain. A provisional diagnosis of oral cancer was considered, and an incisional biopsy was done. Histopathological presentation of the epithelial tumor island, pseudo glandular duct-like structures, and neoplastic cells showing features of dysplasia and keratin pearl formation confirmed the diagnosis as adenoid (acantholytic) squamous cell carcinoma. *Conclusion.* The histopathological presentation of adenoid (acantholytic) squamous cell carcinoma reflects the prognosis and metastatic behavior of the diseases. The knowledge of histopathological features of ASCC would be a guide to the untrained eye for the diagnosis and management of this uncommon variant to minimize the rate of metastasis or reoccurrence.

1. Introduction

Squamous cell carcinoma (SCC) is the most common cancer of the head and neck region. It follows a geographical pattern of incidence which is highest among South Asians [1]. Squamous cell carcinoma has several histopathological variants such as verrucous, spindle, basaloid, adenosquamous, adenoid, and undifferentiated type [2].

The behavioral pattern and prognosis of SCC often can be correlated with molecular analysis for aneuploidy, loss of the tumor suppressor gene, and loss of heterozygosity. However, few histopathological variants of SCC guide the prognosis and biological behavior on its routine microscopic presentation; basaloid and adenoid variants are two among them [3, 4]. Adenoid (acantholytic) squamous cell carcinoma represents 2-4% of SCC which affects mainly the sun-exposed areas of the skin [5]. Goldman et al. in 1977 reported the first case of oral cavity-associated adenoid (acantholytic) squamous cell carcinoma (ASCC). Here, we present a case of a female patient diagnosed with ASCC. This case report is intended to highlight the rare pathology familiarizing its histopathological features in regards to the biological behavior.

2. Case Report

An 80-year-old female presented with a complaint of a nonhealing lesion in the right posterior region of the lower jaw for two months. The lesion was gradually increasing in size associated with moderate, intermediate-type pain with purulent discharge. She had a habit of chewing tobacco with slaked lime for 60 years, 6-7 times per day which she kept for 10-20 minutes at variable sites in the vestibular region and spit. She also had a habit of smoking tobacco for 50 years, 5-6 cigarettes per day, and had no other significant medical history.

On extraoral examination, there was a localized swelling around the body of the mandible on the right side with a single, firm, mobile, and tender lymph node approximately measuring $1 \times 1.5\,cm^2$ in maximum dimension palpable in the submandibular region. Intraoral examination revealed a single, soft, erythematous swelling with ulceration extending from 44 to 48 involving the vestibule, buccal mucosa, edentulous alveolar ridge, and lingual mucosa extending towards the floor of the mouth, measuring approximately 2.5×2.5 c m^2 in maximum dimension. The surface of the lesion shows localized thick purulent discharge and is tender on palpation with peripheral induration. There was a root stump associated with 42-44 and carious exposure on 33-41 with edematous gingiva (Figure 1). The panoramic radiograph revealed a homogenous radiolucent lytic lesion involving the body and angle of the mandible on the right side with irregular cortical margin in the body area extending from 44 to 46.

The clinical diagnosis of oral carcinoma was made, and an incisional biopsy was suggested. A single, soft tissue measuring $13 \times 7 \times 5$ mm in maximum dimension, creamish white in color, and firm in consistency was obtained and fixed in 10% neutral buffered formalin. The fixed tissue was processed, embedded, and sectioned with the soft tissue microtome at a thickness of $3\,\mu m$ and stained with routine hematoxylin and eosin stain. The histopathological section revealed epithelial tumor islands within connective tissue showing the central area of acantholysis. Islands show features of dysplasia in the form of dyskeratosis, mitotic figures, cellular and nuclear pleomorphism, and keratin pearl formation (Figures 2 and 3). Numerous pseudo glandular structures lined by a single layer of flat to polygonal cells were appreciated (Figure 4). Periodic acid-Schiff stain confirmed these structures to be nonglandular without any mucinous components. The lumen shows detached keratinocytes with the intense eosinophilic cytoplasm (Figure 2). Surrounding connective tissue was fibrocellular with inflammatory cell infiltrates. No lymphovascular or perineural invasion was evident. Reviewing the diagnostic criteria, a final diagnosis of adenoid (acantholytic) squamous cell carcinoma was made. The patient was suggested for radiotherapy at the cancer center because of the extensive nature of the lesion and age. However, the patient refused to visit any cancer center and passed away four months following the diagnosis.

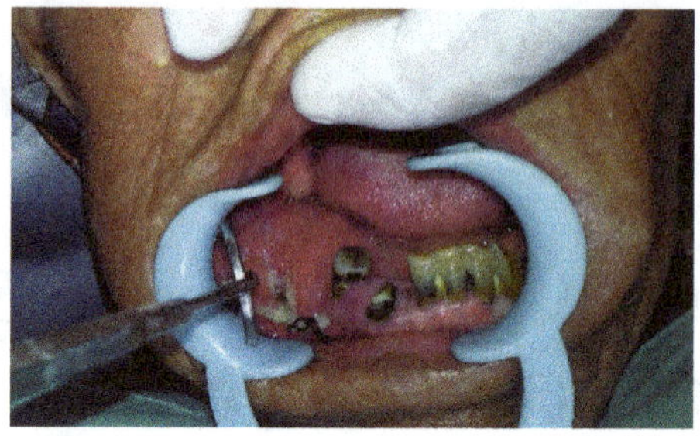

Figure 1: Erythematous ulcerative growth involving the right alveolar ridge and vestibule.

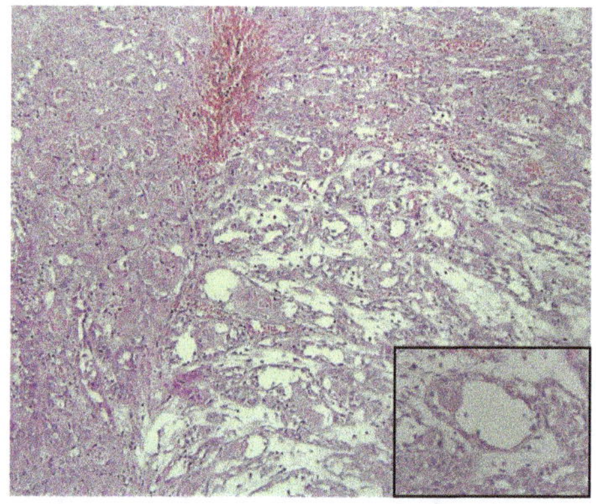

Figure 2: Section showing epithelial tumor islands with keratin pearls and pseudo glandular duct-like structures (H&E, 10x); inset: pseudo glandular duct-like structures lined by a single layer of cells with the dyskeratotic cell within the space (H&E, 40x).

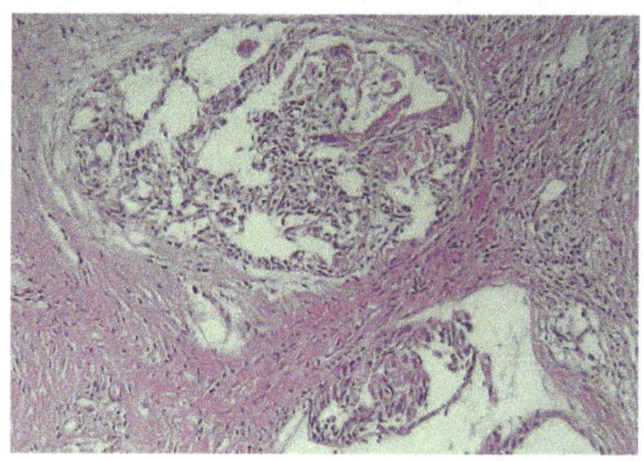

Figure 3: Epithelial tumor islands within connective tissue showing acantholysis and loss of cellular attachment (H&E, 10x).

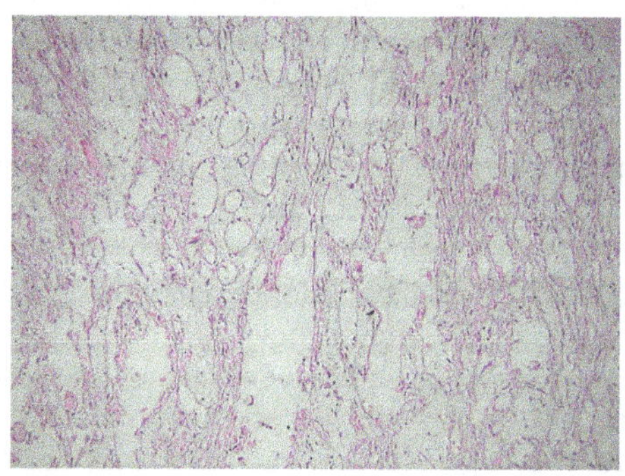

Figure 4: Space giving the pseudo glandular presentation (H&E, 10x).

3. Discussion

Adenoid (acantholytic) squamous cell carcinoma (ASCC), first described by Lever in 1947, is now a well-recognized histopathological variant of squamous cell carcinoma that rarely occurs within the oral cavity [6, 7]. The condition is prevalent in sun-exposed areas of the head and neck region where radiation is claimed to be the etiological agent whereas the intraoral presentation lacks this etiological basis. Sun exposure has also been associated with increased incidence of ASCC in the lower lip [8]. In contrast to conventional OSCC where alcohol and tobacco are the prime etiological agents, no such definitive etiology has been ascribed to ASCC. In the case report of Bhogavaram et al., trauma has been emphasized as the origin of ASCC; however, due to the paucity of its

Table 1: A brief review of the ADSCC cases of the mandible reported in the literature.

Author	Clinical details	Management	Staging	Follow-up
Chandrakala et al. [5] (2018)	63/F Tobacco chew; ulcerated erythematous mass	Radiotherapy suggested	—	No follow-up
Tsuji et al. [17] (2016)	76/M	—	—	—
Pathak et al. [3] (2014)	55/F; ulceroproliferative mass	Surgery, radiotherapy, and chemotherapy	—	Free of disease (6 months)
Vidyavathi et al. [18] (2012)	40/M Tobacco smoke; polypoidal mass	Surgery	T3 N2 M0	—
Terada [19] (2011)	73/F; exophytic papillary mass	Surgery	—	Free of disease (3 months)
Prasad and Kaur [20] (2010)	70/F; exophytic ulcerated mass	—	—	—
Kusafuka et al. [21] (2006)	64/F	Surgery	cT2cN0cM0	5-month follow-up shows no node/distance metastasis
Driemel et al. [22] (2004)	58/F; exophytic mass	Surgery & radiotherapy	pT4 pN0 cM0 R0	Died after 7 months of initial diagnosis
Jones et al. [23] (1993)	58/M Tobacco smoke	Surgery	—	Free of disease (9 months)
Zaatari and Santoianni [16] (1986)	86/M; nodular growth	Surgery	—	—

occurrence, etiopathological basis has not been well identified [9]. O'Shea et al. in their immunofluorescence-based study summarized that the loss of cellular adhesion in ASCC is primarily due to desmosomal defects specifically desmogleins 1 and 2 or desmoplakin or both [10].

Chandrakala et al. in 2018 have summarized a total of 45 cases of ASCC in the oral cavity reported in English language literature to date making this pathology uncommon. The literature shows male predilection and lip to be the predominant site (22 cases) of occurrence which includes 16 cases of the lower lip, 4 cases of the upper lip, and the remaining 2 cases which were not specified. Cases other than the lip were found in the gingiva, tongue, floor of the mouth, and buccal mucosa [5]. After an extensive literature review in year 2018 [5], seven more cases have been added to the literature which includes lesion associated with the upper lip, maxilla, buccal mucosa, and tongue region [8, 9, 11, 12]. The present case is seen within the mandibular jaw. A thorough literature review on the cases of the mandibular jaw revealed a total of 10 published cases to the best of our knowledge (Table 1).

Lasser et al. and Leon et al. summarized the diagnostic criteria for ASCC as follows: (i) the basic cell should be keratinizing squamous type, (ii) adenoid structure consists of a rounded space with a definitive wall, principally of one cell thickness, and (iii) the lumen of the adenoid/ductal structure contains single or group of dyskeratotic acantholytic cells [7]. Based on microscopic features, ASCC has many synonyms such as adenoid SCC, pseudo glandular SCC, SCC with gland-like features, angiosarcoma-like SCC, pseudo vascular adenoid SCC, and epithelioma dyskeratoticum segregans [13, 14]. The combined microscopic features of the duct-like structures with conventional SCC often give a list of histopathological differential diagnosis which includes conventional squamous cell carcinoma, adenosquamous cell carcinoma, mucoepidermoid carcinoma, and angiosarcoma. Conventional SCC lacks duct-like structures lined by a single layer of polygonal cells. Adenosquamous cell carcinoma has both the component similar to ASCC but stains positive for periodic acid-Schiff (PAS), Alcian blue, and mucicarmine. Mucoepidermoid has the characteristic presence of three different types of cells such as mucous, epidermoid, and intermediate type with the positivity of PAS, Alcian blue, and mucicarmine. Angiosarcoma also shows close histopathological resemblance to ASCC where the sections have to be thoroughly evaluated for the presence of dysplastic epithelial tumor islands with keratin pearl formations. Vascular markers, CD31 and CD34 along with Fli-1 protein, would be diagnostic for angiosarcoma [2, 5, 13].

Skin-associated ASCC has poor prognosis [14]; similarly, ASCC of the larynx is also commented for its aggressive behavior showing regional lymphadenopathy and reoccurrence [15, 16]. The biological behavior of ASCC of the oral cavity is considered to have poor prognosis by some author to variable by other which might be due to limited reported cases [2, 5, 6, 13]. Detachment of neoplastic cells due to acantholysis is correlated with its distant metastasizing behavior [10]. Ishikawa et al. in their study found that 46-month survival for ASCC was zero percent whereas 30-month survival was just 20.4% and concluded the ASCC of the oral cavity to have an extremely poor prognosis. The study has also analyzed the treatment protocol opted in various ASCC patients. Out of 13 cases evaluated, 7 were treated with surgery (alone and with radical dissection), in which 6 showed a good postoperative course without evidence of diseases whereas 6 cases were treated with adjuvant (chemotherapy or radiotherapy) along with surgery, all of them showed reoccurrence and died due to diseases within 7-46 months of primary surgery showing poor prognosis. Despite limited cases and a short period of follow-up, the study suggested that radical surgery might be very important in the patient of oral ASCC.

4. Conclusion

The histopathological presentation of adenoid (acantholytic) squamous cell carcinoma reflects the prognosis and metastatic behavior of the diseases. The knowledge of histopathological features of ASCC would be a guide to the untrained eye to avoid misdiagnosis and to opt for the best possible treatment protocol to minimize the rate of metastasis or reoccurrence improving the prognosis.

References

[1] F. Bray, J. Ferlay, I. Soerjomataram, R. L. Siegel, L. A. Torre, and A. Jemal, "Global cancer statistics 2018: GLOBOCAN estimates of incidence and mortality worldwide for 36 cancers in 185 countries," *CA: A Cancer Journal for Clinicians*, vol. 68, no. 6, pp. 394–424, 2018.

[2] S. K. Patil, C. S. Parimala, K. P. Nithin, M. B. R. Ahmed, and R. Naik, "Case report adenoid squamous cell carcinoma on buccal mucosa : a case report," *Journal of Advanced Medical and Dental Sciences Research*, vol. 2, no. 3, pp. 142–145, 2014.

[3] J. Pathak, N. Swain, S. Patel, and L. S. Poonja, "Histopathological variants of oral squamous cell carcinoma-institutional case reports," *Journal of Oral and Maxillofacial Pathology*, vol. 18, no. 1, pp. 143–145, 2014.

[4] B. Perez-Ordoñez, M. Beauchemin, and R. C. K. Jordan, "Molecular biology of squamous cell carcinoma of the head and neck," *Journal of Clinical Pathology*, vol. 59, no. 5, pp. 445–453, 2006.

[5] J. Chandrakala, S. Srinath, G. Giraddi, and R. K. Kendole, "Adenoid squamous cell carcinoma of oral cavity: a case report," *Journal of Dentistry*, vol. 19, no. 1, pp. 68–73, 2018.

[6] K. Kalele, R. Deshmukh, and A. Alsi, "A sneak peep at adenoid/acantholytic variant of oral squamous cell carcinoma," *Journal of Oral Medicine, Oral Surgery, Oral Pathology and Oral Radiology*, vol. 4, no. 3, pp. 128–130, 2018.

[7] S. Ishikawa, H. Ishikawa, T. Kato et al., "Acantholytic squamous cell carcinoma of the maxillary gingiva: case report and literature review," *Journal of Oral and Maxillofacial Surgery, Medicine, and Pathology*, vol. 26, no. 4, pp. 488–491, 2014.

[8] I. Allon, M. Abba, I. Kaplan et al., "Oral variant of acantholytic squamous cell carcinoma–histochemical and immunohistochemical features," *Acta Histochemica*, vol. 121, no. 8, article 151443, 2019.

[9] B. Bhogavaram, R. Sinha, K. Rapolu, and B. P. Boggarapu, "Adenoid squamous cell carcinoma of upper lip, a rare variant of squamous cell carcinoma: a case report," *Journal of Family Medicine and Primary Care*, vol. 9, pp. 5779-5782, 2020.

[10] C. O'Shea, J. E. Fitzpatrick, and P. J. Koch, "Desmosomal defects in acantholytic squamous cell carcinomas," *Journal of Cutaneous Pathology*, vol. 41, no. 11, pp. 873–879, 2014.

[11] X. Han, X. Lin, and X. Shao, "Pseudovascular adenoid squamous cell carcinoma of the tongue: a case report and literature review," *International Journal of Clinical and Experimental Pathology*, vol. 13, no. 5, pp. 1086–1089, 2020.

[12] J. E. Kim, C. Lee, K. Y. Oh, and K. H. Huh, "A rare acantholytic variant of squamous cell carcinoma of the maxilla: a case report and literature review," *Medicine (Baltimore)*, vol. 99, no. 32, article e21631, 2020.

[13] E. Papadopoulou, K. I. Tosios, N. Nikitakis, N. Papadogeorgakis, and A. Sklavounou-andrikopoulou, "Acantholytic squamous cell carcinoma of the gingiva: report of a case and review of the literature," *Oral Surgery, Oral Medicine, Oral Pathology, Oral Radiology, and Endodontics*, vol. 109, no. 6, pp. e67–e71, 2010.

[14] M. Sajin, A. Hodorogea Prisăcaru, M. C. Luchian et al., "Acantholytic squamous cell carcinoma: pathological study of nine cases with review of literature," *Romanian Journal of Morphology and Embryology*, vol. 55, no. 2, pp. 279–283, 2014.

[15] M. C. González-Vela, J. F. Val-Bernal, M. Mayorga, L. Zaldumbide, and M. Báscones, "Adenoid squamous cell carcinoma of the larynx: an uncommon histological variant of squamous cell carcinoma," *APMIS*, vol. 114, no. 6, pp. 470–473, 2006.

[16] G. S. Zaatari and R. A. Santoianni, "Adenoid squamous cell carcinoma of the nasopharynx and neck region," *Archives of Pathology & Laboratory Medicine*, vol. 110, no. 6, pp. 542–546, 1986.

[17] K. Tsuji, M. Wato, Y. Uehara, K. Kurioka, and M. Ueda, "Immunohistochemical study of acantholytic squamous cell carcinomas of head and neck region," *Journal of Osaka Dental University*, vol. 50, no. 1, pp. 41–45, 2016.

[18] K. Vidyavathi, C. S. B. R. Prasad, M. L. Harendra Kumar, and R. P. Deo, "Pseudovascular adenoid squamous cell carcinoma of oral cavity: a mimicker of angiosarcoma," *Journal of Oral and Maxillofacial Pathology*, vol. 16, no. 2, pp. 288–290, 2012.

[19] T. Terada, "Papillary squamous cell carcinoma of the oral cavity with acantholytic and pseudovascular features," *International Journal of Clinical and Experimental Pathology*, vol. 4, no. 8, pp. 794–796, 2011.

[20] K. K. Prasad and S. Kaur, "Acantholytic squamous cell carcinoma of the oral cavity: an uncommon histological variant of squamous cell carcinoma," *Minerva Stomatologica*, vol. 59, no. 6, pp. 377–380, 2010.

[21] K. Kusafuka, M. Ebihara, H. Ishiki et al., "Primary adenoid squamous cell carcinoma of the oral cavity," *Pathology International*, vol. 56, no. 2, pp. 78–83, 2006.

[22] O. Driemel, K. Braxein, H. Pistner, and H. Kosmehl, "Oral adenoid squemous carcinoma. Tumor markers and prognosis," *Mund-, Kiefer- und Gesichtschirurgie*, vol. 8, no. 2, pp. 118–122, 2004.

[23] A. C. Jones, P. D. Freedman, and S. M. Kerpel, "Oral adenoid squamous cell carcinoma: a report of three cases and review of the literature," *Journal of Oral and Maxillofacial Surgery*, vol. 51, no. 6, pp. 676–681, 1993.

21

Ligneous Periodontitis in a Patient with Type 1 Plasminogen Deficiency: A Case Report and Review of the Literature

Arun Sadasivan[1] **Roshni Ramesh**[2] **and Deepu George Mathew**[3]

[1]*Department of Periodontics, Sree Mookambika Institute of Dental Sciences, Kulashekaram, Tamil Nadu, India*
[2]*Department of Periodontics, Government Dental College, Thrissur, Kerala, India*
[3]*Department of Oral and Maxillofacial Pathology, Annoor Dental College, Muvattupuzha, Kerala, India*

Correspondence should be addressed to Arun Sadasivan; sadasivan_arun@hotmail.com

Academic Editor: Mine Dündar

Background. Ligneous periodontitis or destructive membranous periodontal disease is a rare condition involving gingival tissues, which is due to plasminogen deficiency and fibrin deposition. Plasminogen deficiency is an ultrarare autosomal recessive disease. The disease is characterized by gingival enlargement and periodontal tissue destruction that leads to rapid tooth loss despite treatment attempts. A defect in fibrinolysis and abnormal wound healing are the main pathogenesis of this condition. It is caused by mutations in *PLG*, the gene coding for plasminogen, which results in decreased levels and functional activity. *Case Presentation.* In this case report, clinical and histopathological findings of a 26-year-old male patient who presented with generalized membranous gingival enlargement are presented. He was the third child of consanguineous parents and had multicystic congenital hydrocephalus at birth. Besides the gingival enlargement, he also presented ligneous conjunctivitis since childhood. The intraoral examination revealed generalized periodontal breakdown. Radiographs showed alveolar bone loss present in every quadrant. All blood investigations were normal except for plasminogen deficiency. A biopsy sample was excised from affected gingiva and a series of histopathological evaluation was performed. Based on clinical and histopathological evidence, a diagnosis of destructive membranous periodontal disease or ligneous periodontitis was made. A clinical exome assay for the PLG gene was also done. It was confirmed as Type 1 plasminogen deficiency. *Conclusion.* Ligneous periodontitis has been rarely reported in India. The reasons could be because of the rarity of the disease or missed diagnosis. The need to take a proper history and perform a proper clinical examination and histopathologic evaluation has to be stressed when diagnosing and treating gingival enlargements. If a genetic condition is suspected, genetic screening is also needed. All these will help the clinician in correctly diagnosing the disease and formulating a proper treatment plan for managing the condition.

1. Introduction

Gingival enlargements are a common feature seen in patients which present aesthetic, functional, psychological, and periodontal problems. The etiology in most of the cases has an inflammatory, hormonal, drug-induced, idiopathic, or cancerous origin. There are, however, certain rare conditions in which the etiology is obscure. One such condition is destructive membranous periodontal disease or ligneous periodontitis (LP). This condition has been attributed to a plasminogen deficiency. Other possible causes such as autoimmune or hypersensitivity reactions, trauma, and viral or bacterial infections have been reported [1, 2].

Haemostasis depends on many factors like vasoconstriction, formation of blood coagulation factors, and fibrinolysins, especially plasmin. Plasmin is derived from plasminogen (PLG), which is its proenzyme; it is synthesized in the liver and circulates in the plasma. PLG plays an important role in intravascular and extravascular fibrinolysis and wound healing. It is converted to plasmin by cleavage of the Arg561-Val562 peptide bond by either a tissue-type PLG activator (tPA) or a urokinase-type PLG activator (uPA). Activation of PLG by tPA is the major pathway that leads to efficient lysis of fibrin clots in the blood stream, whereas activation of PLG by uPA seems to be mainly responsible for mediating PLG activation in association with cell surfaces especially wound healing and tissue remodelling [3]. Plasmin also acts as a broad spectrum proteolytic factor either directly by degrading extracellular matrix proteins, e.g., laminin, fibronectin, and proteoglycans, or indirectly by activating latent metalloproteinases. Therefore, it plays a crucial role in tissue homeostasis, e.g., remodelling, angiogenesis, and wound healing. Moreover, plasmin has also been found to play an important role in host defence against infections [4, 5].

Plasminogen deficiency is a rare (1.6 in 1 million individuals) autosomal recessive disease caused by homozygote or compound-heterozygote mutations of the plasminogen gene PLG. The PLG gene maps to chromosome 6q26-q27. It spans about 52.5 kilobases (kb) of DNA and consists of 19 exons and 18 introns. The PLG cDNA of 2.7 kb encodes a protein consisting of 791 amino acid residues [6]. There are two types of plasminogen deficiency: (1) hypoplasminogenemia (Type I PLG deficiency), in which there is a marked decrease in the levels of PLG antigen $\leq$ 1.9 mg/dL (normal range 6 to 25 mg/dL) and functional activity of up to 33% (normal range 80 to 120%), and (2) dysplasminogenemia (Type II PLG deficiency), in which the level of immunoreactive PLG is within normal range but the specific activity of PLG is reduced [7–10].

Gingival enlargement in hypoplasminogenemia has been described as "amyloidaceous ulcerated gingival hyperplasia" or destructive membranous periodontal disease (ligneous periodontitis). The term ligneous periodontitis (LP) was first coined by Gunhan et al. to describe a destructive membranous periodontal disease [11]. LP generally starts in childhood with conjunctiva as well as gingival mucosa as its most affected sites [1, 12]. Ligneous periodontitis is characterized by gingival enlargement and severe attachment loss, which is associated with plasminogen deficiency, the accumulation of amyloid-like material in the lamina propria, and deposition of fibrin [5, 11, 13]. Most cases of LP have been reported in association with ligneous conjunctivitis (LC), which suggests that both clinical manifestations may be related. LC is a rare form of chronic conjunctivitis that usually affects children, girls more often than boys (3 : 1), and can occur at any age. It is characterized by fibrin-rich pseudomembranes mainly on tarsal conjunctivae [1, 8]. Type II PLG deficiency patients, however, have never reported developing pseudomembranous lesions.

In this case report, the clinical, histopathological, and genetic evaluation of a 26-year-old male patient who presented with generalized membranous gingival enlargement is presented.

2. Case Presentation

A 26-year-old male patient reported to our clinic with complaints of generalized swelling of gums and pain and bleeding from gums. Gingival enlargement was present since childhood and was slowly increasing in size. The enlargements had been previously localized in sites and had been surgically excised at 8 years of age, but recurrence occurred. He had periodic oral prophylaxis done. He was the third child of second degree consanguineous parents. At birth, he presented with multicystic hydrocephalus which was drained by ventriculoperitoneal shunt. Since an early age, he also presented with profuse granulomatous growth in conjunctiva in both eyes. Corneal involvement and chronic obstruction led to the progressive blindness of the left eye by the age of 15. Histopathological evaluations led to a diagnosis of ligneous conjunctivitis.

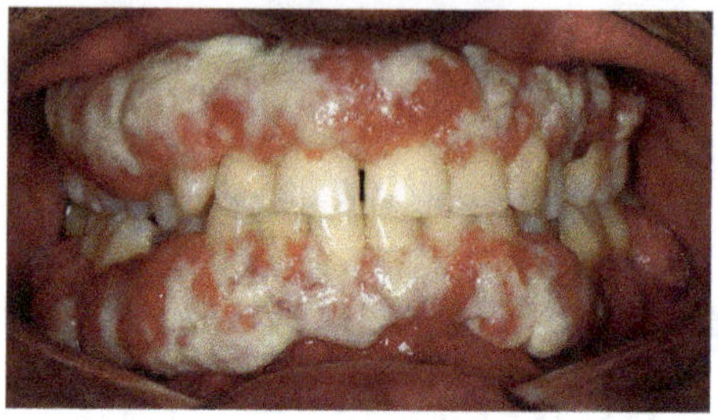

FIGURE 1: Intraoral examination of a 26-year-old male patient with PLG deficiency (Type 1) showing membranous gingival enlargement.

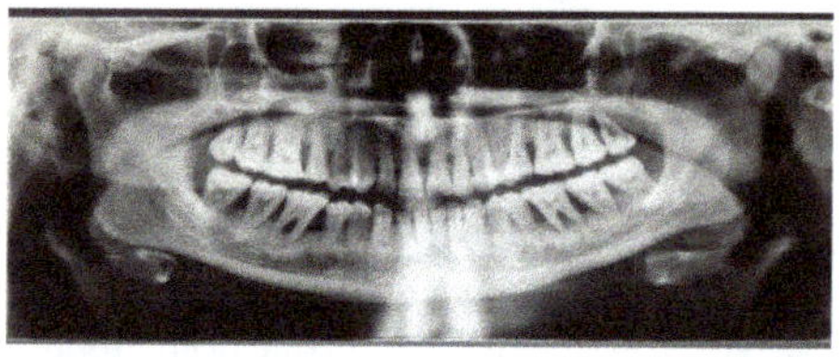

FIGURE 2: Panoramic radiograph showing extensive generalized periodontal breakdown.

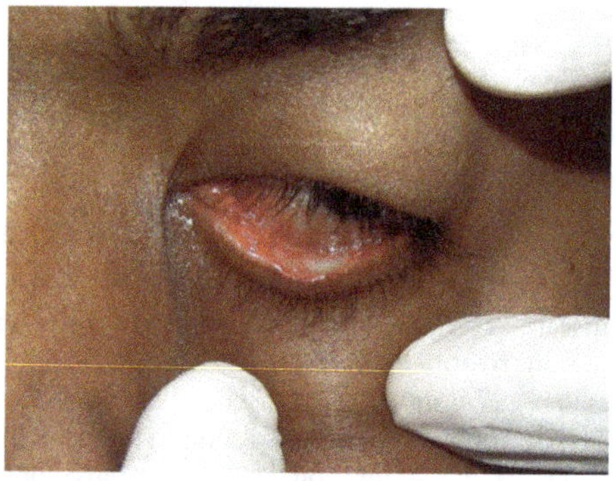

FIGURE 3: Ligneous conjunctivitis.

2.1. Clinical and Radiographic Examination. The intraoral examination revealed solid, nodular, and fragile erythematous and hyperplastic gingival enlargements involving the marginal and attached gingiva in both maxillary and mandibular arches. The periodontal evaluation revealed signs of generalized severe periodontitis, ulceration, and white-yellow fibrinous pseudomembranes (Figure 1). Probing showed increased pocket depths ranging from 8 to 10 mm in many teeth, bleeding on probing in over 30% of sites, and generalized tooth mobility. The panoramic radiograph showed generalized alveolar bone loss of more than 50%, especially in the posterior teeth (Figure 2). Recurrent conjunctivitis was seen as a white membrane in the mucosa of the upper and lower eye lids (Figure 3). The patient's growth and development were within normal limits, and no other family member reported similar findings.

2.2. Laboratory Investigations. Haematological assessment and biochemical tests were done all of which were within normal parameters except for plasma plasminogen activity which showed a level of <5% (biological reference=low, reference interval: 75-140%), a lactate dehydrogenase (LDH) level of 331 IU/L (reference range = 135-214), SGOT/AST levels of 60 IU/L (reference range = 15-37), and SGPT/ALT levels of 66 IU/L (reference range = 30-65). Plasminogen deficiency was diagnosed as due to hypoplasminogenemia which is named Type I PLG plasminogen deficiency. Haematological evaluation and biochemical tests such as liver function tests, serum proteins, azotemia, glycemia, hormonal values, and kidney function tests were within normal limits.

2.3. Histopathological Examination. Under the effect of local anaesthesia, an incisional biopsy of the gingival enlargement was done. The haematoxylin-and-eosin-stained soft tissue section showed a parakeratinised stratified squamous surface epithelium with branching and anastomosing rete ridges in association with a fibrovascular connective tissue. The connective tissue showed subepithelial deposits of homogenous eosinophilic material that resembled amyloid. These areas were relatively acellular. The deeper parts of the connective tissue showed a diffuse mixed inflammatory cell infiltrate comprised predominantly of neutrophils, lymphocytes, and plasma cells. Sections also showed capillary vessels and extravasated red blood cells. Gingival biopsies all stained for fibrin but stained (Congo Red) negatively for amyloid, lipid, keratin, immunoglobulins, and glycogen. Masson's trichrome was negative and PAS variably positive (Figure 4).

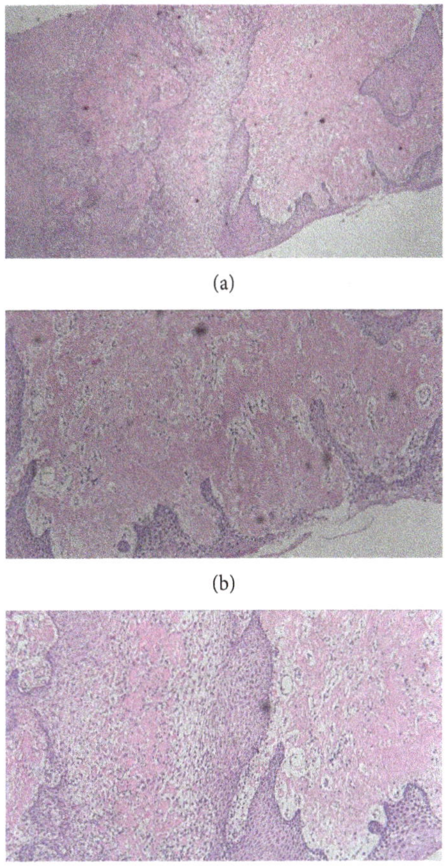

(a)

(b)

(c)

Figure 4: (a) H&E stain; original magnification is ×4, while magnification in (b) is ×10 and magnification in (c) is ×40. Photomicrograph showing parakeratinised stratified squamous surface epithelium with branching and anastomosing rete ridges and connective tissue showing subepithelial deposits of homogenous eosinophilic material that resembled amyloid. The deeper parts show a diffuse mixed inflammatory cell infiltrate comprising predominantly of neutrophils.

2.4. Genetic Testing and Variant Interpretation. After the clinical and histopathological diagnosis of ligneous periodontitis associated with Type 1 plasminogen deficiency was made, DNA tests were done to the patient at MedGenome laboratories, Bangalore, India. The test methodology performed was targeted gene sequencing. Selective capture and sequencing of the protein coding regions of the genome/genes was performed. Mutations identified in the exonic regions are generally actionable when compared to variations that occur in noncoding regions. Targeted sequencing represents a cost-effective approach to detect variants present in multiple/large genes in an individual. DNA extracted from blood was used to perform targeted gene capture using a custom capture kit. The libraries were sequenced to mean > 80-100x coverage on an Illumina sequencing platform. The sequences obtained are aligned to a human reference genome (GRCh37/hg19) using the BWA program [14, 15]. It was analyzed using Picard and GATK version 3.6 to identify variants relevant to the clinical condition [16, 17] (Figure 5).

Variant interpretation was a homozygous missense variation in exon 7 of the PLG gene (chr6:161137712G>A; depth: 50x) that results in the amino acid substitution of histidine for arginine at codon 235 (p.Arg23His; ENST00000308192.9). Inheritance was autosomal recessive. The observed variation lies in the kringle domain of the plasminogen protein [18] and has previously been reported as pathogenic as per ClinVar and SwissVar [19, 20]. The p.Arg235His variant has not been reported in the 1000 Genomes, ExAC, and the internal database of the MedGenome laboratories. The in silico predictions of the variant are probably damaging by PolyPhen-2 (HumDiv) and damaging by SIFT and MutationTaster 2. The reference codon is conserved across species. For the OMIM phenotype, Type 1 plasminogen deficiency (OMIM#217090) is caused by homozygous or compound heterozygous mutations in the PLG gene (OMIM∗173350).

2.5. Treatment Done. After the diagnosis of LP, the management of the dental condition was done. Supra- and subgingival debridement was performed under local anaesthesia. Oral hygiene instructions were given to the patient who was advised to rinse twice daily with 0.2% chlorhexidine digluconate for a period of two weeks. A marked reduction in pocket depth and bleeding on probing was noticed after

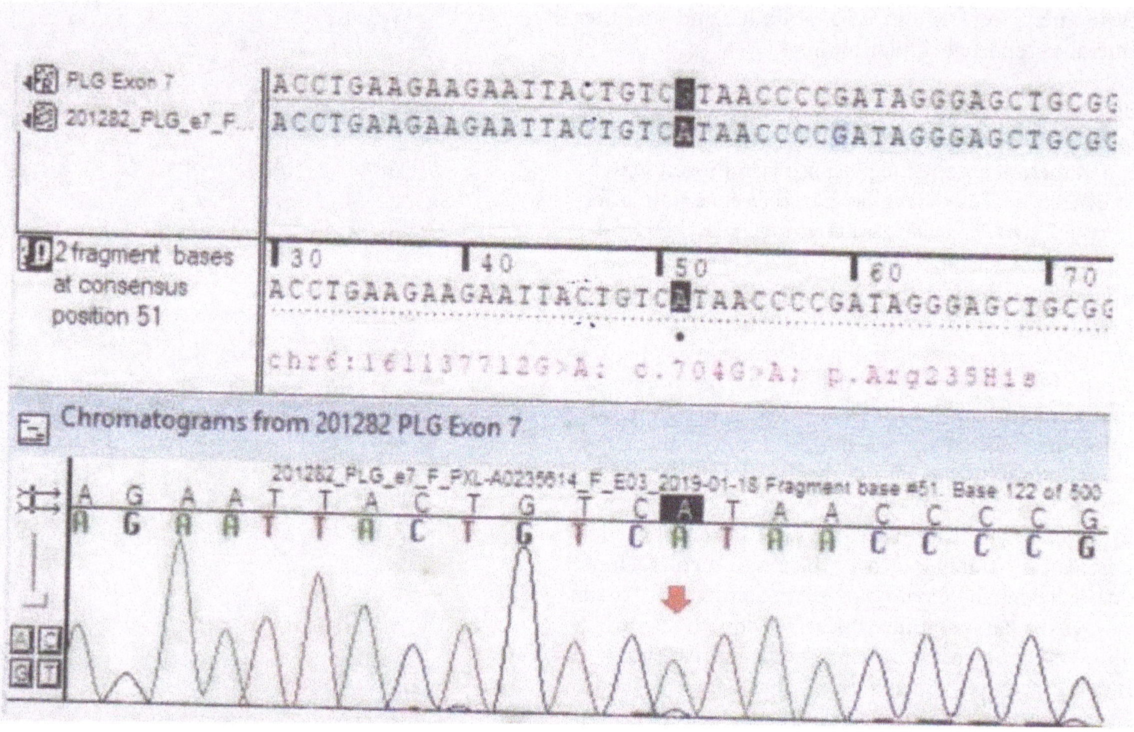

FIGURE 5: Sequence chromatogram and alignment to the reference sequence showing the variation in exon 7of the PLG gene (chr6:161137712G>A; c.704G>A; p.Arg235His) detected in homozygous condition in the patient.

eight weeks, but the enlargements still persisted. Surgical excision of the lesion was done by internal bevel gingivectomy on the upper right quadrant and by a diode laser in the upper left quadrant. However, recurrence of the lesion was seen after 3 months (Figure 6). The patient was also referred to an ophthalmology clinic for the management of ligneous conjunctivitis.

3. Discussion

In this report, a case of LP has been presented along with its corresponding clinical, radiographic, histopathologic, and genetic findings in addition to its management by excision. Only a limited number of cases with plasminogen deficiency and oral lesions have been reported in the literature [5]. Congenital plasminogen deficiency is a rare autosomal recessive disease which is clinically characterized by chronic mucosal pseudomembranous, nodular enlargements in both the maxilla and mandible depending on the subepithelial fibrin deposition and inflammation [11, 21]. It is now well documented that hypoplasminogenemia is a multisystemic disease. Clinical manifestations in a collection of 74 patients with severe (i.e., homozygous or compound-heterozygous) hypoplasminogenemia showed a median age of first clinical manifestation of 9.54 months (range 3 days to 61 years). The female-to-male ratio was 1.43 : 1. The majority of the affected patients suffered from ligneous conjunctivitis (81%) and ligneous gingivitis (30%). Other manifestations included the involvement of the upper and lower respiratory tract (20%), the middle ear (15%), the female genital tract (9%), the gastrointestinal tract (2.7%), the kidneys (4%), and the skin (juvenile colloid milium: 1%). Congenital occlusive hydrocephalus was seen in 12% of the patients. A few (5%) patients exhibited Dandy-Walker malformation, a congenital hypoplasia, and upward rotation of the cerebellar vermis and cystic dilation of the fourth ventricle [7, 22–25]. In the present case, the patient presented with congenital hydrocephalus, ligneous conjunctivitis, and enlargements in both jaws since childhood. Based on the clinical and radiological findings, a provisional diagnosis of LP was considered.

The exact pathophysiology of the clinical presentation seen in LP is still not clear. In vitro data and animal studies indicated that alterations in tissue repair and host defense mechanisms are responsible for the onset and the progression of periodontal destruction [4, 26]. Plasminogen plays an important role in intravascular and extravascular fibrinolysis, wound healing, cell migration, tissue remodelling, angiogenesis, and embryogenesis [27]. Local extracellular fibrinolysis by plasmin is required for the initial removal of the fibrin-rich matrix as well as for the remodelling of the granulation tissue and completion of wound healing [10, 28, 29]. Impairment of the pathway due to hypoplasminogenemia leads to fibrin accumulation and an increased inflammatory reaction. Consequently, the process of wound healing stops at the stage of granulation tissue formation and cellular proteolysis, which may then further support the invasion of pathogens. This process is notably pronounced in mucous membranes such as the periodontal tissues [29, 30]. The fact that only 32% of patients who suffer from PLG Type 1 deficiency develop ligneous periodontitis strongly supports the notion that external triggers, i.e., trauma or infection, may play an

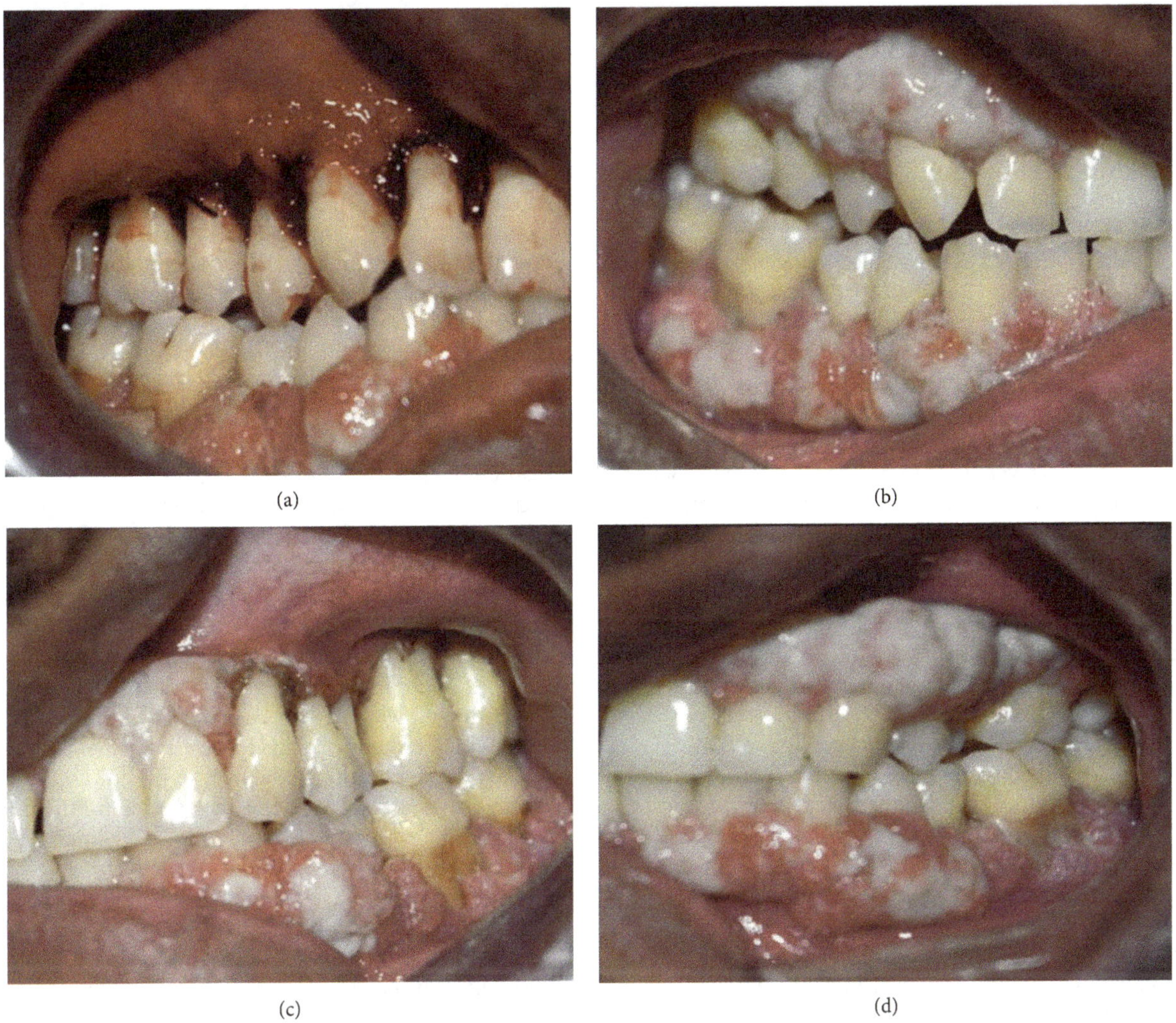

FIGURE 6: (a) Surgical excision by internal bevel gingivectomy on the right maxillary region. (b) 3-Month follow-up shows recurrence of the lesion. (c) Excision by diode laser on left maxillary region. (d) 3-Month follow-up shows recurrence of the lesion.

additional significant role in the pathogenesis of this disease [5, 10, 31]. The average age of patients reported in the literature with ligneous periodontitis is 12-18 years, while isolated cases have been reported in older patients; these differences may reflect variability in PLG activity due to different plasminogen gene mutations [32].

Histopathological examination was done to confirm the diagnosis. Severe acute inflammation and irregular acanthosis of the epithelium with extensive fibrin leakage and the accumulation of an amyloid-like material in the lamina propria is the characteristic feature of this disease at histopathological examination. This condensed fibrin accumulation lacks reticulin fibres [11]. A variety of other hyaline deposits, ranging from classical amyloid to mixtures of immunoglobulins, fibrin, fibrinogen, and albumin, might be found in the gingiva. Indeed, amyloid is itself a nonspecific term for a spectrum of entities, including immunoglobulin light chains, serum amyloid fibrillar proteins, β2-microglobulin, keratin transthyretin, and others [33]. In the present case too, the section showed parakeratinised stratified squamous surface epithelium with branching and anastomosing rete ridges in association with a fibrovascular connective tissue. The connective tissue showed subepithelial deposits of homogenous eosinophilic material that resembled amyloid. These areas were relatively acellular. Gingival biopsies all stained for fibrin but stained (Congo Red) negatively for amyloid, lipid, keratin, immunoglobulins, and glycogen. Masson's trichrome was negative and PAS variably positive. These findings confirmed the diagnosis of LP.

Inherited homozygous or compound-heterozygous hypoplasminogenemia is a very rare disorder (with an incidence estimated at below 1 : 10) which is associated with deficient extravascular PLG-dependent fibrinogen clearance leading to impaired wound healing mainly of mucous membranes. In affected patients, the wound healing capacity seems to be arrested at the stage of granulation tissue formation [8]. Studies suggest that the K19E mutation is the most common molecular genetic defect in patients with hypoplasminogenemia worldwide [25]. A variety of other genetic abnormalities have been identified in the PLG gene in subjects with heterozygous, homozygous, and compound-heterozygous hypoplasminogenemia: missense mutations include T9N, L128P, R134K, G142R, G176D, T181P, R216H, D219N, R234H, P285A, P285T, R306H, N307I, T352I,

P353A, P491R, A505V, R513H, S575P, W597C, A675T, P744S, C765G, and R776H; nonsense mutations include C133X, K378X, Q380X, E460X, R471X, Q540X, and W597X; frameshift mutations include W417fsX432, E455fsX493, V563fsX580, and L650fsX652; and splice site mutations include IVS11-2A/G, IVS11-7T/G, IVS11+1G/A, and IVS17 +1delG as well as amino acid deletion mutation K212del and amino acid insertion mutation T319_N320insN [7, 22–25].

Congenital heterozygous hypoplasminogenemia is a rare condition and was first described in 1982 in a patient with thromboembolic disease [34]. It was earlier thought that heterozygous hypoplasminogenemia might be a risk factor for venous thrombosis; however, a study by Drew et al. has suggested that isolated heterozygous or homozygous/compound-heterozygous hypoplasminogenemia by itself is not a risk factor for deep venous thrombosis [35]. In 1997, Schuster et al. demonstrated distinct homozygous and compound-heterozygous mutations in the PLG gene and confirmed the autosomal-recessive inheritance of this disorder [23]. Studies have shown the incidence rate of hypoplasminogenemia worldwide to be less than 1%. A large epidemiologic study performed in blood donors in the United Kingdom demonstrated an observed rate of heterozygous (asymptomatic) plasminogen deficiency of 25 out of 9611 patients or 0.26% [36]. The incidence rate of (heterozygous) hypoplasminogenemia has been roughly estimated in different geographic regions at 0.35% (only in white subjects) in Minnesota, USA [37], at 0.13% in Southern Germany [38], and at 0.42% in Japan [39].

In our case, the GATK Best Practices framework was followed for the identification of variants in the sample. Gene annotation of the variants was performed using the VEP program against the Ensembl release 87 human gene model [40]. Clinically relevant mutations were annotated using published variants in the literature and a set of disease databases—ClinVar, OMIM, GWAS, HGMD, and SwissVar. Common variants were filtered based on allele frequency in 1000 Genomes phase 3, ExAC, EVS, dbSNP147, 1000 Japanese Genome, and our internal Indian population database. Nonsynonymous variant effects were calculated using multiple algorithms such as PolyPhen-2, SIFT, MutationTaster 2, MutationAssessor, and LRT. Only nonsynonymous and splice site variants found in the clinical exome panel consisting of 8332 genes were used for clinical interpretation. Silent variations that do not result in any change in amino acid in the coding region were not reported. A homozygous missense variation in exon 7 of the PLG gene (chr6:161137712G>A; depth: 50x) that results in the amino acid substitution of histidine for arginine at codon 235 (p.Arg23His; ENST00000308192.9) was detected. Inheritance was autosomal recessive. The observed variation lies in the kringle domain of the plasminogen protein and has previously been reported as pathogenic as per ClinVar and SwissVar [18–20].

The most characteristic features of this destructive periodontal disease are widespread membranous, nodular gingival enlargements in both maxilla and mandible leading to rapid tooth loss despite several treatment attempts [11]. Several therapeutic approaches to reduce the bacterial load to decrease the inflammation and thus the progression of the disease have been attempted; these procedures include scaling and root planing, chlorhexidine rinsing, administration of antibiotics, and periodontal surgery [9, 25, 30]. Neering et al. have reported that patients with PLG-deficiency Type I may benefit from nonsurgical periodontal therapy including full mouth disinfection in combination with adjunctive antibiotic therapy and a strict supportive periodontal therapy regime every three months [32]. Most of the reports have been described as failures due to rapid gingival regrowth and progressive bone loss [5]. Scully et al. suggested that gingival lesions can be controlled by topical heparin or intravenous purified plasminogen [41]. Gunhan et al. stated that systemic fibrinolytic and antithrombotic agents may prove more beneficial than local treatments, because the ligneous lesions tend to involve several mucosal areas [11]. Traditional periodontal treatment options for managing gingival enlargements include either gingivectomy or flap surgeries. The main objective is to excise the enlargements and reestablish healthy gingival margins and contours. The healing pattern in flap surgeries is by primary intention, whereas in gingivectomy, it involves healing by secondary intention. These healing mechanisms involve the formation of a fibrin clot, which creates a framework for normal periodontal tissues to grow back. However, in patients with plasminogen deficiency, the inadequacy of plasmin results in the overgrowth of fibrin. This is the main reason for the failure of conventional periodontal treatment modalities in these patients. A case report indicated that the treatment with warfarin exerts protection against relapsing gingival hyperplasia over an observation period of 3 years in a 54-year-old patient. The authors reported about a combination of gingivectomy, an administration of 20 mg doxycycline daily, and the use of a 0.12% chlorhexidine digluconate mouth rinse. One week after surgery, the patient started with 5 mg warfarin daily for an indefinite time [42]. Silva et al. reported a complete regression of oral mucous lesions after systemic and topical corticosteroids [43]. A recent clinical trial by Shapiro et al. was the first to evaluate the clinical utility of Glu-plasminogen in children and adults with congenital plasminogen deficiency. Human Glu-plasminogen replacement therapy was administered intravenously at 6.6 mg/kg every 2-4 days to 14 patients for a period of 12 weeks. Upon administration, results show the achievement of physiological levels of plasminogen activity that temporally coincided with clinical efficacy and improved disease management [44]. In the present case, the 26-year-old male patient reported with gingival enlargements present since childhood. Excision of the lesion was done with a surgical blade on one side and with a diode laser on the other side. However, recurrences of the lesions were seen within 3 months.

4. Conclusion

This case report discusses the diagnosis of ligneous periodontitis associated with Type 1 plasminogen deficiency in a 26-year-old male patient. The clinical presentation was that of a generalized gingival enlargement. Through this case report, we would like to stress on the importance of a thorough history taking, intraoral clinical evaluation, radiographic evaluation, and haematological examination, as a varied etiopathogenesis is reported for gingival enlargements. A histopathological examination of the biopsy specimen helped in confirming the diagnosis. Genetic testing helped in precisely identifying the gene, location, variant, zygosity, and inheritance pattern. Excision of the enlargements by means of surgical and laser techniques were not successful and recurrence occurred. The lack of efficacious therapy has increased the suffering of affected patients under the burden of this very rare blood disease.

Abbreviations

LP:	Ligneous periodontitis
PLG:	Plasminogen
LC:	Ligneous conjunctivitis
SGOT:	Serum glutamic oxaloacetic transaminase
AST:	Aspartate amino transferase
SGPT:	Serum glutamic pyruvic transaminase
ALT:	Alanine transaminase
PAS:	Periodic acid-Schiff
BWA program:	Burrows-Wheeler aligner program
SIFT:	Scale invariant feature transform
OMIM:	Online Mendelian Inheritance in Man
GATK:	Genome Analysis Toolkit
VEP:	Variant effect predictor
GWAS:	Genome-wide association study
HGMD:	Human Gene Mutation Database.

Consent

The authors certify that they have obtained the appropriate patient consent form. In the form, the patient has given consent for his clinical information to be reported in the journal. The patient understands that his name and initials will not be published, and due efforts will be made to conceal his identity; however, anonymity cannot be guaranteed.

References

[1] A. A. Hidayat and P. J. Riddle, "Ligneous conjunctivitis: A clinicopathologic study of 17 cases," *Ophthalmology*, vol. 94, no. 8, pp. 949–959, 1987.

[2] E. J. Holland, C. C. Chan, T. Kuwabara, A. G. Palestine, J. J. Rowsey, and R. B. Nussenblatt, "Immunohistologic Findings and Results of Treatment with Cyclosporine in Ligneous Conjunctivitis," *American Journal of Ophthalmology*, vol. 107, no. 2, pp. 160–166, 1989.

[3] T. H. Bugge, M. J. Flick, M. J. Danton et al., "Urokinase type plasminogen activator is effective in fibrin clearance in the absence of its receptor or tissue-type plasminogen activator," *Proceedings of the National Academy of Sciences of the United States of America*, vol. 93, no. 12, pp. 5899–5904, 1996.

[4] R. Sulniute, T. Lindh, M. Wilczynska, J. Li, and T. Ny, "Plasmin is essential in preventing periodontitis in mice," *The American Journal of Pathology*, vol. 179, no. 2, pp. 819–828, 2011.

[5] S. Sivolella, M. de Biagi, M. T. Sartori, M. Berengo, and E. Bressan, "Destructive membranous periodontal disease (ligneous gingivitis): a literature review," *Journal of Periodontology*, vol. 83, no. 4, pp. 465–476, 2012.

[6] T. E. Petersen, M. R. Martzen, A. Ichinose, and E. W. Davie, "Characterization of the gene for human plasminogen, a key proenzyme in the fibrinolytic system," *Journal of Biological Chemistry*, vol. 265, no. 11, pp. 6104–6111, 1990.

[7] V. Schuster, S. Seidenspinner, P. Zeitler et al., "Compound-heterozygous mutations in the plasminogen gene predispose to the development of ligneous conjunctivitis," *Blood*, vol. 93, no. 10, pp. 3457–3466, 1999.

[8] V. Schuster and S. Seregard, "Ligneous conjunctivitis," *Survey of Ophthalmology*, vol. 48, no. 4, pp. 369–388, 2003.

[9] I. Kurtulus, A. Gokbuget, A. Efeoglu et al., "Hypoplasminogenemia with ligneous periodontitis: a failed local therapeutic approach," *Journal of Periodontology*, vol. 78, no. 6, pp. 1164–1175, 2007.

[10] V. Schuster, B. Hügle, and K. Tefs, "Plasminogen deficiency," *Journal of Thrombosis and Haemostasis*, vol. 5, no. 12, pp. 2315–2322, 2007.

[11] Ö. Günhan, M. Günhan, E. Berker, C. A. Gürgan, and H. Yildirim, "Destructive membranous periodontal disease (ligneous periodontitis)," *Journal of Periodontology*, vol. 70, no. 8, pp. 919–925, 1999.

[12] Ö. Günhan, B. Celasun, F. Perrini et al., "Generalized gingival enlargement due to accumulation of amyloid like material," *Journal of Oral Pathology & Medicine*, vol. 23, no. 9, pp. 423–428, 1994.

[13] T. Baykul and Y. Bozkurt, "Destructive membranous periodontal disease (ligneous periodontitis): a case report and 3 years follow-up," *British Dental Journal*, vol. 197, no. 8, pp. 467-468, 2004.

[14] H. Li and R. Durbin, "Fast and accurate long-read alignment with Burrows-Wheeler transform," *Bioinformatics*, vol. 26, no. 5, pp. 589–595, 2010.

[15] L. R. Meyer, A. S. Zweig, A. S. Hinrichs et al., "The UCSC genome browser database: extensions and updates 2013," *Nucleic Acids Research*, vol. 41, no. D1, pp. D64–D69, 2012.

[16] A. McKenna, M. Hanna, E. Banks et al., "The Genome Analysis Toolkit: a MapReduce frame work for analyzing next-generation DNA sequencing data," *Genome Research*, vol. 20, no. 9, pp. 1297–1303, 2010.

[17] H. Li, B. Handsaker, A. Wysoker et al., "The Sequence Alignment/Map format and SAMtools," *Bioinformatics*, vol. 25, no. 16, pp. 2078-2079, 2009.

[18] http://pfam.xfam.org/protein/P00747.

[19] http://www.ncbi.nlm.nih.gov/clinvar/RCV000014545.25.

[20] http://web.expasy.org/variantpages/VAR018659.html.

[21] J. B. Bateman, T. H. Pettit, S. J. Isenberg, and K. B. Simons, "Ligneous conjunctivitis: an autosomal recessive disorder," *Journal of Pediatric Ophthalmology and Strabismus*, vol. 23, no. 3, pp. 137–140, 1986.

[22] D. Schott, C. E. Dempfle, P. Beck et al., "Therapy with a purified plasminogen concentrate in an infant with ligneous conjunctivitis and homozygous plasminogen deficiency," *The*

New England Journal of Medicine, vol. 339, no. 23, pp. 1679–1686, 1998.

[23] V. Schuster, A. M. Mingers, S. Seidenspinner, Z. Nüssgens, T. Pukrop, and H. W. Kreth, "Homozygous mutations in the plasminogen gene of two unrelated girls with ligneous conjunctivitis," *Blood*, vol. 90, no. 3, pp. 958–966, 1997.

[24] V. Schuster, P. Zeitler, S. Seregard et al., "Homozygous and compound heterozygous type I plasminogen deficiency is a common cause of ligneous conjunctivitis," *Thrombosis and Haemostasis*, vol. 85, no. 6, pp. 1004–1010, 2001.

[25] K. Tefs, M. Gueorguieva, J. Klammt et al., "Molecular and clinical spectrum of type I plasminogen deficiency: a series of 50 patients," *Blood*, vol. 108, no. 9, pp. 3021–3026, 2006.

[26] Ö. Günhan, A. Avci, Ö. Dereci, Ş. Akgün, and B. Celasun, "Extensive fibrin accumulation and accompanying epithelial changes in the pathogenesis of ligneous mucosal disease (ligneous periodontitis)," *The American Journal of Dermatopathology*, vol. 34, no. 1, pp. 35–40, 2012.

[27] F. J. Castellino and V. A. Ploplis, "Structure and function of the plasminogen/plasmin system," *Thrombosis and Haemostasis*, vol. 93, no. 4, pp. 647–654, 2005.

[28] J. Schaller and S. S. Gerber, "The plasmin—antiplasmin system: structural and functional aspects," *Cellular and Molecular Life Sciences*, vol. 68, no. 5, pp. 785–801, 2011.

[29] E. Zorio, J. Gilabert-Estelles, F. Espana, L. Ramon, R. Cosin, and A. Estelles, "Fibrinolysis: the key to new pathogenetic mechanisms," *Current Medicinal Chemistry*, vol. 15, no. 9, pp. 923–929, 2008.

[30] R. Mehta and A. D. Shapiro, "Plasminogen deficiency," *Haemophilia*, vol. 14, no. 6, pp. 1261–1268, 2008.

[31] S. K. Rao, J. Biswas, R. Rajagopal, G. Sitalakshmi, and P. Padmanabhan, "Ligneous conjunctivitis: a clinicopathologic study of 3 cases," *International Ophthalmology*, vol. 22, no. 4, pp. 201–206, 1998.

[32] S. H. Neering, S. Adyani-Fard, A. Klocke, S. Rüttermann, T. F. Flemmig, and T. Beikler, "Periodontitis associated with plasminogen deficiency: a case report," *BMC Oral Health*, vol. 15, no. 1, 2015.

[33] R. S. Cotran, V. Kumar, and S. I. Robbins, *Robbins Pathologic Basis of Disease*, WB Saunders, 2nd edition, 1989.

[34] D. K. Hasegawa, B. J. Tyler, and J. R. Edson, "Thrombotic disease in three families with inherited plasminogen deficiency," *Blood*, vol. 60, 1982.

[35] A. F. Drew, A. H. Kaufman, K. W. Kombrinck et al., "Ligneous conjunctivitis in plasminogen deficient mice," *Blood*, vol. 91, no. 5, pp. 1616–1624, 1998.

[36] R. C. Tait, I. D. Walker, J. A. Conkie, S. I. Islam, and F. McCall, "Isolated familial plasminogen deficiency may not be a risk factor for thrombosis," *Thrombosis and Haemostasis*, vol. 76, no. 6, pp. 1004–1008, 1996.

[37] D. Dykes and H. Polesky, "Incidence of PLG∗Q0 allele in human populations," in *Advanced in Forensic Haemogenetics*, W. Mayr, Ed., pp. 261–264, Berlin, Springer, 1988.

[38] S. Weidinger, W. Patutschnick, and F. Schwarzfischer, "Further evidence of a silent plasminogen (PLG) allele in two paternity cases," *Zeitschrift für Rechtsmedizin*, vol. 101, no. 2, pp. 99–104, 1988.

[39] A. Okamoto, T. Sakata, T. Mannami et al., "Population-based distribution of plasminogen activity and estimated prevalence and relevance to thrombotic diseases of plasminogen deficiency in Japanese: the Suita Study," *Journal of Thrombosis and Haemostasis*, vol. 1, no. 11, pp. 2397–2403, 2003.

[40] W. McLaren, B. Pritchard, D. Rios, Y. Chen, P. Flicek, and F. Cunningham, "Deriving the consequences of genomic variants with the Ensembl API and SNP Effect Predictor," *Bioinformatics*, vol. 26, no. 16, pp. 2069-2070, 2010.

[41] C. Scully, A. Y. Gokbuget, C. Allen et al., "Oral lesions indicative of plasminogen deficiency (hypoplasminogenemia)," *Oral Surgery, Oral Medicine, Oral Pathology, Oral Radiology, and Endodontology*, vol. 91, no. 3, pp. 334–337, 2001.

[42] G. Fine, K. Bauer, M. al-Mohaya, and S.-B. Woo, "Successful treatment of ligneous gingivitis with warfarin," *Oral Surgery, Oral Medicine, Oral Pathology, Oral Radiology, and Endodontology*, vol. 107, no. 1, pp. 77–80, 2009.

[43] G. B. Silva, C. Bariani, E. F. Mendonça, and A. C. Batista, "Clinical manifestations due to severe plasminogen deficiency: a case report," *Journal of Dentistry for Children*, vol. 73, no. 3, pp. 179–182, 2006.

[44] A. D. Shapiro, C. Nakar, J. M. Parker et al., "Plasminogen replacement therapy for the treatment of children and adults with congenital plasminogen deficiency," *Blood*, vol. 131, no. 12, pp. 1301–1310, 2018.

22

Proliferative Verrucous Leukoplakia of the Gingiva: An Early Lesion Refractory to Surgical Excision

Dhanushka Leuke Bandara,[1] **Primali Rukmal Jayasooriya**,[2] **and Ruwan Duminda Jayasinghe**[1]

[1]*Department of Oral Medicine & Periodontology, Faculty of Dental Sciences, University of Peradeniya, Peradeniya 20400, Sri Lanka*
[2]*Department of Oral Pathology, Faculty of Dental Sciences, University of Peradeniya, Peradeniya 20400, Sri Lanka*

Correspondence should be addressed to Dhanushka Leuke Bandara; dhanulb@pdn.ac.lk

Academic Editor: Rui Amaral Mendes

This report describes a case of proliferative verrucous leukoplakia (PVL) of the gingiva with no discernible aetiology, which presented in a 36-year-old female. The initial nonscrapable gingival lesion was treated with CO_2 laser ablation, and the histopathological evaluation was carried out. The presence of koilocytic cells in the superficial epithelium led to immunohistochemical investigations with p16 antibody, which showed strong nuclear positivity and slight cytoplasmic positivity in >50% of the cells with >25% confluency. However, it was not possible to confirm the presence of HPV infection with further investigations due to logistic reasons. The lesion recurred twice within a short time despite the surgical resection following the first recurrence. Thus, this paper presents a case of proliferative verrucous leukoplakia, which demonstrated a significant resistance to routine treatment protocols recommended in the management of such lesions.

1. Introduction

White lesions in the oral cavity could represent a variety of aetiological factors including increased or abnormal keratin production in the oral epithelium, which is denoted by the term "keratosis" [1].

In addition to keratotic lesions that occur due to tobacco use, they may also occur due to frictional, chemical, or thermal irritations as well as due to inflammation. Frictional keratosis is usually seen in areas of recurring mild mechanical trauma or irritation while chemical keratosis may occur as the result of the compounds in smokeless tobacco, certain toothpastes, inappropriately used acidic medications, and alkaline liquids [2, 3]. Usually, keratotic lesions cannot be scrapped off and may differ in texture depending on the cause [3].

Oral leukoplakia (OL) is defined as a "white plaque of questionable risk having excluded (other) known diseases or disorders that carry no increased risk for cancer" [4]. Proliferative verrucous leukoplakia (PVL) is a rare form of oral leukoplakia with a malignant transformation rate of 70% [5]. It develops initially as a white plaque of hyperkeratosis that eventually becomes a multifocal disease with confluent, exophytic, and proliferative features showing different degrees of dysplasia. PVL is more commonly a disease of the elderly females which can develop in both tobacco users and nontobacco users [5, 6].

Recently, Woo et al. have reported a subset of lesions, with the majority clinically presenting as OL, harbouring high-risk HPV subtypes and positive for p16 [7]. In addition, clinicopathological spectrums of these lesions are similar to tobacco-induced leukoplakia that occurs more often in adult males on the tongue and floor of the mouth [7]. According to Barasch et al., when interpreting p16 positivity, the presence of p16 positivity in >50% of cells with >25% confluence or >70% positivity could be considered as the threshold to determine a positive reaction [8].

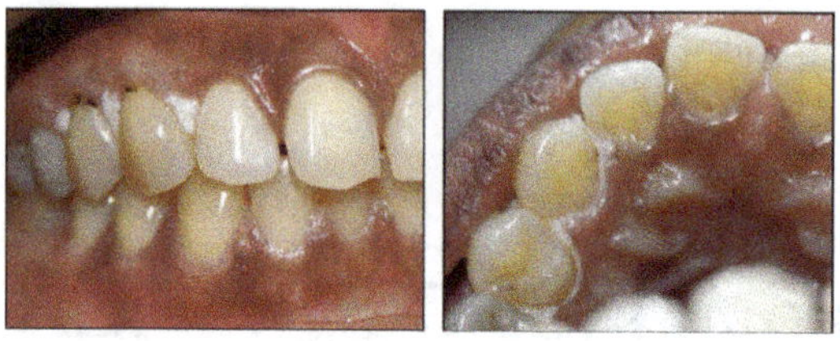

FIGURE 1: Linear, plaque-like whitish lesion on the palatal and buccal gingiva of 13, 14, and 15.

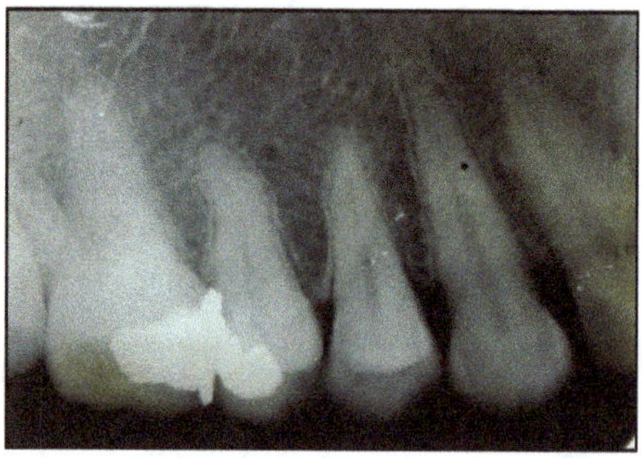

FIGURE 2: IOPA radiograph of 13–15 region.

This case report describes a rare case of early stage of PVL with no apparent aetiology that developed in a relatively young patient.

2. Case Presentation

A 36-year-old female presented with an asymptomatic whitish lesion, on the gingiva in relation to 13, 14, and 15. The lesion had existed for more than one year in duration which had initiated during her second pregnancy. She was otherwise healthy except for having mild hypochromic microcytic anaemia due to being a carrier for thalassemia trait. However, her serum ferritin levels were within the normal range. Her plaque control measures revealed brushing twice daily with a fluoridated toothpaste although supplementary tools were not used. Furthermore, the patient did not practice any risk habits such as betel chewing, smoking, or alcohol consumption.

Intraoral examination revealed a linear, plaque-like whitish lesion on the palatal and buccal free gingiva of 13, 14, and 15 (Figure 1). No verrucous/papillary appearance was evident, and the lesion was nonscrapable.

She had no other significant extraoral or intraoral findings, and the radiological examination in relation to the site was normal (Figure 2). As baseline investigations, an incisional biopsy was performed together with the necessary haematological investigations.

2.1. The Histological Findings. The histopathological analysis revealed a hyperorthokeratinized stratified squamous epithelium which showed cytological atypia in the lower part amounting to mild epithelial dysplasia with numerous koilocytes in the stratum spinosum (Figures 3 and 4).

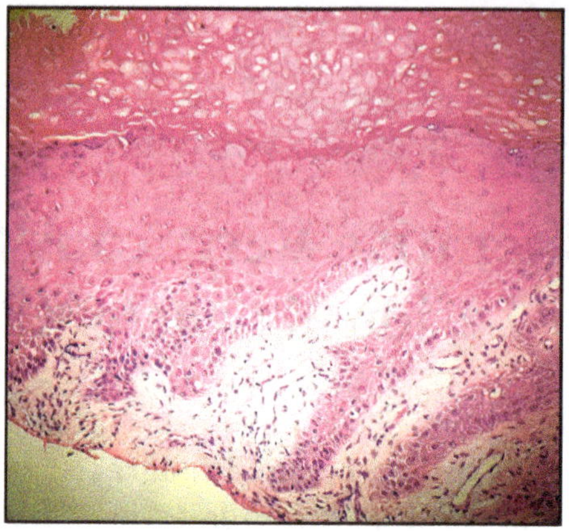

FIGURE 3: Keratosis with mild epithelial dysplasia under H&E staining.

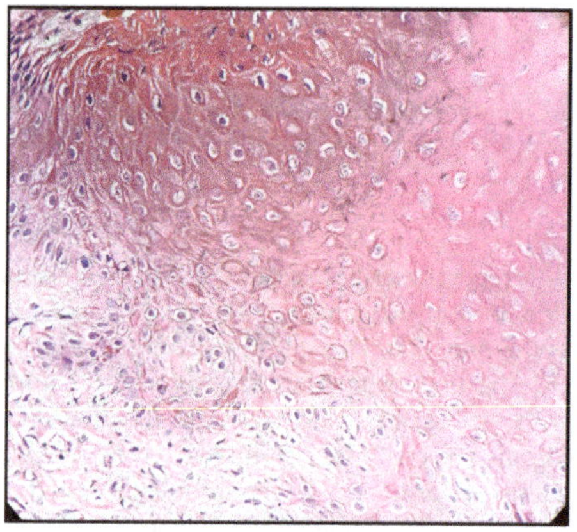

FIGURE 4: Koilocytic cells under ×40 magnification.

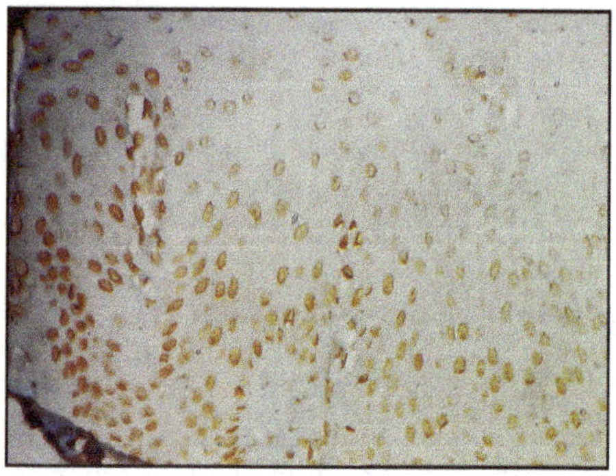

FIGURE 5: Immunohistochemical assay with p16 showing positive staining in >50% of the cells with >25% cell confluency.

Furthermore, due to the presence of koilocytosis, immunohistochemical evaluation was carried out with p16 antibody which clearly revealed positivity in >50% of the cells with >25% confluency (Figure 5). It is also worthwhile to mention that in the present lesion, nuclear staining was stronger compared to cytoplasmic staining.

However, as p16 is only a surrogate marker, it was not possible to confirm the high-risk HPV infection as the etiological factor for the present lesion due to the absence of adequate amount of fresh tissue. Therefore, considering the histological findings together with the clinical features, early stage of PVL was derived as the possible diagnosis.

2.2. Management. Thus, following informing the patient regarding the findings, she was referred for HIV and gynecological screening. The HIV test was negative, and she had no abnormalities detected with the gynecology screening.

However, despite the thorough probing into the possible causative factors including behavioural risk factors and habits, no aetiological factor for this oral lesion was revealed, except for p16 positivity, which could not be confirmed as due to a high-risk HPV infection with further investigations.

For the management of the lesion, resection of the lesion with adequate margins using CO_2 laser was carried out following improving the oral hygiene. Nevertheless, the lesion reappeared within few weeks at the same sites which led to perform a surgical resection with an adequate margin in the second attempt.

However, the lesion recurred similar to the initial presentation showing its resistance to excision. Thus, within a period of nearly six months, it recurred thrice despite electrosurgical interventions. Considering the diagnosis of PVL, currently, the patient is being followed up with short recall intervals and the lesion remains same with no significant change in size compared to the initial presentation.

3. Discussion

As the lesion described in the present report is a rare occurrence, difficulties were encountered when naming the lesion, especially with references to the terms "keratosis" and "leukoplakia." According to literature, similar lesions have been named as linear gingival keratosis [3] as well as linear gingival leukoplakia [9]. When linear gingival keratosis/leukoplakia reported in literature [10] was compared with the present lesion, it did not show bone erosion. In contrast to lesions reported in literature [9, 10], the present lesion showed dysplasia and p16 positivity. However, in this case, the lesion was diagnosed as an early stage of PVL rather than linear gingival keratosis, due to the fact that it occurred in a female in the gingiva and also as it was refractory to surgical management.

In frictional keratosis histology of the spinous layer often demonstrate intraepithelial edema and occasional vacuolated cells with pyknotic nuclei resembling koilocytes [3]. The diagnosis of frictional keratosis typically consists of a detailed clinical examination, considering the possible oral habits and the agents that may involve in the chronic trauma of the oral mucosa [10]. However, in the present case, no aetiological factor was found indicating frictional irritation. Furthermore, the patient did not reveal any possibility of chemical irritation. A minority of keratotic lesions show dysplastic changes [1]. In this case, although the dysplastic changes were mainly observed in the lower part of the epithelium, dyskeratosis and koilocytosis were mainly observed in the upper layers of the epithelium. Though, it was not possible to confirm the presence of high-risk HPV infection in the present lesion, it would be worthwhile to explore the contribution of HPV in future studies.

When considering the management, PVL is commonly treated with conventional surgery, electrocautery, laser ablation, and cryosurgery [11]. Except in conventional surgery where resection of the lesion is targeted, in other methods, the tissue destruction is obtained via intercellular and extracellular freezing, denaturing lipid-protein complexes, and cell dehydration. There are several advantages of using CO_2 lasers for oral lesions, particularly less intraoperative bleeding, minimal damage to adjacent tissue, delayed acute inflammatory reaction, and reduced myofibroblast activity, leading to reduced wound contraction and scarring [11]. In addition, though generally lesions that are diagnosed as mild epithelial dysplasia are followed up [1, 4, 12], surgical excision was planned due to aesthetic concerns of the patient.

PVL is a progressive disease and may not respond to traditional treatment [5] similar to the present case which showed a high recurrence rate despite the early interventions carried out in the management.

When there is no obvious aetiology for oral PVL, the lesions may be considered as leukoplakia and managed accordingly [12]. Furthermore, in the present case, histological diagnosis of koilocytic dysplasia was not excluded completely, though the lesion displayed histologic features of HPV infection such as koilocytosis and multinucleated keratinocytes.

4. Conclusion

The key feature in the case presented was the high recurrence rate showed despite the various treatment methods. Therefore, the patient should be followed up with close monitoring to detect any further increase in dysplastic changes which could follow with the presence of koilocytic cells and with PVL lesions. In addition, occurrence of early PVL lesions as gingival keratosis should be further explored.

Acknowledgments

We acknowledge the immense support given by the patient and the clinical staff of the respective clinics during the management.

References

[1] S. Warnakulasuriya, N. W. Johnson, and I. van der Waal, "Nomenclature and classification of potentially malignant disorders of the oral mucosa," *Journal of Oral Pathology & Medicine*, vol. 36, no. 10, pp. 575–580, 2007.

[2] V. C. Carrard and I. van der Waal, "A clinical diagnosis of oral leukoplakia; a guide for dentists," *Medicina Oral, Patología Oral y Cirugía Bucal*, vol. 23, no. 1, pp. e59–e64, 2017.

[3] M. D. Mignogna, G. Fortuna, S. Leuci et al., "Frictional keratoses on the facial attached gingiva are rare clinical findings and do not belong to the category of leukoplakia," *Journal of Oral and Maxillofacial Surgery*, vol. 69, no. 5, pp. 1367–1374, 2011.

[4] S. S. Napier and P. M. Speight, "Natural history of potentially malignant oral lesions and conditions: an overview of the literature," *Journal of Oral Pathology & Medicine*, vol. 37, no. 1, pp. 1–10, 2008.

[5] A. Munde and R. Karie, "Proliferative verrucous leukoplakia: an update," *Journal of Cancer Research and Therapeutics*, vol. 12, no. 2, pp. 469–473, 2016.

[6] S. Gandolfo, R. Castellani, and M. Pentenero, "Proliferative verrucous leukoplakia: a potentially malignant disorder involving periodontal sites," *Journal of Periodontology*, vol. 80, no. 2, pp. 274–281, 2009.

[7] S. B. Woo, E. C. Cashman, and M. A. Lerman, "Human papilloma virus-associated oral intraepithelial neoplasia," *Modern Pathology*, vol. 26, no. 10, pp. 1288–1297, 2013.

[8] S. Barasch, P. Mohindra, K. Hennrick, G. K. Hartig, P. M. Harari, and D. T. Yang, "Assessing p16 status of oropharyngeal squamous cell carcinoma by combined assessment of the number of cells stained and the confluence of p16 staining: a validation by clinical outcomes," *The American Journal of Surgical Pathology*, vol. 40, no. 9, pp. 1261–1269, 2016.

[9] N. Sapna and K. L. Vandana, "Idiopathic linear leukoplakia of gingiva: a rare case report," *Journal of Indian Society of Periodontology*, vol. 14, no. 3, pp. 198–200, 2010.

[10] T. Nagao, S. Warnakulasuriya, S. Hasegawa et al., "Elucidating risk factors for oral leukoplakia affecting gingivae in Japanese subjects," *Translational Research in Oral Oncology*, vol. 1, 2016.

[11] C. S. Farah and N. W. Savage, "Cryotherapy for treatment of oral lesions," *Australian Dental Journal*, vol. 51, no. 1, pp. 2–5, 2006.

[12] I. van der Waal, K. P. Schepman, E. H. van der Meij, and L. E. Smeele, "Oral leukoplakia: a clinicopathological review," *Oral Oncology*, vol. 33, no. 5, pp. 291–301, 1997.

23

The Creeping Attachment Induced Technique (CAIT) in Natural and Restored Teeth: Case Reports with 24 Months of Follow-Up

Michele Perelli,[1,2] Roberto Abundo,[1,2] Giuseppe Corrente,[1,2] and Paolo Giacomo Arduino[3]

[1]*Private Practice, Turin, Italy*
[2]*Department of Periodontology, University of Pennsylvania, PA, USA*
[3]*Department of Surgical Sciences, CIR-Dental School, University of Turin, Turin, Italy*

Correspondence should be addressed to Michele Perelli; micperelli@yahoo.it

Academic Editor: Sukumaran Anil

This article describes a nonsurgical approach for treating gingival recessions and increasing gingival thickness around the natural teeth. Two female patients, presenting gingival recessions at the maxillary frontal teeth, were treated. Patient #1 had a discrepancy among the central maxillary incisors' gingival margin, and tooth UL1 needed to be restored. Patient #2 presented a buccal gingival recession at tooth UL3. In both cases, the sulcular gingival margin was gently disephitelized with a diamond bur leaving the soft tissue healing by itself. After 4 weeks, the procedure was reperformed. After 6 months, the gingival margins appeared thicker and a creeping attachment was achieved in both cases, obtaining gingival symmetry, related to the adjacent or contralateral teeth, and root coverage. Gingival asymmetry, gingival recessions, and gingival thickness may be improved by means of a guided gentle nonsurgical stimulation, providing creeping attachment in the natural and also restored teeth, with a healthy and stable tissue after 24 months of follow-up.

1. Introduction

In a healthy periodontium, the free gingival margin is normally located 1-2 mm coronally to the cementum-enamel junction (CEJ) and follows her convex contour around the tooth [1]. When gingival recession occurs, the free gingival margin is positioned apically, with the root's surface exposed to the oral environment. Every single patient has a personal gingival biotype which determines the thickness of the keratinized tissue. According to Rasperini's report, gingival thickness can be easily recorded by means of dedicated probes [2]. A well-known classification of gingival recessions is based on their coronoapical extension (with or without involvement of the mucogingival junction) and on the interproximal periodontal support [3]. Gingival recessions may have different causes, often associated with cervical defects of the dental enamel, radicular dentin, or both, due to caries, mechanical abrasions, chemical erosions, or abfractions [4]. If possible, root coverage could be obtained with a mucoperiosteal coronally or lateral-coronally advanced flap [5]. Histological data provides that healing of this modality of treatment may lead to a new connective attachment in the inner part of the flap and a long junctional epithelium in the coronal part [6]. Clinical study also reported the decreasing of gingival recession (REC) and physiological probing pocket depth (PD) in treated teeth [7]. The authors also describe that the adjunct of a connective tissue graft may thicken the gingival biotype and improve the performance in root coverage [8]. Recently, some authors have described the BOP (Biologically Oriented Preparation) technique, developed to shape the gingival tissue around a prepared tooth with a nonsurgical approach, which enables, by means of an induced coagulum and a provisional crown adapted to protect it under and along the gingival margin, to obtain gingival regrowth with a stability of its position over time [9].

The aim of the present manuscript is to describe the healing capacity of the periodontal tissue, when properly stimulated, in the presence of a gingival recession with a modified nonsurgical technique. REC, biotype, and free gingival margin stability were also recorded in this 2-year follow-up prospective clinical study.

2. Case Presentation

Two female patients, not smokers, presenting gingival recessions at the maxillary teeth, were recruited and treated in the same private practice in Turin, Italy. Treatments were both performed in 2016 by the same clinician (M.P.). Patients did not report any contraindication to dental treatment. Patient #1 presented various maxillary gingival recessions; in particular, the left central incisor's free gingival margin was strongly misaligned compared to the contralateral tooth's gingival margin. Moreover, UL1 has been previously endodontically treated with an esthetical defect due to discoloration and radicular abrasion, having a buccal gingival margin almost 3 mm more apical than the contralateral (REC 3 mm), a 3 mm PD and showing a medium biotype (Figure 1). The treatment plane is aimed at reaching a pink and white aesthetic success by aligning the gingival parables of the central incisors and restoring the tooth with a ceramic crown.

Patient #2 presented a single I Miller class recession in correspondence with the maxillary left canine. No radicular abrasion or abfraction were noticed, while a small coronal abrasion in correspondence with the cementum-enamel junction (CEJ) was noticed. REC was 4 mm, PD was 2 mm, and a gingival biotype was detailed as a medium (Figure 2). The treatment plane is aimed at a complete root coverage.

Both subjects initially received nonsurgical periodontal therapy, including oral hygiene instructions and supra- and subgingival scaling as required. Oral hygiene instructions were given by experienced dental hygienists. During each visit, subjects were instructed about oral hygiene maintenance at home. Such instructions were reinforced at each visit and were personalised when necessary. Instructions included modified bass technique with soft brushes (for 1 month) and a subsequent switch to medium brushes associated with interdental brushes. The patients were advised to change brushes every month and to change interdental brushes every 2 weeks.

2.1. Patient #1. Tooth UL1 had endodontic retreatment; when tooth reconstruction and delivery of the provisional crown were performed, the full-mouth plaque score (FMPS) and the full-mouth bleeding score (FMBS) indexes were both less than 25%.

The tooth had vertical preparation, and temporary crown margins were adapted at first at the free gingival margin position (Figures 3 and 4). One week later after local anaesthesia, bone sounding was performed. The temporary crown buccal margin was 2 mm shortened, and the gingival epithelial components (sulcus and the upper part of the junctional epithelium) were gently disephitelized with a diamond flame bur (120-micron granulometry) and the root surface exposed to the oral environment planed and smoothed with manual curettes and washed with saline solution (Figures 5 and 6). The patient was

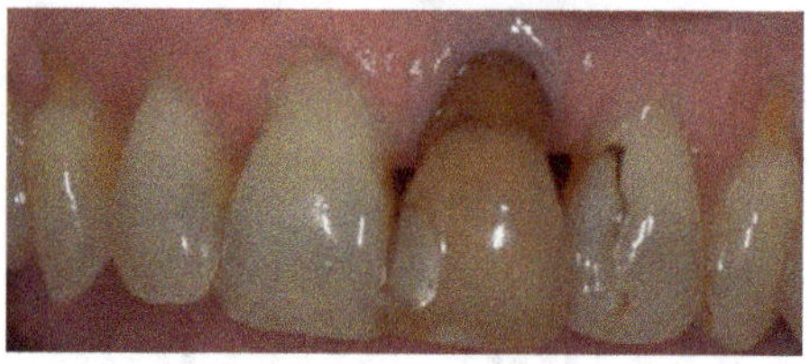

FIGURE 1: Patient #1: tooth UL1 presents an anaesthetic discoloration, cervical abrasion, thin gingival biotype, and free gingival margin discrepancy compared to the contralateral tooth.

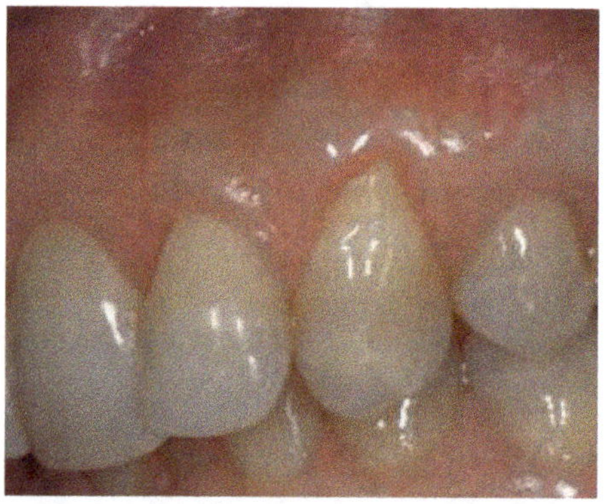

FIGURE 2: Patient #2: a buccal gingival recession of more than 2 mm is noticed in correspondence with UL3.

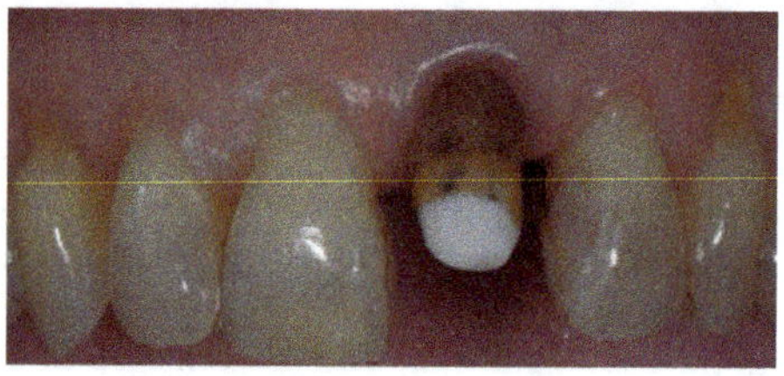

FIGURE 3: Central incisor was endodontically treated, restored with a composite post, and prosthetically prepared with a vertical finishing line.

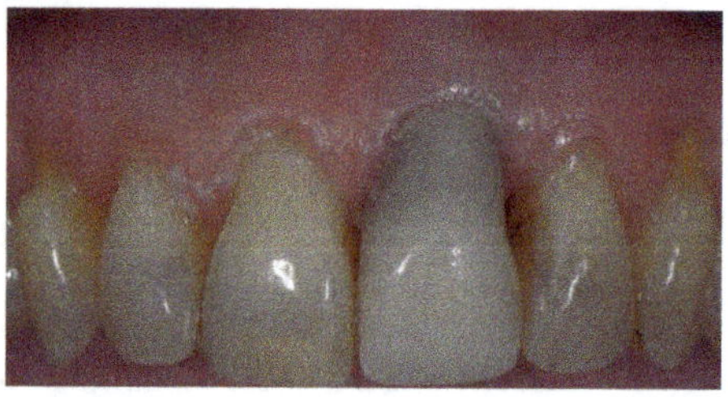

FIGURE 4: Temporary crown was delivered, and its cervical margin was located at the free gingival baseline position.

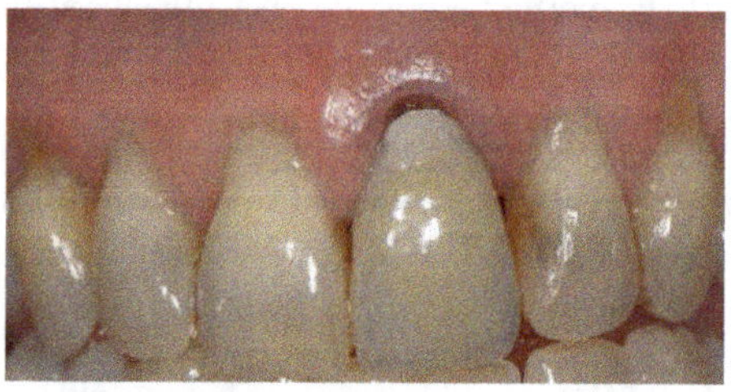

FIGURE 5: Temporary crown margin was 2 mm shortened.

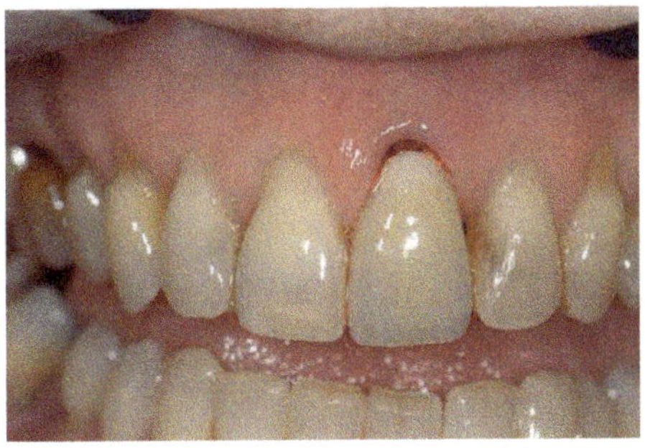

Figure 6: With diamond bur sulcus, junctional epithelium was gently removed, thus creating an induced inflammation.

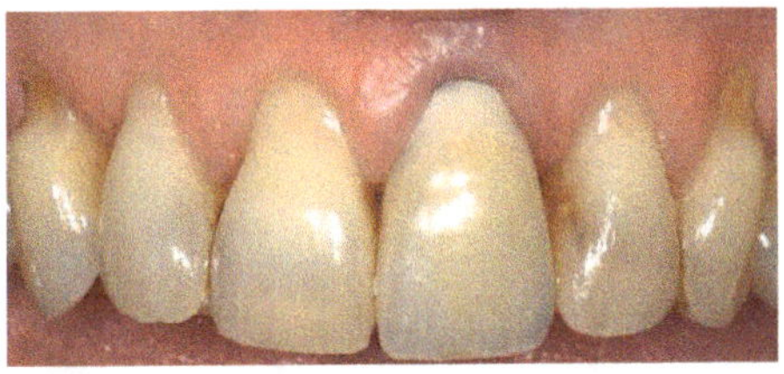

Figure 7: After 6 weeks, free gingival margin appeared thicker and an initial creeping can be noticed.

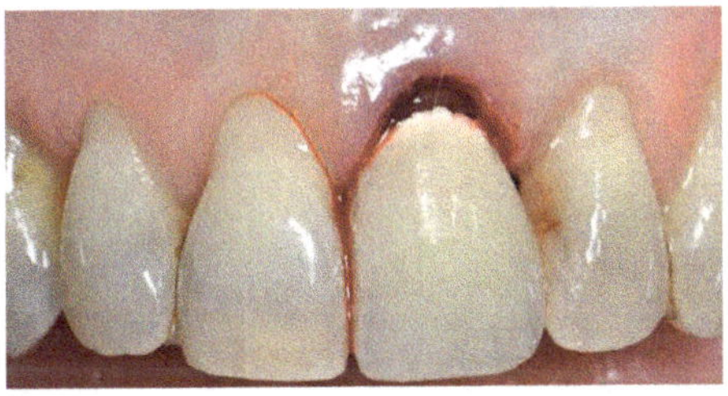

Figure 8: Temporary crown cervical margin was reshaped, mirroring the contralateral, and "stimulation" was performed again.

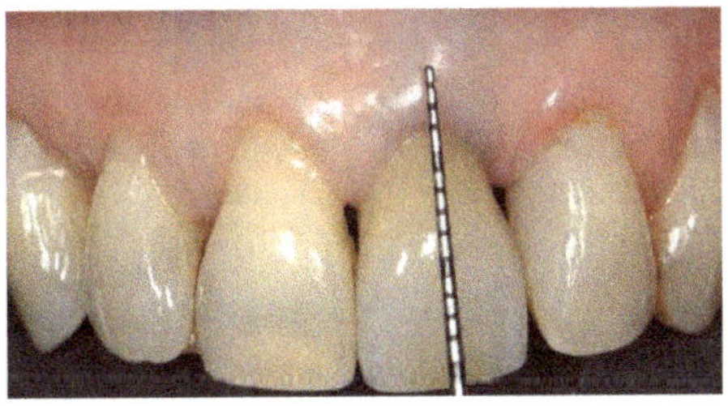

Figure 9: 10 month picture: central incisors free gingival margin was at the same level; creeping occurred on UL1, with the thickening of the biotype.

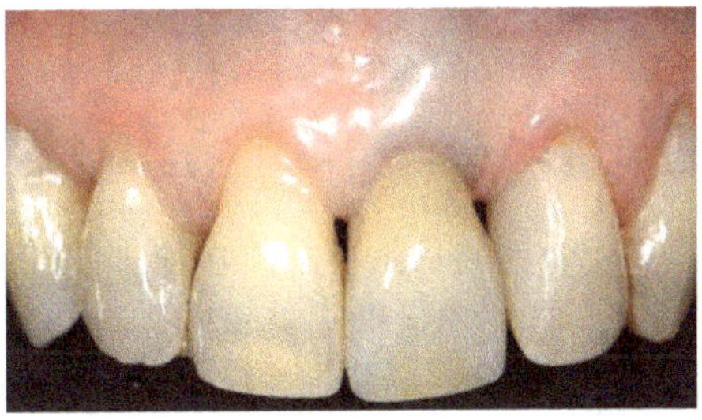

Figure 10: A definitive zirconia-ceramic crown was cemented (note the scalloped gingival architecture without scars or color mismatching). Control at 24 months of follow-up.

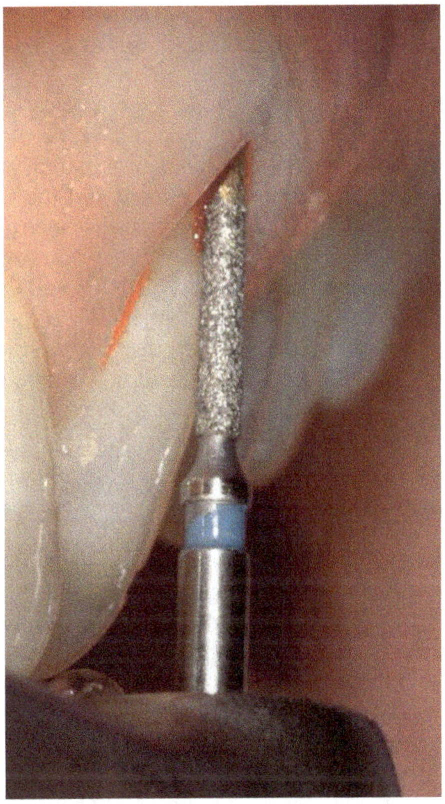

Figure 11: Radicular exposed surface was manually cleaned, and gingival epithelial components adjacent to the tooth were gently removed with a diamond bur.

instructed to clean the area with a 0.2% chlorhexidine spray solution twice a day for 4 weeks and not brushing the area. After 4 weeks, the gingival tissue appeared thicker, not inflamed, and an initial creeping was noticed. At this time, the patient started brushing with a soft toothbrush using the recommended technique. After 6 months, the gingival margin reached the temporary crown (Figure 7). Her buccal margin was shortened and aligned to the contralateral CEJ level, and the gingival margin was stimulated as before with the same postop chemical plaque control (Figure 8).

After 10 months, the maxillary central incisors presented free gingival margin at the same level with a different biotype, thicker on the treated gingiva. Impressions were taken and a zirconia-ceramic definitive crown was cemented to the tooth (Figure 9). At 2-year control, the free gingival margin's position was stable and the gingiva was in good health (Figure 10).

2.2. Patient #2. After professional scaling and root planning, FMBS and FMPS indexes were both less than 25%. After local anaesthesia, bone sounding was done. Using the same previous reported protocol, dental sulcus and coronal portion of the junctional epithelium were disephitelized with a diamond flame bur (120-micron granulometry), and the radicular surface was planed and smoothed with a manual curette (Figures 11 and 12). The patient was instructed not to brush the tooth for 4 weeks, using a 0.2% chlorhexidine spray twice a day for 4 weeks. Cold beverage and cold food were discouraged, in order to eventually prevent hypersensitivity. After 4 weeks, the free gingival margin appeared thicker with a slight creeping starting. In this second appointment, after local anaesthesia, the gingival margin was again stimulated as described before (Figure 13). The patient was instructed to start brushing the teeth after 4 weeks from this appointment. After 6 months, root coverage was reached, with a thick gingival margin and no pathological probing or inflammation (Figure 14). No dentin hypersensitivity was reported by the patient during this period.

In both patients, this technique demonstrated to be effective in gaining keratinized tissue and thickening the gingival biotype. In patient #1, the treated gingival margin had a coronal growth at the end of the treatment and the soft tissue marginal discrepancy among the incisors solved, with a creeping of almost 3 mm. There were no scars or tissues' blending; coverage of the exposed brown root and thickening of the gingiva were obtained. In patient #2, complete root coverage was achieved with a creeping of more than 2 mm also in this case. There was no dentin postop sensibility, and the PD was 2 mm. Results were stable at the 2-year follow-up (Figures 10 and 15).

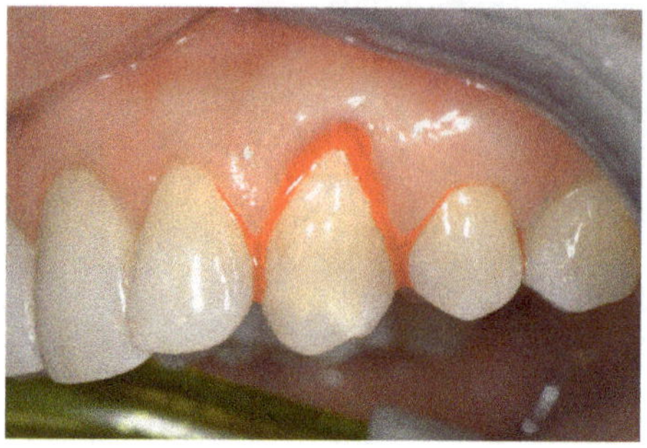

Figure 12: Marginal bleeding occurred with blood clot formation and stabilization.

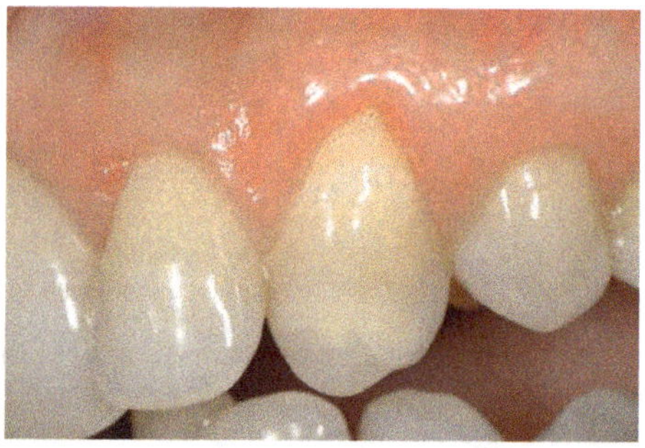

Figure 13: Gingival margin was thicker and again stimulated with the same protocol (4 weeks of follow-up).

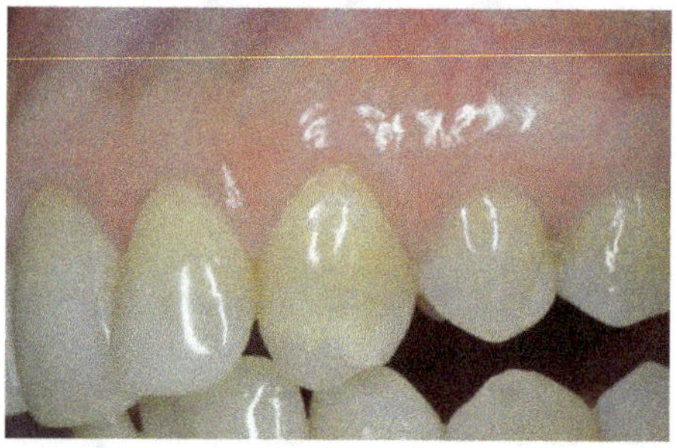

Figure 14: Complete root coverage was achieved by means of an induced creeping attachment at 6 months of follow-up; no scars and no tissue blending could be appreciated.

3. Discussion

Gingival wound healing is a complex and dynamic process, usually involving different cellular types and metabolic mediators. In this process, epithelial and connective tissues interact and stimulated each other. The blood clot organization and stabilization is the first important phase described. Blood clot contains growth factors and defensive cells and is self-sustaining on the cleaned root surface. It is followed by the granulation phase [10]. During this step, the connective tissue, which is the sustaining component of the soft tissues, may thicken because the cells contained in the coagulum can promote its formation. To confirm this, the first observation in the study was the thickening of the gingival biotype, acting as a "connective" response to the technique. The last phase is tissue maturation which can hesitate to creeping attachment [11, 12], even with more than 2 mm growth in coronoapical dimension with the establishment of a physiological healthy probing depth. This is probably linked to a tissue rebound due to a new, healthy, and stronger connective tissue which ensures a firm contact between junctional epithelium and the root surface and "pushes" the gingival margin coronally.

In literature, the term "creeping attachment" has been described occurring during the second month after surgery [13] and continuing for 12 months and more, sometimes without a constant progression pattern, and recently has been reported also around implants [14, 15].

Most of the studies available in the literature involving the creeping attachment are related to the use of free gingival autografts [16, 17]. Matter mentioned that the factors that seem to have a definite influence on the phenomenon of creeping attachment around the teeth are the width of the recession, the position of the graft, the bone resorption, the position of the tooth, and the hygiene of the patient [12]. The physiologic mechanism behind creeping attachment on the natural teeth has not yet been fully elucidated, and it seems to be a multifactorial and unpredictable phenomenon. The proliferation of periosteum-derived connective tissue cells in response to surgical trauma, the characteristics of the donor tissue, its ability to bridge over the root surface and proliferate, and mature once transplanted seem to be crucial in determining whether the gingival margin will ultimately creep in a coronal direction [13].

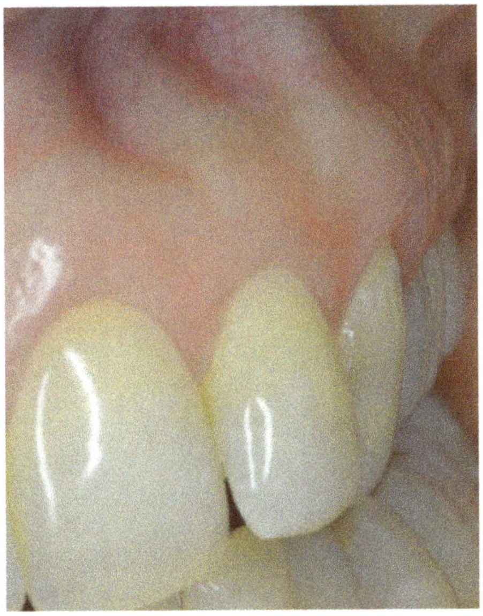

FIGURE 15: Stability of the root coverage on UL3 after 24 months.

It might be speculated that creeping attachment over the natural teeth might be more predominant due to the positive and favourable cellularity provided by the periosteum, and the capacity of the periodontal ligament to proliferate over a denuded root surface.

The reported stimulated nonsurgical biological approach may be useful to help clinicians in restoring dentogingival harmony and architecture both in the natural and restored teeth with good stability over time without any complications. An also important achieved result was the gingival thickening. In the present article, we have measured it with a dedicated probe and the results are in accordance with those reported by Agustin-Panadero and coworkers [18], describing a mean gingival thickening of 0.41 ± 0.28 mm for one-piece crowns and 0.38 ± 0.36 mm for FPD's, with gingival margin stability in all cases.

The findings of these two case reports must be investigated by studies with a larger number of patients, longer follow-up, and an evaluation in different gingival biotype and different clinical settings.

References

[1] J. Zweers, R. Z. Thomas, D. E. Slot, A. S. Weisgold, and F. G. A. van der Weijden, "Characteristics of periodontal biotype, its dimensions, associations and prevalence: a systematic review," *Journal of Clinical Periodontology*, vol. 41, no. 10, pp. 958–971, 2014.

[2] G. Rasperini, R. Acunzo, P. Cannalire, and G. Farronato, "Influence of periodontal biotype on root surface exposure during orthodontic treatment: a preliminary study," *The International Journal of Periodontics & Restorative Dentistry*, vol. 35, no. 5, pp. 665–675, 2015.

[3] P. D. Miller and E. P. Allen, "The development of periodontal plastic surgery," *Periodontology 2000*, vol. 11, no. 1, pp. 7–17, 1996.

[4] N. Guttiganur, S. Aspalli, M. V. Sanikop, A. Desai, R. Gaddale, and A. Devanoorkar, "Classification systems for gingival recession and suggestion of a new classification system," *Indian Journal of Dental Research*, vol. 29, no. 2, pp. 233–237, 2018.

[5] U. Pagliaro, M. Nieri, D. Franceschi, C. Clauser, and G. Pini-Prato, "Evidence-based mucogingival therapy. Part 1: a critical review of the literature on root coverage procedures," *Journal of Periodontology*, vol. 74, no. 5, pp. 709–740, 2003.

[6] K. Al-Hamdan, R. Eber, D. Sarment, C. Kowalski, and H. L. Wang, "Guided tissue regeneration-based root coverage: meta-analysis," *Journal of Periodontology*, vol. 74, no. 10, pp. 1520–1533, 2003.

[7] J. L. Wennstrom and G. Zucchelli, "Increased gingival dimensions. A significant factor for successful outcome of root coverage procedures? A 2-year prospective clinical study," *Journal of Clinical Periodontology*, vol. 23, no. 8, pp. 770–777, 1996.

[8] P. Cortellini, M. Tonetti, C. Baldi et al., "Does placement of a connective tissue graft improve the outcomes of coronally advanced flap for coverage of single gingival recessions in upper anterior teeth? A multi-centre, randomized, double-blind, clinical trial," *Journal of Clinical Periodontology*, vol. 36, no. 1, pp. 68–79, 2009.

[9] I. Loi and A. Di Felice, "Biologically oriented preparation technique (BOPT): a new approach for prosthetic restoration of periodontically healthy teeth," *The European Journal of Esthetic Dentistry*, vol. 8, no. 1, pp. 10–23, 2013.

[10] C. H. F. Hämmerle, W. V. Giannobile, and Working Group 1 of the European Workshop on Periodontology, "Biology of soft tissue wound healing and regeneration-consensus report of group 1 of the 10th European Workshop on Periodontology," *Journal of Clinical Periodontology*, vol. 41, pp. S1–S5, 2014.

[11] A. Santos, G. Goumenos, A. Pascual, and J. Nart, "Creeping attachment after 10 years of treatment of a gingival recession with acellular dermal matrix: a case report," *Quintessence International*, vol. 42, no. 2, pp. 121–126, 2011.

[12] J. Matter, "Free gingival grafts for the treatment of gingival recession. A review of some techniques," *Journal of Clinical Periodontology*, vol. 9, no. 2, pp. 103–114, 1982.

[13] A. Borghetti and J. P. Gardella, "Thick gingival autograft for the coverage of gingival recession: A clinical evaluation," *The International Journal of Periodontics & Restorative Dentistry*, vol. 10, no. 3, pp. 216–229, 1990.

[14] L. A. Bell, T. A. Valluzzo, J. J. Garnick, and B. M. Pennel, "The presence of "creeping attachment" in human gingiva," *Journal of Periodontology*, vol. 49, no. 10, pp. 513–517, 1978.

[15] C. Parra and D. Capri, "Peri-implant mucosal creeping: two case reports," *The International Journal of Periodontics & Restorative Dentistry*, vol. 38, no. 2, pp. 227–233, 2018.

[16] P. M. Camargo, P. R. Melnick, and E. B. Kenney, "The use of

free gingival grafts for aesthetic purposes," *Periodontology 2000*, vol. 27, no. 1, pp. 72–96, 2001.

[17] F. J. Otero-Cagide and M. F. Otero-Cagide, "Unique creeping attachment after autogenous gingival grafting: case report," *Journal of the Canadian Dental Association*, vol. 69, no. 7, pp. 432–435, 2003.

[18] R. Agustin-Panadero, B. Serra-Pastor, A. Fons-Font, and M. F. Sola-Ruiz, "Prospective clinical study of zirconia full-coverage restorations on teeth prepared with biologically oriented preparation technique on gingival health: results after two-year follow-up," *Operative Dentistry*, vol. 43, no. 5, pp. 482–487, 2018.

24

Actinomycosis as a Rare Local Manifestation of Severe Periodontitis

Moody Kaldas,[1,2] **André Barghorn,**[3] **and Patrick R. Schmidlin**[2]

[1]*Private Practice, Oetwil am See, Switzerland*
[2]*Clinic of Conservative and Preventive Dentistry, Center of Dental Medicine, University of Zurich, Switzerland*
[3]*Institute of Pathology Medica, Zurich, Switzerland*

Correspondence should be addressed to Patrick R. Schmidlin; patrick.schmidlin@zzm.uzh.ch

Academic Editor: Jose López-López

Actinomycosis is a chronic suppurative infection primarily caused by anaerobic gram-positive filamentous bacteria, primarily of the genus Actinomyces. Oral-cervicofacial actinomycosis is the localization found most often, presenting as a soft tissue swelling, an abscess, a mass lesion, or sometimes an ulcerative lesion. Periodontitis-like lesions, however, are rare findings. This report describes the case of a 41-year-old healthy female patient (nonsmoker), who was referred to the clinic with dull and throbbing pain in the second quadrant. Tooth 25 showed increased mobility and probing pocket depths up to 10 mm, with profuse bleeding upon probing. Radiographically, considerable interproximal horizontal bone loss was found, and the diagnosis of periodontitis stage 3, grade C was made. The situation was initially stabilized with adhesive splinting and local anti-infective therapy. Two weeks later, the bone defect was treated with guided tissue regeneration (GTR) using a xenogenic filler material (BioOss Collagen) and a resorbable membrane (Bio-Gide). Due to a suspicious appearance of the excised granulation tissue, the collected fragments were sent for histopathological evaluation. This evaluation revealed a chronic granulomatous inflammation with the presence of filamentous bacterial colonies, consistent with Actinomyces. The patient was successfully treated. While there are only few reports in the literature, actinomycotic lesions represent a rare but possible finding in cases with localized periodontal destruction. In conclusion, systematic biopsy of the infrabony tissue in localized periodontal lesions may help to provide a more accurate counting of Actinomyces-associated lesions, thereby improving diagnosis, therapy, and prevention.

1. Introduction

Actinomycosis is a chronic infectious disease, usually characterized by abscess formation and draining sinuses. It is known for more than a century to be caused mainly by gram-positive filamentous bacteria, which have a fungus-like histomorphological appearance. Typical intertwining bacterial filamentous colonies can be found, which are called sulfur granules because they macroscopically appear as yellowish specks [1]. Since these bacteria are frequently found in the mouth, nose, and throat regions, it is not surprising that actinomycosis mostly affects the face and neck regions. Cervicofacial actinomycosis accounts for about 50-60% of the cases [2]. Parotid and submandibular glands and the mandible are mostly affected [3]. The so-called "lumpy jaw" includes both soft and hard tissue of the head and neck regions [4]. Other localizations include the chest (pulmonary actinomycosis), abdomen, and pelvis. The bacterial infection always involves several genera of bacteria, which synergistically interact. However, the disease may not be diagnosed correctly unless the tissue is biopsied and the Actinomyces colonies are identified [4]. Actinomycosis is four times more common in men than in women and affects especially men between 20 and 60 years of age [5].

For disease establishment, bacteria must be able to enter and colonize tissues; for instance, due to trauma, surgery, or other common infection pathways. If an abscess occurs, the infection drains mostly through the skin and generates a sinus tract. Common accompanying symptoms are fever, mild or no pain, swelling or a hard, red to reddish-purple lump on the affected site. It is noteworthy that different Actinomyces strains exist in the physiologic and pathogenic oral flora [6]. Studies have shown coaggregations between strains of *A. viscosus* and *A. naeslundii* with oral streptococci-like *S. mitis* [7–9]. Specific morphological arrangements in the form of corncobs have also been observed [10, 11], which are mainly mediated by cell-surface interactions between bacterial receptors [8, 9]. Under physiological symbiotic conditions, these bacteria are commensals and do not cause pathologies. However, given specific dysbiotic circumstances, tissues may be damaged, invaded and opportunistic chronic or aggressive inflammatory processes may be initiated. In general, the functional integrity of the mucosal barrier or the periodontal ligament must be somehow compromised, allowing for access to the underlined tissues [12, 13]. Among the isolated Actinomyces species, *A. israelii* is the most common identified strain in actinomycosis. Coaggregated cells are more resistant to phagocytosis and killing by neutrophils and are therefore linked with pathogenicity [14].

In this report, we present a rare case of localized periodontal destruction between teeth 25 and 26, which was ultimately diagnosed as an actinomycosis (or Actinomyces-associated lesion) based on histopathology, although the clinical presentation resembled a simple localized severe periodontitis. It is noteworthy that approximately 14 percent of rare diseases with orofacial involvement also show manifestations in the form of gingivitis, periodontitis, and gingival hyperplasia in connection with the underlying disease [15]. However, the new classification of periodontal and peri-implant diseases and conditions does not consistently mention or classify them. Also, actinomycosis was not included and discussed. Therefore, we aim to highlight and describe the characteristics of this particular lesion, discussing the relevant literature and potential implications for future research.

2. Materials and Methods

2.1. Case Report. A 41-year-old female patient was referred by her private dentist to our clinic for a second opinion and treatment of a localized interdental periodontal bone defect between teeth 25 and 26. The patient was systemically healthy and a nonsmoker. Over the course of the previous two years, she had regularly attended maintenance appointments with her dentist and dental hygienist. A little over one year ago, a loss of bone level was observed; however, local therapy (scaling and root planning under local anesthesia) neither brought stagnation nor improvement. At this point, the periodontal referral was initiated.

At the time of the first evaluation, the patient was not suffering from acute pain. However, the patient reported an intermittent throbbing sensation in the interdental space and a feeling of pressure.

The patient displayed overall excellent oral hygiene (very minute visible plaque and calculus, if any), but—as a secondary sign of accentuated brushing habits—some recession, on the buccal surfaces, as well as initial noncarious cervical lesions (mixed erosions/abrasions). Intermittently, the patient noted some gingival bleeding, especially when using dental floss at this site. Tooth 25 showed increased tooth mobility (Grade 3) and probing pocket depths up to 10 mm, with profusive bleeding upon probing. Neither tooth 25 nor 26 had probable furcations. The periodontal screening indices (PSI) of the other sextants displayed values of a maximum of 2, which corresponded to no probing pocket depths greater than 3 mm and maybe some bleeding and even minute calculus (Figures 1(a) and 1(b)). In this context, some interdental attachment loss of the other teeth was up to 4 mm (>5 mm in the affected area).

The percussion test for teeth 25 and 26 was negative, and their vitality test positive (CO_2). Clinically, a missing papilla was noted. The col area was keratinized, and no signs of ulceration or necrosis were visible. The loss of tissue was radiographically corroborated, where a clear bone deficiency was visible (Figure 2(a)).

2.1.1. Diagnosis, Prognosis, and Treatment Plan. A localized severe periodontitis stage 3, grade C was diagnosed (formerly known as "localized aggressive periodontitis"). Since the patient was highly motivated, displayed good oral hygiene, had no furcation involvements, and was in good systemic health, with no history of smoking, the overall prognosis for therapy was considered to be good. The fact that an experienced dental hygienist had already performed subgingival scaling without any clinical success and subgingival calculus was not identifiable, we put a surgical intervention and focus to open inspection. A root fracture could also not be excluded, and therefore, explorative flap surgery was discussed with the patient. She was informed about all therapeutic options, i.e., primary, an open flap debridement, potentially with a regenerative procedure, materials, and costs. The regeneration of the defect was mainly dependent on the bony characteristics of the lesion (defect architecture, depth, and containing walls). A treatment plan consisting of xenogenic filler material application in combination with enamel matrix proteins and possibly fixing a membrane, if applicable, was determined. Intra- and postoperative risks were highlighted (mainly, infection and incomplete regeneration). The patient agreed to a surgical intervention with a regenerative approach (details of the respective intervention as actually performed will follow below). No bacterial test was performed due to the local characteristics of the lesion, and since a prescription of antibiotics has inherent risk factors, as such, the test was not planned at that stage.

2.1.2. Treatment. Due to the tooth mobility and functional overload of the involved teeth, an interdental splinting with composite resin material including occlusal adjustment was indicated and performed 2 weeks before surgery. Tooth 25 was even left in slight infraocclusion. Preoperatively, the patient received 500 mg mefenamic acid (Ponstan, Pfizer, Zurich, Switzerland). Under local anesthesia, a modified papilla preservation flap at the interdental papilla on the palatal site was prepared (surgery: PRS; Figure 1(c)). In order to avoid vertical incisions, the flap was extended to the mesial and distal aspects with a semilunar incision at the buccal site. A mucoperiosteal flap was prepared, and the defect thoroughly debrided of granulation tissue. The latter was found to be of a very unique consistency as compared to excised/removed periodontal granulation tissue, which normally consists merely of soft tissue. However, the removed material

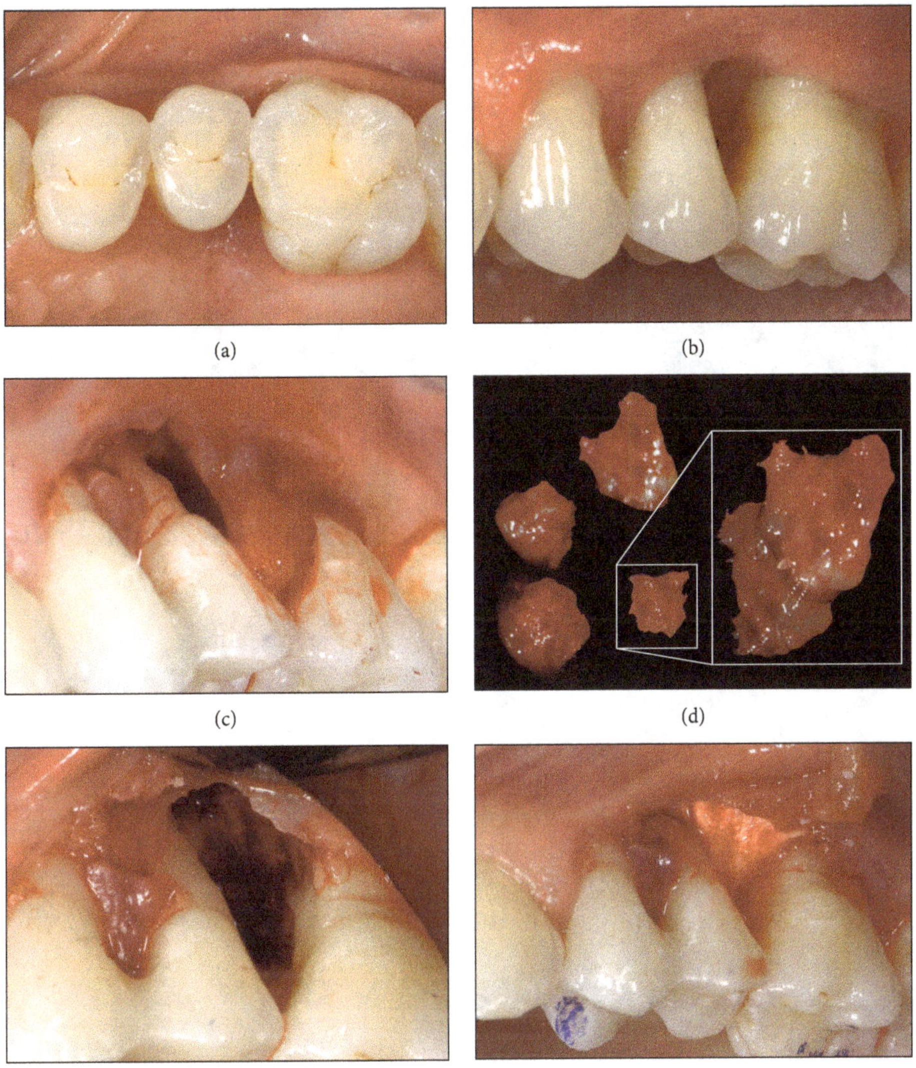

(a) (b) (c) (d) (e) (f)

FIGURE 1: Clinical images of the case before therapy (a, b). A periodontal flap was raised (c), and granulation tissue was removed (d). The defect (e) was filled with a xenogenic material and covered with a resorbable membrane (f).

contained filamentous and relatively hard granular particles (Figure 1(d)). Therefore, a histological analysis of the solid collectable tissues was deemed advisable and this tissue was transferred to a biopsy vial. Afterwards, the tooth surfaces were thoroughly cleaned and the defects abundantly rinsed with PVP iodine (Betadine, Mundipharma) [16]. Afterwards, the defect was inspected for tissue and calculus remnants (Figure 1(e)). A fracture of the root or other hard tissue-related complications such as cemental tears were excluded [17]. The area was rinsed with sterile saline solution and dried with swabs. Then, enamel matrix derivatives (EMD, Straumann, Basel, Switzerland) were added to the dry tooth surface and a mixture of 90% bovine bone granules with the addition of 10% porcine collagen (Bio-Oss Collagen, Geistlich, Wolhusen, Switzerland) was filled into the defect and adapted. The latter had been soaked with EMD before application for 5 minutes. Finally, a resorbable collagen membrane (Bio-Gide, Geistlich) was applied to cover the filled defect (Figures 1(f) and 2(b)) and the defect closed. For prophylactic measures, clindamycin (Dalacin C, Pfizer, Zurich, Switzerland) was prescribed for 7 days with a suggested intake 3 times 300 mg per day. Pain killers (mefenamic acid, Ponstan) were prescribed for the first two days, if needed.

The biopsy samples were fixed in 4% neutral-buffered formalin solution and processed according to standard protocols. The slides were stained with hematoxylin and eosin (H&E), elastica van Gieson (EvG), periodic acid Schiff's reaction (PAS), Gram, and Giemsa using a Tissue-Tek Prisma stainer module (Sakura Seiki, Nagano, Japan) and commercial staining solutions. Additional stains included Grocott and Ziehl-Neelsen executed on a VENTANA BenchMark Special Stains stainer module (Roche Diagnostics, Risch-Rotkreuz, Switzerland) using the manufacturers' GMS II Staining Kit and AFB III Staining Kit, respectively.

After one week of uneventful healing, sutures were removed, proper oral hygiene was reinforced, and the patient was instructed to continue rinsing with antiseptic up to 6 weeks.

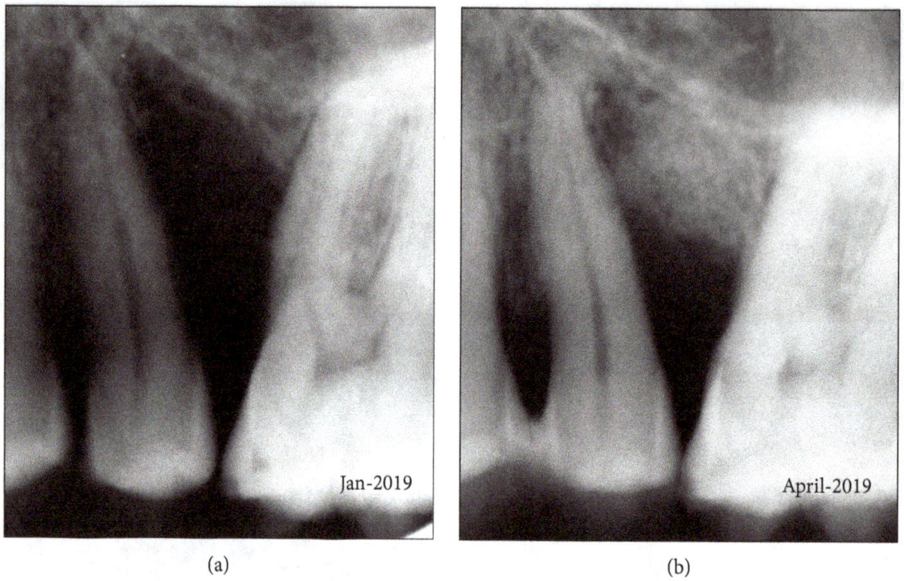

FIGURE 2: Radiographs before (a) and after surgery (b).

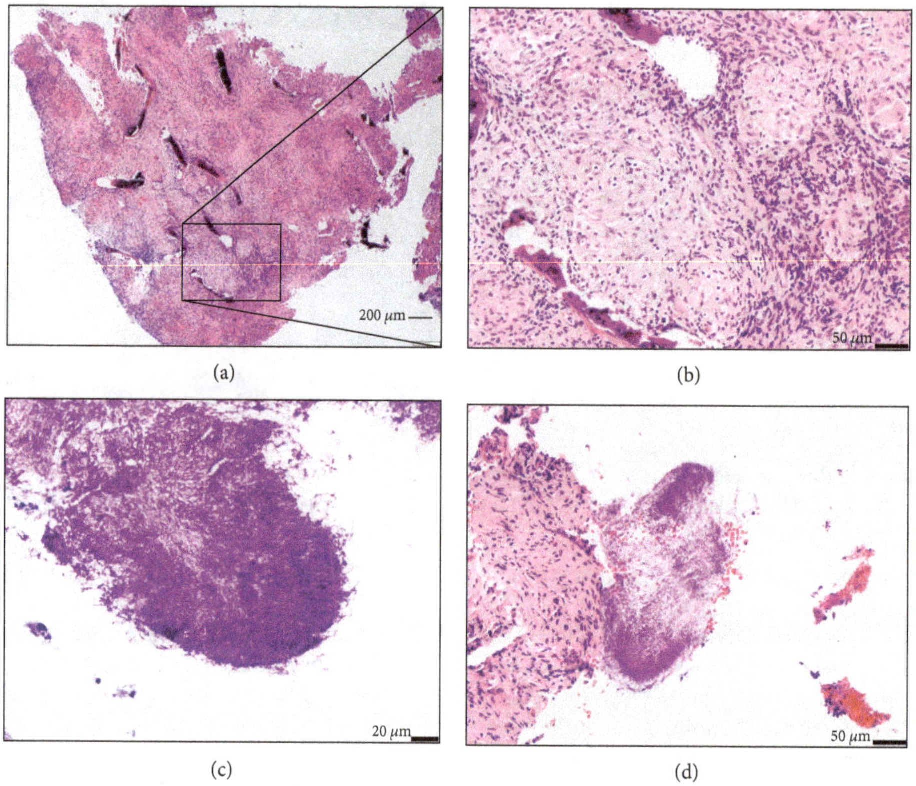

FIGURE 3: Histology of a representative tissue fragment with clearly visible bone trabeculae and neutrophil infiltration (a), at higher magnification (b). Also visible were different colonies of bacteria (mainly Actinomyces spp.) between and adherent between the tissue fragments (c, d).

3. Results

3.1. Histologic Evaluation. The biopsy samples showed an extensive epithelioid granulomatous reaction with Langhans giant cells, fibrosis and 4n destruction and focal remodeling (Figures 3(a) and 3(b)). Fragments with squamous epithelium demonstrated intraepithelial neutrophilic infiltration and subepithelial aggregations of lymphocytes and abundant plasma cells. On the surface of the biopsy, colonies of filamentous bacteria were identified (Figures 3(c) and 3(d)). These were positive for gram and PAS stains but not for Ziehl-Neelsen' stain, consistent with Actinomyces spp. Acid fast bacteria were not detected.

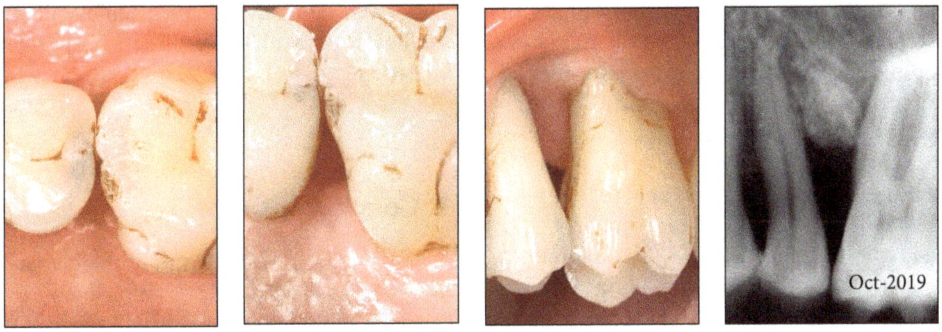

(a) (b) (c) (d)

Figure 4: Clinical outcome revealed no residual pockets > 3 mm and no bleeding on probing; some staining was visible due to rinsing with chlorhexidine (a–c). The radiograph showed a densification of the grafted site and stable conditions (d).

Table 1: Overview on the available case reports.

Study	Clinical diagnosis	Histology	Age/sex	Tooth/teeth	Systemic diseases	Therapy
[2]	Adult periodontitis, local abscess	Yes	60/f	33/34	n.a.	Debridement, doxycycline, chlorhexidine
[18]	Localized periodontitis	Yes/no images shown	38/f	26/27	Depression	Debridement, excision, amoxicillin
[19]	Chronic periodontitis	Yes	46/f	46	Rheumatic mitral insufficiency	Scalin & root planning, flap surgery with GTR, amoxicillin with clavulanate
[20]	Juvenile periodontitis	Yes	14/f	33/34	Epilepsy	Excision, penicillin
This study	Localized severe periodontitis stage 3 and grade C	Yes	41/f	25/26	Healthy	Flap surgery and GTR

n.a.: not available; f: female; GTR: guided tissue regeneration.

3.2. Clinical Outcome. No probing was performed until six months postoperative. At this reevaluation point, no probing depths exceeding 3 mm were found and no bleeding upon probing was observed. The interdental soft tissues displayed adequate keratinization, with no signs of inflammation (Figures 4(a)–4(c)). The radiograph showed a consolidation of the implanted material, with some accentuated mineralization (Figure 4(d)).

4. Discussion

The case presented showed clinical features which were diagnosed as a severe periodontitis stage 3, grade C. Extensive localized attachment and bone loss were apparent and were corroborated by radiographs. A histologic evaluation of the excised granulation tissue ultimately revealed the presence of gram-positive filamentous bacterial colonies, consistent with Actinomyces spp. The question as to whether local trauma and/or infection caused disease initiation and progression between the two teeth in the absence of actual systemic or environmental risk factors remains speculative. Lesions related to actinomycosis have been described previously in a few periodontitis case reports (Table 1) [2; 18-20].

Despite previous data showing that actinomycosis is more common in men than in women [5], all identified publications reported on cases in females, with one case in a very young patient, but all clinically diagnosed with periodontitis. Unfortunately, the new classification of periodontal and peri-implant diseases and conditions does not mention it. It seems, therefore, important to have actinomycosis as a potential distinct pathway of localized periodontitis in mind, which could be—at least—considered an atypical presentation of local tissue destruction resembling periodontitis. It may even be a distinct disease entity. Oral actinomycosis is not a common disease, but it can cause massive destruction. Interestingly, implant failure mimicking peri-implantitis associated with actinomycosis has also been reported in the literature as well [21].

As always—when looking at isolated destructive processes—the question arises as to which specific (local) causes can explain such devastating tissue involvement. Several explanations for isolated defects have been described in the literature: vertical root fractures [22], endoperiolesions [23], functional overload [24], foreign body reactions [25], and cemental tears [16, 26]. Clinicians must always be aware of such potential implications, but a clear identification of the causative agent is sometimes very difficult clinically. Periodontitis in younger patients, formerly known as early-onset, juvenile, or aggressive periodontitis also reveals distinct patterns of local or generalized, but sometimes symmetric involvement of teeth and sites. The reason for this remains unclear; however, age at onset, the duration, and the frequency of systemic factors give rise to a possible distinction between localized or more generalized forms [27]. Obviously, bacterial colonization of the tissues remains the primary or major cause for attachment loss. The composition and grade of infection may be influenced by systemic, environmental and local factors as mentioned above [28]. Especially when facing local infestations, the role of a true infective process becomes more prominent [29]. Actinomycosis, a chronic infection primarily caused by gram-positive anaerobic bacteria, can display acute and chronic infective features.

The organisms may histologically display a number of fungus-like characteristics, i.e., a tendency to grow as mass of rounded bodies (clubs) and filaments. Due to a rather low intrinsic virulence, a chronic granulomatous tissue response is frequent. Acute forms normally display a rather sudden onset and one or more multiple pus discharging sinuses containing sulphur granules. In the case of periodontitis-like lesions, the sulcus and pocket may be considered a draining surrogate and the progression and clinical presentation may be completely different.

Our case should be considered a gradual onset with typical signs of inflammation, which led to bone involvement and loss with fibrosis rather than suppuration, which renders a proper clinical diagnosis even more difficult. Actinomycosis is considered one of the most "misdiagnosed diseases" and is listed as a "rare disease "by the National Institute of Health (NIH) [30]. Its implication in periodontitis has been vastly neglected so far.

However, reports of cases are growing—given a global look at actinomycosis according to a systematic review of pediatric cases—which showed 10 reports were made during the past 11 years, while only 20 cases were described in a 48-year period [31]. This was mainly attributed to more modern diagnostic techniques.

When it comes to treatment of Actinomyces-associated lesions, removal of the foci of infection including the excision of all involved granular soft tissue and sequestrated bone is mandatory. Penicillin administration has also recommended and showed better in vitro activity as compared to other antibiotics including clindamycin [32]. In the case of periodontitis, the sole prescription of penicillin is not a frequent therapeutic scheme; however, it is frequently prescribed in orofacial infections [33, 34]. As this case showed, removal of the affected tissues and proper debridement resulted in an adequate healing response. In the present case, clindamycin was mainly prescribed as a bacteriostatic agent in order to avoid (re) infection of the implanted materials. Since chronic infections may include aerobes and anaerobes, clindamycin may have a role in the therapy of these infections; however, the spectrum against the main putative periodontopathogens remains rather low, but it has been described as an alternative for treatment of several head and neck infections.

One important question remains, namely, how the diagnosis of "actinomycosis-" or "Actinomyces-associated lesion" can actually influence the treatment, since it can only be provided after tissue removal during surgery and after histological evaluation, which may take some time. This implies that at the day of surgery, important information may still be missing. If there is a difference in selective treatment options, i.e., the standard protocol of localized periodontal destruction with or without Actinomycosis infection remains to be elaborated and more epidemiological data on potential implications of this rare disease in periodontology have to be gathered.

5. Conclusions

Actinomycosis infection should be considered in case of an uncommon localized destruction in the periodontium, and biopsies including histopathologic evaluations should be envisaged.

Acknowledgments

This work was funded by the Clinic of Conservative and Preventive Dentistry, Center of Dental Medicine, University of Zurich, Switzerland, as part of a Master thesis.

References

[1] R. A. Smego Jr. and G. Foglia, "Actinomycosis," *Clinical Infectious Diseases*, vol. 26, no. 6, pp. 1255–1261, 1998.

[2] U. Sakallioglu, G. Acikgoz, T. Kirtiloglu, and F. Karagöz, "Rare lesions of the oral cavity: case report of an actinomycotic lesion limited to the gingiva," *Journal of Oral Science*, vol. 45, no. 1, pp. 39–42, 2003.

[3] J. K. Park, H. K. Lee, H. K. Ha, H. Y. Choi, and C. G. Choi, "Cervicofacial actinomycosis: CT and MR imaging findings in seven patients," *American Journal of Neuroradiology*, vol. 24, no. 3, pp. 331–335, 2003.

[4] S. Tortorlci, F. Burruano, M. L. Buzzanca, P. Difalco, D. Cabibi, and E. Maresi, "Cervico-facial actinomycosis: epidemiological and clinical comments," *American Journal of Infectious Diseases*, vol. 4, no. 3, pp. 203–208, 2008.

[5] G. Pulverer, H. Schütt-Gerowitt, and K. P. Schaal, "Human cervicofacial actinomycoses: microbiological data for 1997 cases," *Clinical Infectious Diseases*, vol. 37, no. 4, pp. 490–497, 2003.

[6] I. Kaplan, K. Anavi, Y. Anavi et al., "The clinical spectrum of _Actinomyces_ -associated lesions of the oral mucosa and jawbones: correlations with histomorphometric analysis," *Oral Surgery, Oral Medicine, Oral Pathology, Oral Radiology, and Endodontology*, vol. 108, no. 5, pp. 738–746, 2009.

[7] G. Borgeau and B. C. McBride, "Dextran-mediated interbacterial aggregation between dextran-synthesizing streptococci and Actinomyces viscosus," *Infection and Immunity*, vol. 13, no. 4, pp. 1228–1234, 1976.

[8] J. O. Cisar, P. E. Kolenbrander, and F. C. McIntire, "Specificity of coaggregation reactions between human oral streptococci and strains of Actinomyces viscosus or Actinomyces naeslundii," *Infection and Immunity*, vol. 24, no. 3, pp. 742–752, 1979.

[9] F. C. McIntire, A. E. Vatter, J. Baros, and J. Arnold, "Mechanism of coaggregation between Actinomyces viscosus T14V and streptococcus sanguis 34," *Infection and Immunity*, vol. 21, no. 3, pp. 978–988, 1978.

[10] S. J. Jones, "A special relationship between spherical and filamentous microorganisms in mature human dental plaque," *Archives of Oral Biology*, vol. 17, no. 3, pp. 613–616, 1972.

[11] M. A. Listgarten, H. Mayo, and M. Amsterdam, "Ultrastructure of the attachment device between coccal and filamentous microorganisms in "corn cob" formations of dental plaque," *Archives of Oral Biology*, vol. 18, no. 5, pp. 651–IN5, 1973.

[12] M. M. Curi, L. L. Dib, L. P. Kowalski, G. Landman, and C. Mangini, "Opportunistic actinomycosis in osteoradionecrosis of the jaws in patients affected by head and neck cancer : incidence and clinical significance," *Oral Oncology*, vol. 36, no. 3, pp. 294–299, 2000.

[13] D. De, S. Dogra, A. J. Kanwar, and U. N. Saikia, "Actinomycosis presenting as a destructive ulcerated plaque on the palate and gingiva," *Journal of the American Academy of Dermatology*, vol. 65, no. 6, pp. 1235-1236, 2011.

[14] K. Ochiai, T. Kurita-Ochiai, Y. Kamino, and T. Ikeda, "Effect of co-aggregation on the pathogenicity of oral bacteria," *Journal of Medical Microbiology*, vol. 39, no. 3, pp. 183–190, 1993.

[15] M. Hanisch, "Rare diseases with periodontal manifestations," *International Journal of Environmental Research and Public Health*, vol. 16, no. 5, p. 867, 2019.

[16] P. Sahrmann, T. Imfeld, V. Ronay, T. Attin, and P. R. Schmidlin, "Povidone-iodine gel and solution as adjunct to ultrasonic debridement in nonsurgical periodontitis treatment: an RCT pilot study," *Quintessence International*, vol. 45, no. 4, pp. 281–290, 2014.

[17] P. R. Schmidlin, "Regenerative treatment of a cemental tear using enamel matrix derivatives: a ten-year follow-up," *The Open Dentistry Journal*, vol. 6, no. 1, pp. 148–152, 2012.

[18] R. Rodan, "Unusual presentation of Actinomycosis misdiagnosed as severe periodontal destruction," *Journal of the Royal Medical Services*, vol. 19, no. 1, pp. 53–56, 2012.

[19] N. R. Kim, J. B. Park, and Y. Ko, "Differential diagnosis and treatment of periodontitis-mimicking actinomycosis," *Journal of Periodontal Implant Science*, vol. 42, no. 6, pp. 256–260, 2012.

[20] R. M. Nagler, Y. Ben-Arieh, and D. Laufer, "Case report of regional alveolar bone actinomycosis: a juvenile periodontitis-like lesion," *Journal of Periodontology*, vol. 71, no. 5, pp. 825–829, 2000.

[21] C. X. Sun, J. M. Henkin, C. Ririe, and E. Javadi, "Implant failure associated with actinomycosis in a medically compromised patient," *Journal of Oral Implantology*, vol. 39, no. 2, pp. 206–209, 2013.

[22] R. E. Walton, "Vertical root fracture: factors related to identification," *Journal of the American Dental Association*, vol. 148, no. 2, pp. 100–105, 2017.

[23] W. H. Christie and A. F. Holthuis, "The endo-perio problem in dental practice: diagnosis and prognosis," *Journal of the Canadian Dental Association*, vol. 56, no. 11, pp. 1005–1011, 1990.

[24] R. V. Murali, P. Rangarajan, and A. Mounissamy, "Bruxism: conceptual discussion and review," *Journal of Pharmacology and Bioallied Sciences*, vol. 7, no. 5, pp. 267–270, 2015.

[25] M. N. Al-Qutub, "Orthodontic elastic band-induced periodontitis - a case report," *The Saudi Dental Journal*, vol. 24, no. 1, pp. 49–53, 2012.

[26] P. Y. Jeng, A. L. Luzi, R. M. Pitarch, M. C. Chang, Y. H. Wu, and J. H. Jeng, "Cemental tear: to know what we have neglected in dental practice," *Journal of the Formosan Medical Association*, vol. 117, no. 4, pp. 261–267, 2018.

[27] L. Blomlöf, L. Hammarstrom, and S. Lindskog, "Occurrence and appearance of cementum hypoplasias in localized and generalized juvenile periodontitis," *Acta Odontologica Scandinavica*, vol. 44, no. 5, pp. 313–320, 1986.

[28] T. Larsen and N. E. Fiehn, "Dental biofilm infections - an update," *APMIS Journal of Pathology, Microbiology and Immunology*, vol. 125, no. 4, pp. 376–384, 2017.

[29] A. Mira, A. Simon-Soro, and M. A. Curtis, "Role of microbial communities in the pathogenesis of periodontal diseases and caries," *Journal of Clinical Periodontology*, vol. 44, no. 18, pp. S23–S38, 2017.

[30] O. P. Talwar, A. Ghosh, S. Pradhan, R. M. Swami, and K. C. Shivraj, "A prospective and retrospective study of actinomycosis in last five years at Manipal Teaching Hospital, Pokhara, Nepal," *Kathmandu University medical journal (KUMJ)*, vol. 5, no. 4, pp. 488–491, 2007.

[31] S. Oppenheimer, G. S. Miller, K. Knopf, and H. Blechman, "Periapical actinomycosis: An unusual case report," *Oral Surgery, Oral Medicine, Oral Pathology*, vol. 46, no. 1, pp. 101–106, 1978.

[32] D. W. LeCorn, F. J. Vertucci, M. F. Rojas, A. Progulske-Fox, and M. Bélanger, "In Vitro Activity of Amoxicillin, Clindamycin, Doxycycline, Metronidazole, and Moxifloxacin Against Oral Actinomyces," *Journal of Endodontics*, vol. 33, no. 5, pp. 557–560, 2007.

[33] N. Dar-Odeh, H. T. Fadel, S. Abu-Hammad, R. Abdeljawad, and O. A. Abu-Hammad, "Antibiotic prescribing for orofacial infections in the paediatric outpatient: a review," *Antibiotics*, vol. 7, no. 2, p. 38, 2018.

[34] A. Mombelli, "Microbial colonization of the periodontal pocket and its significance for periodontal therapy," *Periodontology 2000*, vol. 76, no. 1, pp. 85–96, 2018.

25

Symptomatic Apical Periodontitis of the Mandibular First Molar with the Accessory Canal in the Furcation Area Mimicking Furcation Perforation

Alexei Bolyachin[1] **Zurab Khabadze**[2] **Oleg Mordanov**[2] **Magomed Gasbanov**[1,2] **and Takhir Teberdiev**[1]

[1]*Iceberg Dental Trauma Center, Moscow, Russia*
[2]*RUDN University (People's Friendship University of Russia), Moscow, Russia*

Correspondence should be addressed to Oleg Mordanov; mordanov19@gmail.com

Academic Editor: Konstantinos Michalakis

Apical periodontitis frequently presents as a chronic disease. To arrive at a true diagnosis, in addition to the clinical examination, it is mandatory to undertake radiographic examinations and evaluate the clinical presentation. Knowledge of the root canal morphology is a prerequisite for effective nonsurgical endodontic treatment. The internal morphological features of the pulp chamber are variable and complex. This case report describes the treatment and outcome of symptomatic apical periodontitis of a mandibular first molar with the accessory (chamber) canal. The applied treatment fully contributed to the periapical lesion regression as shown in the four-year recall periapical radiography.

1. Introduction

Apical periodontitis is mainly a root canal infection, characterized by inflammation and destruction of periapical and periradicular tissues resulting from the interaction between microbial factors and the host immune response [1, 2]. Destruction of the periodontal ligament is triggered by degradation of the extracellular matrix by metalloproteinases (MMPs) [3] involving periradicular inflammation and bone destruction mediated by proinflammatory cytokines [4].

Normal oral microorganisms and bacteria may give rise to opportunistic pathogens if access to dental pulp tissues appears. Openings in the physical dentin barriers (enamel and cementum) by means of caries, cracks, or traumatic injuries create pathways for bacteria into the pulp chamber and root canal system consequently [5].

Communication between the pulp and the periodontal ligament may occur via the apical foramen and lateral and accessory canals in the apical and coronal parts of the root. Despite careful selection of cases and the use of correct procedures, endodontic treatment occasionally fails, and it can be due to the presence of communications between the pulp tissues and periodontal tissues [6].

Accessory canals result due to a localized failure in the formation of Hertwig's sheath during the embryonic stages of tooth formation. This defect is probably due to the persistence of abnormally placed blood vessels reaching the pulp, which is more common in the furcation region [6].

These canals are also known as interradicular canals [7]. In 2018, Ahmed et al. [8] suggested a new accessory canal classification. The proposed classification provides an accurate description of the position and configuration of the accessory and chamber canals. By chamber canals, the authors mean small canals leaving the pulp chamber that (usually) communicates with the external surface of the root (including the furcation) (Figure 1).

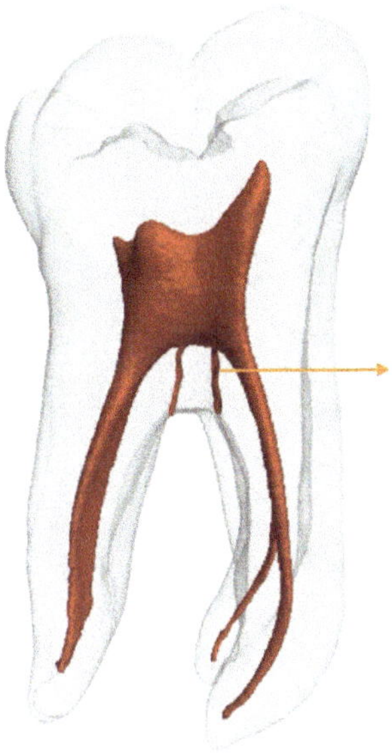

Figure 1: Schematic representation showing chamber canals.

The aim of this case report is to present the treatment and healing of apical chronic periodontitis with isolated furcation bone and apical bone destruction.

2. Case Report

A 27-year-old female patient with noncontributory general medical history presented and was referred to the dental practice in Moscow, Russia. The patient presented to the clinic with the complaint that included nonacute pain forcing on the tooth load during mastication from tooth # 46.

Pulp testing with carbon dioxide did not show any expressive reaction. Percussion was positive. Periodontal probing depth was 3 mm in average.

Periapical radiograph revealed a deep carious lesion in the distal surface of the tooth, communicating with the pulp chamber; there is presence of a radiolucency in the furcation region, not connected with the apical bone lesions present in both roots. No endodontic treatment had been previously performed (Figure 2).

The pulp chamber floor examination with the operative microscope (Carl Zeiss Meditec AG, Jena, Germany) with different zooming revealed no furcation, perforation, or fracture.

The following treatment strategy was applied. Coronal root canal portion was instrumented with Protaper SX (Dentsply Maillefer, Ballaigues, Switzerland) following a glide path development with C-Pilot (VDW, Munich, Germany) 6-15 ISO sizes. The shaping was provided with FlexMaster (Vereinigte, Dentalwerke, Munich, Germany) 15-35 ISO sizes, 4% tapered.

Irrigation protocol included the following: 3% NaOCl, 19% EDTA with the EndoActivator System (Dentsply Tulsa Dental Specialties, Tulsa, OK, USA). Pulp chamber irrigant solution was intensively activated with the ultrasound E4 tip, 3 cycles. Every cycle time was 30 seconds with 30% of ultrasound power in the general mode.

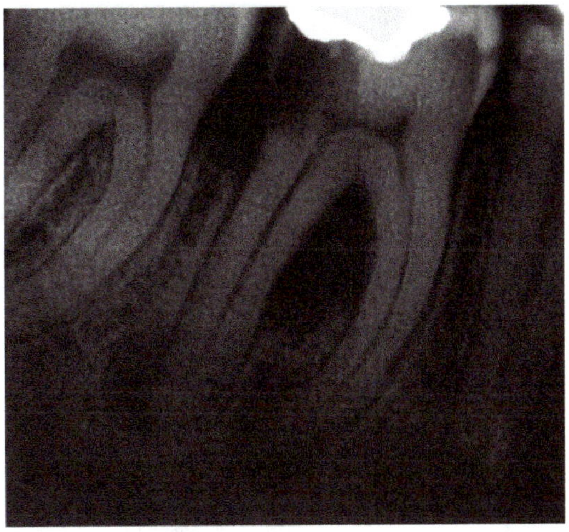

Figure 2: Apical radiograph of tooth # 46. Isolated furcation bone and apical bone destruction in the mesial and distal roots.

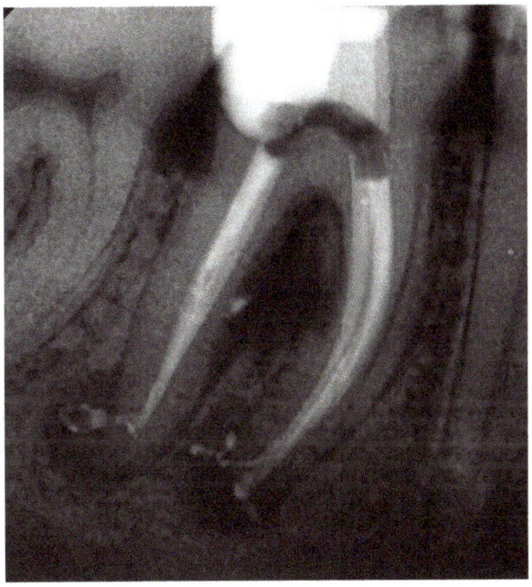

Figure 3: Apical radiograph of tooth # 46 after obturation.

The first appointment was finished placing a calcium hydroxide-based medication on the working length (Ultra-Cal XS paste; Ultradent Products, Inc., South Jordan, UT, USA). The floor of the pulp was covered with polytetrafluoroethylene (PTFE) and retained with the thin composite resin layer (Filtek Flow, 3M ESPE, Saint Paul, MN, USA) for the better sealing and retention. The outer part of the cavity was restored with intermediate restorative material (IRM) according to the double seal technique [9].

After two weeks, the medication was removed with the instrumentation with FlexMaster and irrigation with 3% NaOCl. As the patient was asymptomatic, the canals were dried and filled. The obturation was performed using continuous wave technique with gutta-percha and AH Plus (Dentsply International Inc., York, PA, USA) (Figure 3).

After obturation, the patient was referred to the restorative treatment. The tooth was restored with a lithium

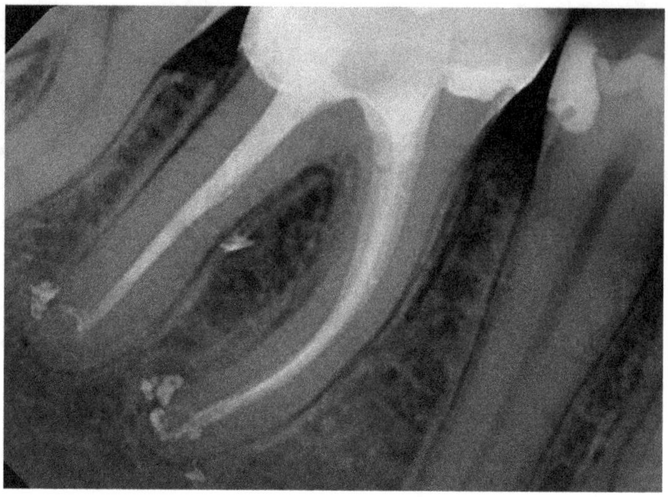

FIGURE 4: Two-year follow-up visit. Full healing was observed in the furcation and the periapical areas of tooth # 46.

disilicate full crown. The patient was recalled after 6, 12, 24, and 48 months (Figure 4). Total periapical and furcation healing was observed after 12 months and confirmed by the Cone Beam Computed Tomography (CBCT) scan 48 months after obturation (Figure 5).

3. Discussion

Different researches aimed at observing interradicular canals in lower molars have reported similar or different results, methodologies, terminology definition, and sample numbers [10].

Wolf et al. [10] observed 9 (7.7%) interradicular canals communicating the pulp chamber floor with the bifurcation area using dye in extracted teeth. The authors investigated the pulp chamber floor and the bifurcation area surface of 117 mandibular first molars. Access cavities were prepared; the pulp chambers were flooded with methylene blue and then centrifuged. An average of 4.2 (0.145 ± 0.03 mm thickness) slices per tooth were obtained by means of a diamond band saw. The presence of interradicular canals and diverticula was investigated using a light microscope (125x). Perlich et al. [11] found 3 canals (4.8%) using scanning electron microscopy and 22 canals (64.5%) using light microscopy in the pulp chamber floor of 62 human maxillary and mandibular molars. Chouchi et al. [12] studied accessory canals in 57 extracted permanent human teeth with micro-CT and revealed 7% ($n = 4$) and 21% ($n = 12$) furcation canals in the first and second mandibular molars, respectively.

Furcation perforation is an injury that leads to a communication between the root canal and the periodontal tissues or the oral cavity. It can be caused by resorption or dental caries or can have an iatrogenic cause including the misaligned use of rotary burs during access, preparation, and search for the root canals [13]. Furcation involvement refers to the condition when periodontal disease has caused bone resorption at the bifurcation or trifurcation of a multirooted tooth [14, 15]. Clinical examination with magnification, vital tests, and no previous endodontic treatment can help to exclude furcation impairment by periodontal disease.

Successful endodontic treatment depends on the thorough debridement of the entire root canal system. Difficult canal anatomy could be one of the causes of improper cleansing of the canal system, with the permanence of microorganisms [16, 17].

Irrigation of the root canals plays an important role in the disinfection process. From a microbiological standpoint, an irrigant should be able to demonstrate antimicrobial and antibiofilm activities and inactive endotoxins [18]. Activation of the irrigant helps to improve root canal cleanliness [19, 20]. Al-Jadaa et al. [21] demonstrated that ultrasonic irrigation causes a rise in the irrigant temperature in the accessory canals to 53.5 ± 2.7°C after the fifth minute, which could improve the irrigation effectiveness. No significant influence of accessory canal position or angulation was found.

Temporary restorative materials are often used during endodontic treatment to seal the root chamber between sessions or until a permanent restoration is placed. An ideal temporary restorative material should exhibit no leakage, good abrasion and compression resistance, lack of porosity, and lack of dimensional changes, and it must also be easily manipulated or removed while being effective in a moist environment [22]. PTFE is also an inexpensive material and previously used in dentistry in different fields. PTFE tape did not provide an avenue for bacterial contamination as temporary spacer materials [23]; however, PTFE retained by friction and may not be applicable in some other conditions, so it needs to be retained with stable material, such as the lite-cured composite resins [24]. E. faecalis grows on and penetrates through PTFE significantly more than it does with IRM (the most commonly used temporary restorations among specialists [24]), revealing its comparably reduced overall antimicrobial sealing ability when placed as the base part of temporary restorations [25]. Furthermore, research has shown that IRM has a poor marginal seal, performs poorly under stress, and exhibits bacterial penetration through the bulk of the material [26]; that is why composite

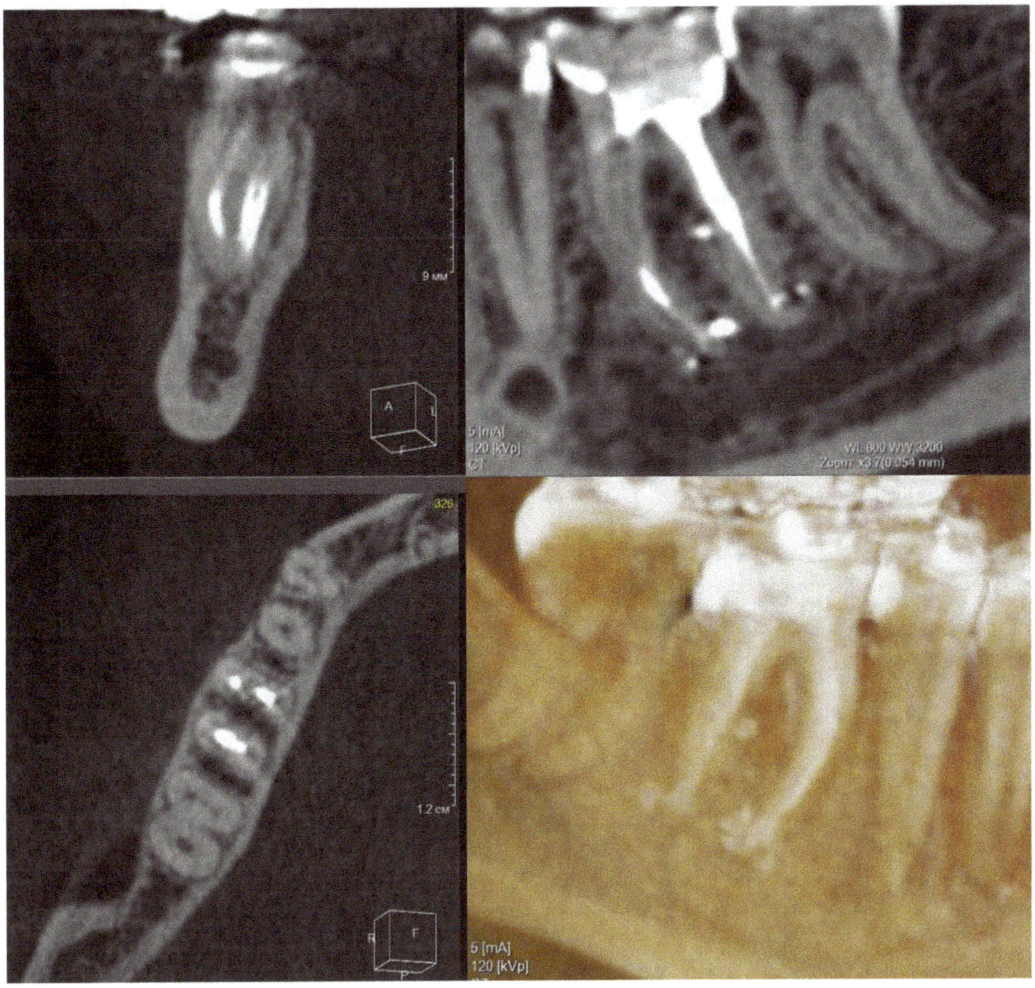

FIGURE 5: CBCT scan of tooth # 46 in 48 months after obturation. Full bone recovery is noticed.

resin creates extra the protection layer from leakage. The use of the composite resin as a full external layer increases the cost of the endodontic treatment.

The "double seal" technique [9] involves placing composite resin as the deeper layer material inside the pulp chamber and access cavity. The IRM is then used as the outer layer which is exposed to loading and the oral cavity. This double layer functions in several ways: the outer layer of IRM is an antibacterial agent; the inner layer of composite resin prevents liquids from the oral cavity to reach the root canal system if it has been able to penetrate through the IRM margins. The white colour of the IRM is readily visible when the clinician needs to remove it. The IRM is also a cheap material that is easily and quickly mixed and placed in the tooth. It sets quickly, and therefore, there is no "waiting time" after placement before the rubber dam can be removed.

4. Conclusion

Activation of the irrigant associated with the instrumentation and the use of the intracanal medication could explain the repair of the furcation and periapical lesions after endodontic treatment.

References

[1] P. N. Nair, "Pathogenesis ofApicalPeriodontitis and theCauses ofEndodonticFailures," *Critical Reviews in Oral Biology and Medicine*, vol. 15, no. 6, pp. 348–381, 2004.

[2] J. J. Segura-Egea, J. Martín-González, and L. Castellanos-Cosano, "Endodontic medicine: connections between apical periodontitis and systemic diseases," *International Endodontic Journal*, vol. 48, no. 10, pp. 933–951, 2015.

[3] T. Sorsa, L. Tjäderhane, Y. T. Konttinen et al., "Matrix metalloproteinases: contribution to pathogenesis, diagnosis and treatment of periodontal inflammation," *Annals of Medicine*, vol. 38, no. 5, pp. 306–321, 2006.

[4] N. Kawashima and P. Stashenko, "Expression of bone-resorptive and regulatory cytokines in murine periapical inflammation," *Archives of Oral Biology*, vol. 44, no. 1, pp. 55–66, 1999.

[5] I. Prada, P. Micó-Muñoz, T. Giner-Lluesma, P. Micó-Martínez, N. Collado-Castellano, and A. Manzano-Saiz, "Influence of microbiology on endodontic failure. Literature review," *Medicina Oral, Patología Oral y Cirugía Bucal*, vol. 24, no. 3, pp. e364–e372, 2019.

[6] P. Poornima and V. V. Subba Reddy, "Comparison of digital radiography, decalcification, and histologic sectioning in the

detection of accessory canals in furcation areas of human primary molars," *Journal of the Indian Society of Pedodontics and Preventive Dentistry*, vol. 26, no. 2, pp. 49–52, 2008.

[7] A. L. Anderegg, D. Hajdarevic, and T. G. Wolf, "Interradicular Canals in 213 Mandibular and 235 Maxillary Molars by Means of Micro-computed Tomographic Analysis: An _Ex Vivo_ Study," *Journal of Endodontia*, vol. 48, no. 2, pp. 234–239, 2022.

[8] H. M. A. Ahmed, P. Neelakantan, and P. M. H. Dummer, "A new system for classifying accessory canal morphology," *International Endodontic Journal*, vol. 51, no. 2, pp. 164–176, 2018.

[9] A. L. Jensen, P. V. Abbott, and S. J. Castro, "Interim and temporary restoration of teeth during endodontic treatment," *Australian Dental Journal*, vol. 52, 1 Suppl, pp. S83–S99, 2007.

[10] T. G. Wolf, S. Wentaschek, R. J. Wierichs, and B. Briseño-Marroquín, "Interradicular Root Canals in Mandibular First Molars: A Literature Review and *Ex Vivo* Study," *Journal of Endodontia*, vol. 45, no. 2, pp. 129–135, 2019.

[11] M. A. Perlich, A. Reader, and D. W. Foreman, "A scanning electron microscopic investigation of accessory foramens on the pulpal floor of human molars," *Journal of Endodontia*, vol. 7, no. 9, pp. 402–406, 1981.

[12] D. Chouchi, A. Berberoğlu, K. Orhan, I. Etikan, H. Tümer, and N. Bağlış, "The location and incidence of patent accessory pulpal canals in permanent molars with periodontal lesion by using micro-computed tomography," *Journal of Medical Imaging and Health Informatics*, vol. 11, no. 1, pp. 85–88, 2021.

[13] S. D. Huamán, M. G. Brito Aragão, A. P. Dias Moreno et al., "Accuracy of conventional periapical radiography in diagnosing furcation repair after perforation treatment," *Journal of Endodontia*, vol. 46, no. 6, pp. 827–831, 2020.

[14] W. Zhang, K. Foss, and B. Y. Wang, "A retrospective study on molar furcation assessment via clinical detection, intraoral radiography and cone beam computed tomography," *BMC Oral Health*, vol. 18, no. 1, p. 75, 2018.

[15] E. S. Gusmão, A. C. Picarte, M. B. Ben Barbosa, C. K. Rösing, and R. Cimoes, "Correlation between clinical and radiographic findings on the occurrence of furcation involvement in patients with periodontitis," *Indian Journal of Dental Research*, vol. 25, no. 5, pp. 572–575, 2014.

[16] S. Gautam, S. R. Galgali, H. S. Sheethal, and N. S. Priya, "Pulpal changes associated with advanced periodontal disease: a histopathological study," *Journal of Oral and Maxillofacial Pathology*, vol. 21, no. 1, pp. 58–63, 2017.

[17] E. M. Weinberg, A. E. Pereda, S. Khurana, P. P. Lotlikar, C. Falcon, and C. Hirschberg, "Incidence of middle mesial canals based on distance between mesial canal orifices in mandibular molars: a clinical and cone-beam computed tomographic analysis," *Journal of Endodontia*, vol. 46, no. 1, pp. 40–43, 2020.

[18] P. R. Shenoi, E. S. Morey, C. S. Makade, M. K. Gunwal, R. T. Khode, and S. S. Wanmali, "In vitro evaluation of the antimicrobial efficacy of chitosan and other endodontic irrigants against Enterococcus faecalis," *General Dentistry*, vol. 64, no. 5, pp. 60–63, 2016.

[19] X. Guo, H. Miao, L. Li et al., "Efficacy of four different irrigation techniques combined with 60 °C 3% sodium hypochlorite and 17% EDTA in smear layer removal," *BMC Oral Health*, vol. 14, p. 114, 2014.

[20] C. Rico-Romano, Á. Zubizarreta-Macho, M. R. Baquero-Artigao, and J. Mena-Álvarez, "An analysis in vivo of intracanal bacterial load before and after chemo-mechanical preparation: a comparative analysis of two irrigants and two activation techniques," *Journal of Clinical and Experimental Dentistry*, vol. 8, no. 1, pp. e9–e13, 2016.

[21] A. Al-Jadaa, F. Paqué, T. Attin, and M. Zehnder, "Necrotic pulp tissue dissolution by passive ultrasonic irrigation in simulated accessory canals: impact of canal location and angulation," *International Endodontic Journal*, vol. 42, no. 1, pp. 59–65, 2009.

[22] A. Ciftçi, D. A. Vardarli, and I. S. Sönmez, "Coronal microleakage of four endodontic temporary restorative materials: an in vitro study," *Oral Surgery, Oral Medicine, Oral Pathology, Oral Radiology, and Endodontics*, vol. 108, no. 4, pp. e67–e70, 2009.

[23] A. Paranjpe, S. Jain, K. J. Alibhai, C. P. Wadhwani, R. P. Darveau, and J. D. Johnson, "In vitro microbiologic evaluation of PTFE and cotton as spacer materials," *Quintessence International*, vol. 43, no. 8, pp. 703–707, 2012.

[24] K. Olcay, L. Steier, H. Erdogan, and S. Belli, "Polytetrafluoroetylene tape as temporary restorative material: a fluid filtration study," *Journal of Istanbul University Faculty of Dentistry*, vol. 49, no. 3, pp. 17–22, 2015.

[25] M. Solomonov, D. H. Levy, A. Yaya, J. Ben Itzhak, and D. Polak, "Antimicrobial evaluation of polytetrafluoroethylene used as part of temporary restorations: an ex vivo study," *Australian Endodontic Journal*, vol. 48, no. 1, pp. 98–104, 2022.

[26] T. AlSwayyed, R. Bin Nafesah, M. Alqutub et al., "Restorative treatment patterns after root canal obturation in public hospitals in Riyadh," *Clinical, Cosmetic and Investigational Dentistry*, vol. Volume 13, pp. 389–394, 2021.

26

Combined Periodontal and Endodontic Management of Palatal Radicular Groove with Platelet-Rich Fibrin and Biodentine®

Arjun Hari Rijal,[1] **Bhageshwar Dhami**,[2] **and Pratistha Ghimire**[3]

[1]*Department of Periodontology and Oral Implantology, Kathmandu University School of Medical Sciences, Dhulikhel, Kavrepalanchok, Nepal*
[2]*Department of Periodontology and Oral Implantology, Kantipur Dental College and Hospital, Basundhara, Kathmandu, Nepal*
[3]*Dental Department, Methinkot Hospital, Kavrepalanchok, Nepal*

Correspondence should be addressed to Arjun Hari Rijal; rajrijal27@gmail.com

Academic Editor: Konstantinos Michalakis

Palatal radicular groove (PRG) is developmental anomaly of root, which when present is associated with periodontal and endodontic problems. Different treatment modalities are available for its management, such as periodontal flap surgery, endodontic management, sealing of PRG with various cements, bone graft procedure for intrabony defect, extraction with intentional replantation after sealing or removal of a PRG, and endodontic treatment as well as the use of various growth factors. Success of the therapy depends on the type, depth, and extent of PRG, presence or absence of intrabony defect, vitality of involved tooth, and types of materials used to seal PRG. This study reports management of PRG with Biodentine® and platelet-rich fibrin in a 44-year-old systemically healthy female patient.

1. Introduction

Different morphological variations associated with maxillary anteriors include congenital absence of tooth, supernumerary tooth, dens invaginatus, Eagle's talon, peg-shaped lateral incisor, gemination, fusion, accessory root, and palatal gingival grooved incisors [1, 2]. Palatal radicular groove (PRG) is a developmental anomaly usually on the palatal surface of maxillary lateral incisors either mesially or distally on the root. It was first described as radicular groove by Black [3], whereas the term 'palatogingival groove' was first coined by Lee et al. [4]. Several technical terms have been proposed to describe the PRG, such as distolingual groove, coronoradicular groove, radicular lingual groove, vertical developmental radicular groove, cingulo-radicular groove, developmental radicular anomaly, interruption groove, PRG, and palatoradicular groove [4–7]. Various hypothesis proposed for the development of PRG include failed attempt to form new root [5, 8], infoldings of Hertwigs epithelial root sheath and inner enamel epithelium [4], or change in the genetic mechanism [9]. Most commonly followed classification for PRG is based on the extent of groove on the surface of root, which was given by Gu [10].

Type I: the groove is short (not beyond the coronal third of the root).

Type II: the groove is long (beyond the coronal third of the root) but shallow, corresponding to a normal or simple root canal.

Type III: the groove is long (beyond the coronal third of the root) and deep, corresponding to a complex root canal system.

Entrance of PRG acts as a site for plaque accumulation, leading to gingivitis and bleeding on probing. In advance cases, PRG allows passage of microorganisms throughout its length, leading to the loss of periodontal attachment and intrabony defects. This is presented as a combined type of primary periodontal lesion with secondary involvement of the pulp. The periodontal breakdown and root surface contamination result in retrogenic pulp necrosis even though PRGs do not reach the apex and are not very deep. Accessory foramina or dentinal tubules along the grooves have been regarded as the possible pathway between the pulp canal and the groove [11, 12].

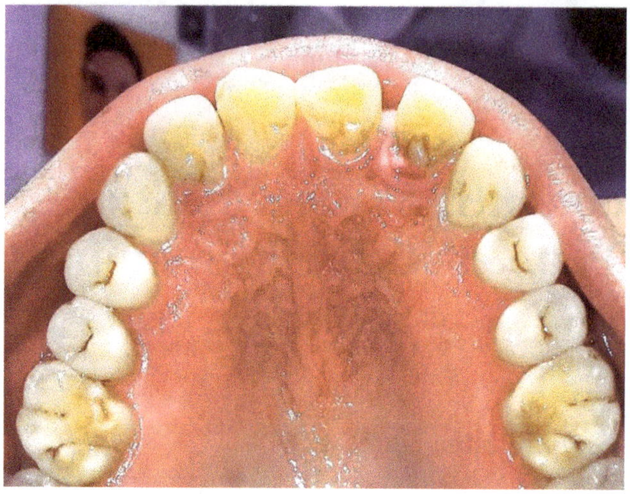

FIGURE 1: Palatal radicular groove with reference to 22.

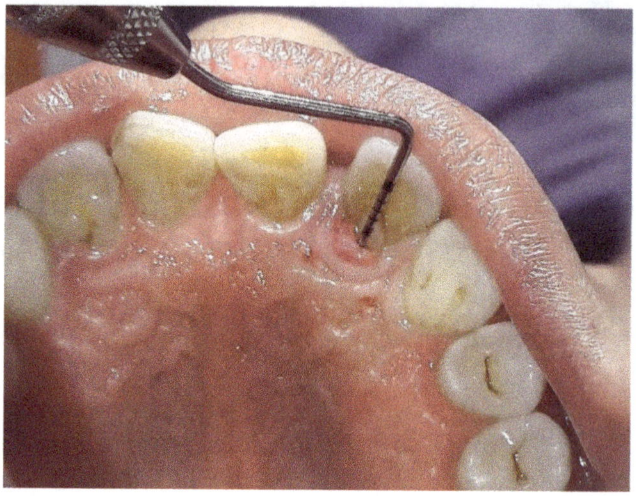

FIGURE 2: Preoperative pocket probing depth of 10 mm with reference to 22.

Different treatment modalities available for the management of PRG include simple gingival curettage of inflamed gingival tissues, saucerization of shallow groove with diamond bur, root canal therapy of involved tooth, and various surgical procedures (periodontal flap with sealing of groove with cement, guided tissue/bone regeneration if intrabony defect present, intentional root canal therapy, and reimplantation). In this study, we have reported successful management of primary periodontal secondary endodontic lesion complicated by class II PRG with Biodentine® and platelet-rich fibrin (PRF).

2. Case Presentation

A 44-year-old female visited the Department of Periodontology and Oral Implantology, Kantipur Dental College Teaching Hospital and Research Centre, Basundhara, Kathmandu, Nepal, with a chief complaint of pain and swelling of gingiva in upper left front region of the jaw for one month. The pain was mild, dull, and continuous in nature. There was no history of trauma, swelling, and pain with respect to the concerned tooth. General examination revealed that the patient was moderately built and nourished. Clinical examination revealed intact crown with no carries or fracture. Vitality testing was negative, whereas positive response was elicited to vertical percussion. There was presence of localized circumscribed gingival inflammation on palatal aspect with respect to the mesio-palatal line angle of 22 (i.e., maxillary left lateral incisor) with pocket probing depth of 10 mm, whereas there was only 3 mm of pocket probing depth on labial aspect of the involved tooth (Figures 1 and 2). Intraoral periapical radiograph of the tooth showed a periapical radiolucency as well as a radiopaque line extending from cingulum of crown to the middle third of the root. No intrabony vertical defect was noted. Cone-beam computed tomography (CBCT) revealed extension of groove up to the middle third of root with interdental bone loss (Figure 3).

Based on these clinical and radiographic examination and findings, it was diagnosed to be the primary periodontal and secondary endodontic lesions.

For the management of the case, non-surgical periodontal therapy (scaling and root planning) was done initially. Patient was referred to the endodontist for root canal treatment, and root canal therapy was completed (Figure 4). One month after completion of endodontic therapy, sealing of PRG with Biodentine® and PRF was planned. Prior to surgery, mouth rinse with 0.2% chlorohexidine gluconate for one minute was advised to the patient. Adequate anaesthesia was achieved with local infiltration of 2% lidocaine with adrenaline in 1:200,000 concentration. Full thickness envelope flap was raised on palatal aspect (Figure 5). Complete debridement was done with removal of granulation tissue. The PRG was smoothened with diamond bur under copious sterile saline irrigation. Conditioning of root was done with 24% ethylenediaminetetraacetic acid (EDTA) for two minutes and removed with sufficient amount of sterile saline solution (Figure 6). Then, the PRG was sealed with Biodentine® (Biodentine® Bioactive Dentin Substitute Septodont; Figure 7). Intravenous blood (by venipuncturing of the antecubital vein) was collected in a 10 ml sterile glass tube (BD Vacutainer® blood collection tubes, 10 ml) without anticoagulant and immediately centrifuged (IntraSpin® system by INTRA-LOCK, Biodentine: Septodont North America Medical Equipment ManufacturingLancaster, PABDVacutainer: JIANGSU HXRT MD CO., LTD. Jiangyan District, 225500, Taizhou City, Jiangsu Province, ChinaIntraspin: Biohorizon Birmingham, AL 35244 USA) at 3,000 rpm for 10 minutes. PRF was separated from red corpuscles base (preserving a small RBC layer) using sterile tweezers just after removal of platelet-poor plasma and then transferred into a sterile dappen dish. PRF was squeezed between two gauze pieces to remove excess of plasma. PRF was placed above the root surface (Figure 8). Finally, flap was approximated with 4-0 silk suture (ETHILON®, Ethicon Inc., Johnson & Johnson, Piscataway, NJ, USA) using simple interrupted suturing technique (Figure 9).

Postsurgically, the surgical area was covered with periodontal dressing (COE-PAK™, (De Trey/Denstply, Konstanz, Germany) Automix Surgical Dressing & Periodontal

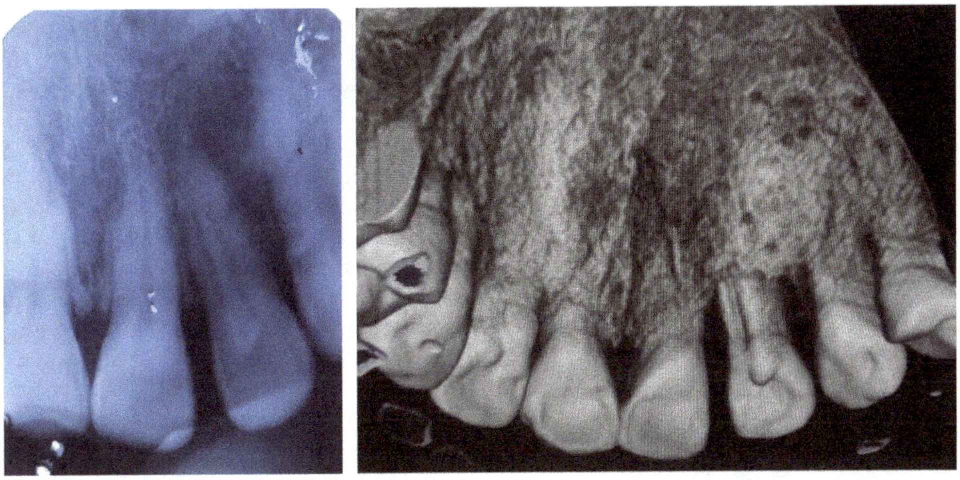

Figure 3: Preoperative periapical radiograph and cone-beam computed tomography.

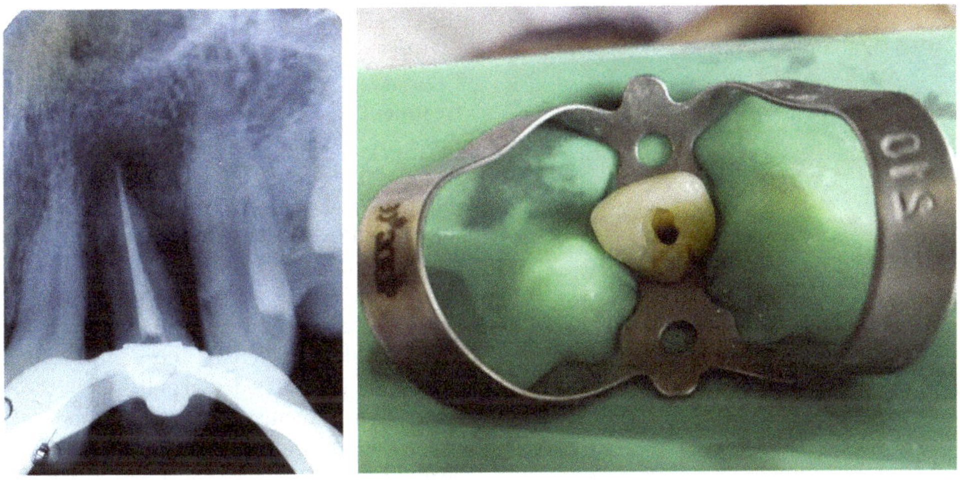

Figure 4: Endodontic management of involved tooth before surgery.

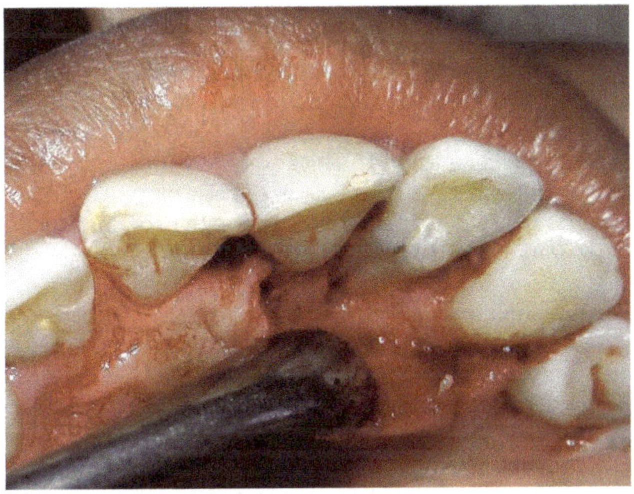

Figure 5: Flap reflection and debridement of the defect.

Pack). Postsurgical instructions were given to the patient. Non-steroidal anti-inflammatory drugs (NSAIDS) (Ibuprofen 400 mg and Paracetamol 375 mg, Flexon Tablet, Aristo Pharmaceuticals Pvt. Ltd.), (23-A, Shah Industrial Estate, Off Veera Desai Road, Andheri (West), Mumbai - 400 053, India.) three times daily for three days) for inflammation control and pain relief and 0.2% chlorhexidine gluconate (CHX oral rinse—100 ml mouth wash) two times a day for 2 weeks were prescribed. After two weeks of surgery, periodontal dressing was removed, and gingival healing was found to be satisfactory and uneventful. Patient was kept on regular follow-up (Figures 10 and 11). Complete examination after 2-year follow-up showed reduction in PPD to 3 mm, and tooth was asymptomatic endodontically though there was presence of periapical lesion, which might be because of healing by scar formation (Figures 12 and 13). In addition, there was reduction in size of radiolucency as compared to preoperative CBCT image (Figures 13 and 14).

3. Discussion

PRG is morphological as well as developmental anomaly, which begins from or near cingulum and extend along the various length of root of maxillary anteriors. There is wide variation in prevalence of PRG. The variation in prevalence

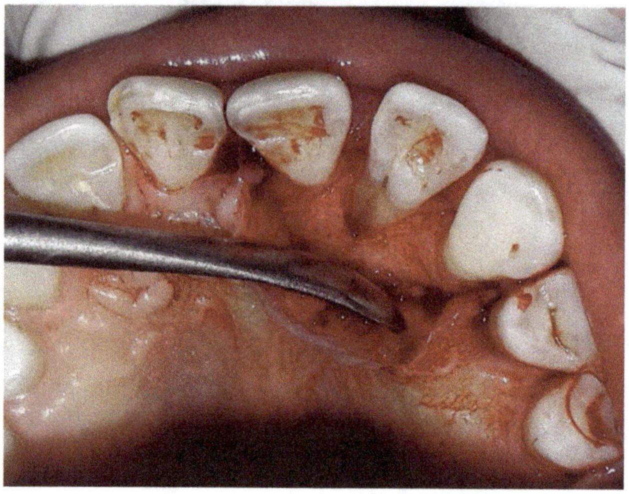

Figure 6: Root conditioning with 24% EDTA.

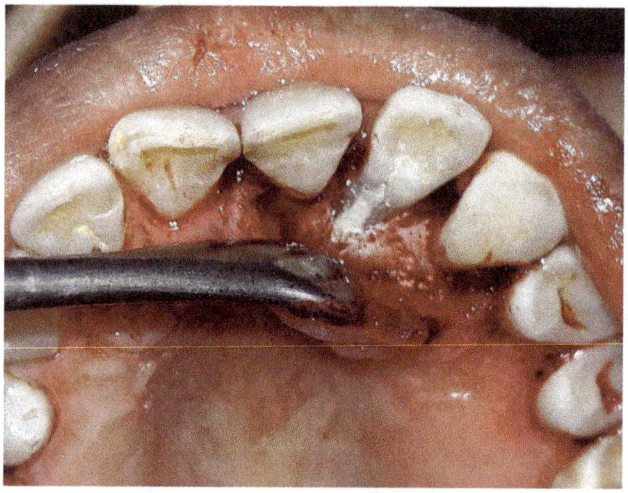

Figure 7: Sealing of groove with Biodentin.

may be due to difference in diagnostic criteria or examination methodologies used, for example, evaluation of extracted teeth versus clinical examination, and clinical examination versus CBCT study (Table 1).

Diagnosis of PRG is very difficult because of its morphological similarity with other anomalies like dens invaginatus, Tomes' root, and extra root variation. In addition, history provided by the patients are non-specific that may resemble with other clinical conditions (e.g., primary or secondary endodontic lesion). Therefore, diagnosis of PRG is mainly done by taking proper patient history, clinical examination, and advanced radiography (CBCT) [21]. Patient usually complaints of continuous dull or acute pain, gingival swelling, and mobility of teeth, which is not associated with dental caries, trauma, or discoloration of the teeth, whereas in some cases, patient may be asymptomatic. In the current case, the patient presented with dull continuous pain along with swelling of gingiva.

Clinical examination may reveal funnel shaped hollow grooves with an accumulation of plaque and calculus, increased pocket probing depth, loss of epithelial attachment, swollen gingiva, and bleeding on probing [21]. Diagnosis of either periodontal or primary endodontic lesion can be made by electric pulp testing, heat test, or cold test. Advanced cases with deep groove, loss of attachment, and increased pocket do not respond to electric or thermal pulp testing [22, 23]. Intraoral periapical radiographs can be used to diagnose PRG associated with periodontal or endodontic lesion. Widening of periodontal ligament space can be seen in primary periodontal lesion, whereas tear-drop shaped radiolucency may be observed in the case of primary endodontic infection [5]. Due to superimposition of various structures, it is difficult to diagnose PRG with two-dimensional radiographs [6]. Therefore, to avoid such difficulty and for proper diagnosis, CBCT was advised in the current case. In this case, increase in pocket probing depth, attachment loss, periapical radiolucency, and para-pulpal line signifies primary periodontal infection with secondary endodontic lesion complicated by PRG. Other differential diagnoses, such as vertical root fracture, gemination, and fused roots, were ruled out based on the clinical examination and CBCT findings.

Previously, if patient had presented with clinical findings of PRG along with draining sinus and advanced periodontitis, treatment of choice would be extraction because of poor prognosis [5]. However, with the development of advanced diagnostic tool, better sealing material, and regenerative material, different treatment options are available for patient with periodontal and endodontic infection complicated by PRG. Basic principles for the management of PRG are complete removal of microorganism, sealing of groove with cement to prevent communication between root canal and periodontium and periodontal regeneration, and complete healing of the periodontium [21]. If the dental pulp is involved, endodontic treatment is recommended before the periodontal approach.

Different treatment modalities, such as periodontal flap surgery, endodontic management, sealing of PRG with various cements, bone graft procedure for intrabony defect, extraction with intentional replantation after sealing or removal of a PRG, and endodontic treatment, and various growth factors are available for the management. In case of mild PRG, odontoplasty in conjunction with periodontal treatment like curettage and root planning and saucerization of groove with diamond round bur can be performed [24]. Similarly, in complex PRG with advanced periodontal infection, various treatment options have been proposed, which includes removal of granulation tissue with periodontal flap, saucerization of groove and sealing with different materials, guided tissue regeneration with or without bone graft, intentional reimplantation, and extraction [25].

Several sealing materials including amalgam, glass ionomer cement, composite resin, calcium silicate-based cement like mineral trioxide aggregate, and Biodentine® have been used to seal moderate-to-deep PRG [21].

Biodentine® is tricalcium-based cement, which is available as powder and liquid. Components of powder are tricalcium silicate, dicalcium silicate, calcium carbonate and oxide, iron oxide, and zirconium oxide. Components of liquid are calcium chloride and water-soluble polymer. Biodentine® has several advantages like easy manipulation during mixing and sealing, short setting time of 9–12 minutes,

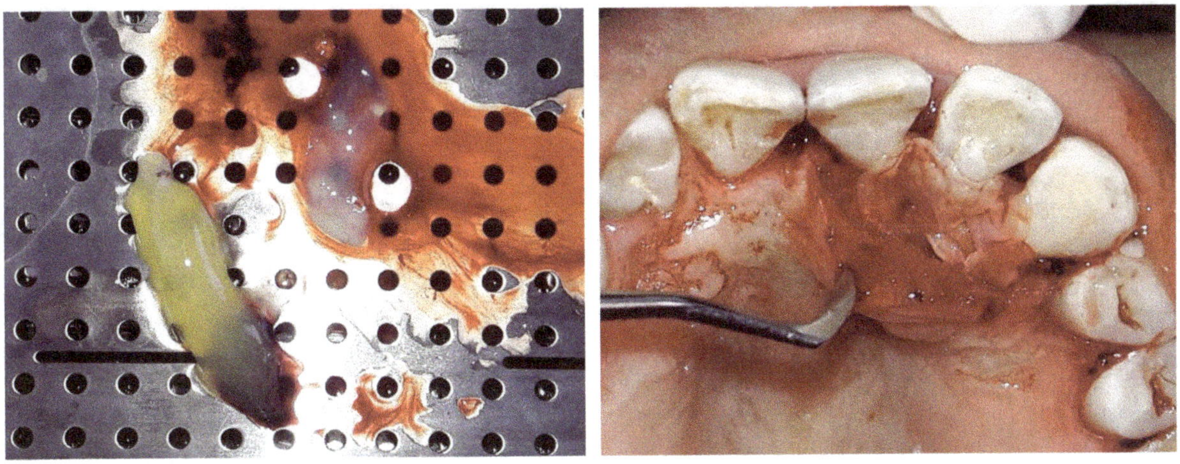

FIGURE 8: Preparation and placement of platelet-rich fibrin.

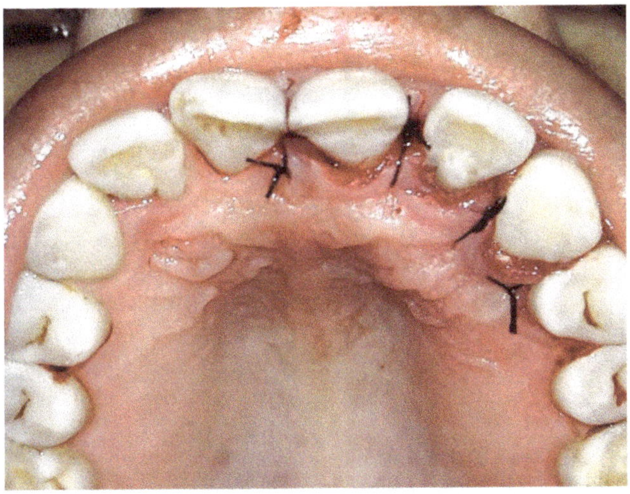

FIGURE 9: Simple interrupted suturing with 4-0 silk suture.

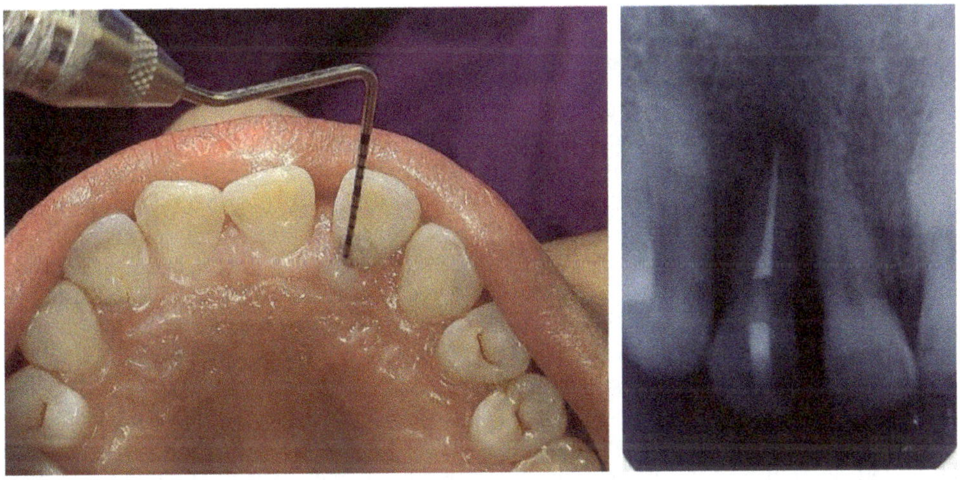

FIGURE 10: Postoperative six months follow-up with pocket probing depth of 4 mm with reference to 22.

improved mechanical properties, good biocompatibility, and regenerative potential [2, 26, 27]. In addition, tricalcium silicate-based cements are considered as the best sealing material for grooves since it does not leach any contaminants [27]. Because of significant advantages of Biodentine®, we used this material to seal moderate type of PRG.

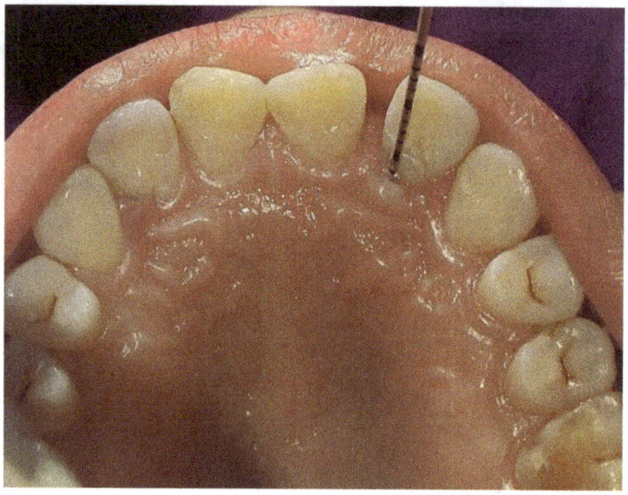

FIGURE 11: Postoperative one year follow-up with pocket probing depth of 4 mm with reference to 22.

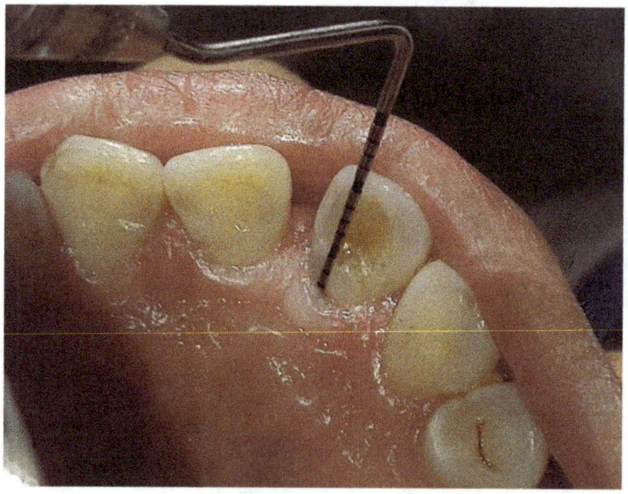

FIGURE 12: Postoperative two years follow-up with pocket probing depth of 3 mm with reference to 22.

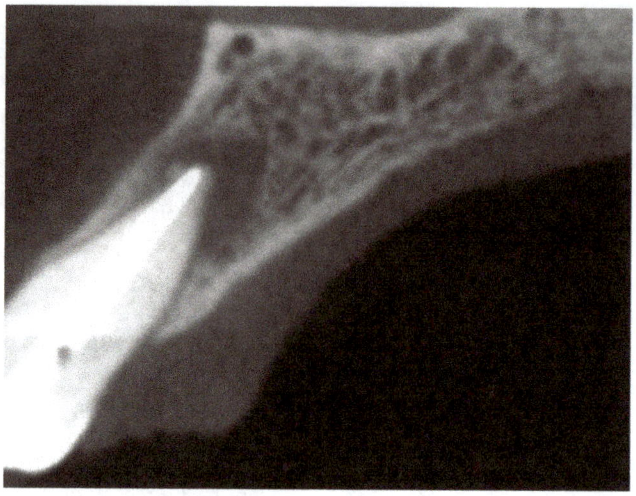

FIGURE 13: Postoperative CBCT showing healing of lesion on the labial aspect.

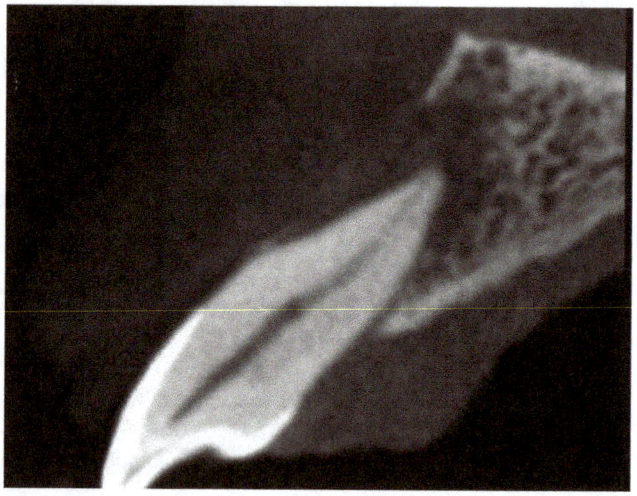

FIGURE 14: Preoperative CBCT showing extensive loss of bone on the labial aspect.

In cases of complex PRG with advanced periodontal infection, various regenerative processes and materials are required for successful management. Guided tissue/bone regeneration with membranes, bone grafts, PRF [27], and enamel matrix proteins [28, 29] has been used for successful management of complex cases. PRF is autologous material, which have various growth factors that help in various regenerative procedures. PRF consists of a fibrin matrix polymerized in a tetra molecular structure, with the incorporation of platelets, leukocyte, and cytokines, and circulating stem cells [30]. Growth factors present in PRF are transforming growth factor type beta 1, platelet-derived growth factor-AB, vascular endothelium growth factor , and glycoproteins (such as thrombospondin-1) [31]. PRF contains cytokines, and cells are entrapped in a matrix, which is released after a short period and can serve as a resorbable membrane. The rationale behind the use of PRF membrane is that the platelet α-granules are a reservoir of many growth factors that are known to play a definitive role in tissue repair [30].

Johns et al. [27] reported successful management of PRG with advanced periodontal infection with root canal therapy, apicectomy, sealing of groove with Biodentin, and bone defect management with bone graft and PRF membrane. After two years, there was significant reduction in PPD, patient was asymptomatic with a 3 mm non-bleeding sulcus, and there was reduction in size of radiolucency radiographically. Dhanyakumar and Devasia [32] treated PRG with combined endodontic–periodontal approach, and Biodentine® was used to seal PRG. Patient was asymptomatic, and significant reduction in PPD and size of radiolucency was noted after three months. Our case reports confirmed that PRF alone could be successfully used for the treatment of PRG-related periodontal infection and Biodentine® to seal the shallow-to-moderate PRG, when an adequate primary closure was obtained.

Table 1: Prevalence of palatal radicular groove.

S.No.	References	Evaluation methods	Prevalence
1	Everett and Kramer [6]	Survey of 625 extracted maxillary lateral incisors	<2%
2	Withers et al. [13]	Clinical examination of 531 maxillary incisor	Overall 8.5%
			2.33%
		Total 2,099 maxillary incisor examined	Maximum 93.8% in maxillary lateral incisors
3	Kogon [7]	3,168 extracted maxillary incisors	Overall 4.6%
			Central incisors 5.6%
			Lateral incisors 3.4%
4	Storrer et al. [14]	73 extracted maxillary lateral incisors	9.58%
5	Al-Rasheed [15]	Clinical examinations of 552 maxillary lateral incisors in 276 Saudi adults	10.3%
6	Hou and Tsai [16]	Clinical examinations of 404 maxillary incisors in 101 individuals	18.1%
7	Shreshta et al. [17]	Clinical examination of 1,362 maxillary anterior teeth	0.88% for lateral incisors
8	Khan et al. [18]	250 patients examined	7.6% of central incisors and 13.4% of lateral incisors
9	Neves et al. [19]	1,668 extracted maxillary central incisors	1.61%
10	Aksoy et al. [20]	CBCT examinations of 993 teeth (330 canines, 315 lateral incisors, and 348 central incisors)	0.57% of central incisors and 2.22% of lateral incisors

4. Conclusion

This case report described a management technique that resulted in clinical and radiographic resolutions of PRG-related periodontal attachment loss by a periodontal regenerative approach with PRF. Also, sealing of PRG with Biodentine® which is a biocompatible material eliminates the risk of adverse tissue response. Biodentine® also has outstanding sealing properties that reduces the risk of clinical failures through bacterial percolation. Biodentine® needs no surface conditioning or bonding and sets quickly, making it simple and easy to use. Currently, no other major disadvantage of the use of PRF has been reported. Therefore, combination of these materials was chosen to treat the complications that would arise due to the presence of PRG. Early diagnosis and suitable treatment plan of PRG-related defect can modify the prognosis and successful treatment of involved tooth.

Acknowledgments

This case report is self-funded.

References

[1] N. Iqbal, S. M. Tirmazi, H. A. Majeed, and M. B. Munir, "Prevalence of palatogingival groove in maxillary lateral incisors," *Pakistan Oral & Dental Journal*, vol. 31, pp. 424–426, 2011.

[2] S. Sharma, P. Deepak, S. Vivek, and D. S. Ranjan, "Palatogingival groove: recognizing and managing the hidden tract in a maxillary incisor: a case report," *Journal Of International Oral Health*, vol. 7, no. 6, pp. 110–114, 2015.

[3] G. V. Black, *Pathology of the Hard Tissues of the Teeth, Oral Diagnosis*, Medico Dental Publishing Company, 1936.

[4] K. W. Lee, E. C. Lee, and K. Y. Poon, "Palato-gingival grooves in maxillary incisors. A possible predisposing factor to localised periodontal disease," *British Dental Journal*, vol. 124, no. 1, pp. 14–18, 1968.

[5] J. H. Simon, D. H. Glick, and A. L. Frank, "Predictable endodontic and periodontic failures as a result of radicular anomalies," *Oral Surgery, Oral Medicine, and Oral Pathology*, vol. 31, no. 6, pp. 823–826, 1971.

[6] F. G. Everett and G. M. Kramer, "The disto-lingual groove in the maxillary lateral incisor; a periodontal hazard," *Journal of Periodontology*, vol. 43, no. 6, pp. 352–361, 1972.

[7] S. L. Kogon, "The prevalence, location and conformation of palato-radicular grooves in maxillary incisors," *Journal of Periodontology*, vol. 57, no. 4, pp. 231–234, 1986.

[8] M. D. Peikoff, J. B. Perry, and L. A. Chapnick, "Endodontic failure attributable to a complex radicular lingual groove," *Journal of Endodontia*, vol. 11, no. 12, pp. 573–577, 1985.

[9] M. Mittal, P. Vashisth, R. Arora, and S. Dwivedi, "Combined endodontic therapy and periapical surgery with MTA and bone graft in treating palatogingival groove," *BML Case Reports*, vol. 2013, p. bcr2013009056, 2013.

[10] Y. C. Gu, "A micro-computed tomographic analysis of maxillary lateral incisors with radicular grooves," *Journal of Endodontia*, vol. 37, no. 6, pp. 789–792, 2011.

[11] W. W. Goon, W. M. Carpenter, N. M. Brace, and R. J. Ahlfeld, "Complex facial radicular groove in a maxillary lateral incisor," *Journal of Endodontics*, vol. 17, no. 5, pp. 244–248, 1991.

[12] Z. R. Gao, J. N. Shi, Y. Wang, and F. Y. Gu, "Scanning electron microscopic investigation of maxillary lateral incisors with a radicular lingual groove," *Oral Surgery, Oral Medicine, and Oral Pathology*, vol. 68, no. 4, pp. 462–466, 1989.

[13] J. A. Withers, M. A. Brunsvold, W. J. Killoy, and A. J. Rahe, "The relationship of palato-gingival grooves to localized periodontal disease," *Journal of Periodontology*, vol. 52, no. 1, pp. 41–44, 1981.

[14] C. M. Storrer, P. L. Sanchez, G. A. Romito, and F. E. Pustiglioni, "Morphometric study of length and grooves of maxillary lateral incisor roots," *Archives of Oral Biology*, vol. 51, no. 8, pp. 649–654, 2006.

[15] A. Al-Rasheed, "Relationship between palato-radicular groove and periodontal health in maxillary lateral incisors," *Pakistan Oral & Dental Journal*, vol. 31, pp. 154–157, 2011.

[16] G. L. Hou and C. C. Tsai, "Relationship between palato-radicular grooves and localized periodontitis," *Journal of Clinical Periodontology*, vol. 20, no. 9, pp. 678–682, 1993.

[17] D. Shreshta, M. Humagain, and S. Swastika, "Prevalence of palate-gingival groove in patients of Dhulikhel Hospital," *Journal of College of Medical Sciences*, vol. 10, no. 1, pp. 32–36, 2014.

[18] A. M. Khan, S. A. Shah, F. Alam et al., "Frequency of palato-gingival groove in maxillary incisors," *Pakistan Oral & Dental Journal*, vol. 39, no. 1, 2019.

[19] F. L. Neves, C. A. Silveira, and H. Faig-Leite, "Anatomical study of palato-gingival groove in maxillary central incisors," *Brazilian Dental Science*, vol. 18, no. 3, pp. 59–67, 2015.

[20] U. Aksoy, F. Kermeoğlu, A. Kalender, H. Eren, M. E. Kolsuz, and K. Orhan, "Cone-beam computed tomography evaluation of palatogingival grooves: a retrospective study with literature review," *Oral Radiology*, vol. 33, no. 3, pp. 193–198, 2017.

[21] H. J. Kim, Y. Choi, M. K. Yu, K. W. Lee, and K. S. Min, "Recognition and management of palatogingival groove for tooth survival: a literature review," *Restorative Dentistry & Endodontics*, vol. 42, no. 2, pp. 77–86, 2017.

[22] P. Castelo-Baz, I. Ramos-Barbosa, B. Martín-Biedma, A. B. Dablanca-Blanco, P. Varela-Patiño, and J. Blanco-Carrión, "Combined endodontic-periodontal treatment of a palatogingival groove," *Journal of Endodontics*, vol. 41, no. 11, pp. 1918–1922, 2015.

[23] K. Al-Hezaimi, J. Naghshbandi, J. H. Simon, and I. Rotstein, "Successful treatment of a radicular groove by intentional replantation and Emdogain therapy: four years follow-up," *Oral Surgery, Oral Medicine, Oral Pathology, Oral Radiology, and Endodontology*, vol. 107, no. 3, pp. e82–e85, 2009.

[24] J. H. Jeng, H. K. Jackson Lu, and L. T. Hou, "Treatment of an osseous lesion associated with a severe palato-radicular groove: a case report," *Journal of Periodontology*, vol. 63, no. 8, pp. 708–712, 1992.

[25] J. Forero-López, L. Gamboa-Martínez, L. Pico-Porras, and J. L. Niño-Barrera, "Surgical management with intentional replantation on a tooth with palato-radicular groove," *Restorative Dentistry & Endodontics*, vol. 40, no. 2, pp. 166–171, 2015.

[26] M. P. Liji and M. J. Rameshkumar, "Integration of PRF and Biodentine® in palatogingival groove case," *IOSR Journal of Dental and Medical Sciences*, vol. 6, no. 4, pp. 26–30, 2013.

[27] D. A. Johns, V. Y. Shivashankar, K. Shobha, and M. Johns, "An innovative approach in the management of palatogingival groove using Biodentine®™ and platelet-rich fibrin membrane," *Journal of Conservative Dentistry*, vol. 17, no. 1, p. 75, 2014.

[28] M. P. Rethman, "Treatment of a palatal-gingival groove using enamel matrix derivative," *Compendium of Continuing Education in Dentistry*, vol. 22, no. 9, pp. 792–797, 2001.

[29] G. Zucchelli, M. Mele, and L. Checchi, "The papilla amplification flap for the treatment of a localized periodontal defect associated with a palatal groove," *Journal of Periodontology*, vol. 77, no. 10, pp. 1788–1796, 2006.

[30] D. M. Dohan Ehrenfest, G. M. de Peppo, P. Doglioli, and G. Sammartino, "Slow release of growth factors and thrombospondin-1 in Choukroun's platelet-rich fibrin (PRF): a gold standard to achieve for all surgical platelet concentrates technologies," *Growth Factors*, vol. 27, no. 1, pp. 63–69, 2009.

[31] J. Choukroun, A. Diss, A. Simonpieri et al., "Platelet-rich fibrin (PRF): a second-generation platelet concentrate. Part IV: clinical effects on tissue healing," *Oral Surgery, Oral Medicine, Oral Pathology, Oral Radiology, and Endodontics*, vol. 101, no. 3, pp. e56–e60, 2006.

[32] N. M. Dhanyakumar and S. R. Devasia, "Management of palatogingival groove using the innovative tricalcium silicate material Biodentine®™," *CODS Journal of Dentistry*, vol. 8, no. 1, pp. 54–58, 2016.

27

Severe, Treatment-Refractory Periodontitis and Vitamin D Deficiency: A Multidisciplinary Case Report

Figliuzzi Michele Mario, Parentela Luca, Aiello Domenico, and Altilia Simone

Department of Health Sciences, "Magna Graecia" University, Catanzaro 88100, Italy

Correspondence should be addressed to Figliuzzi Michele Mario; figliuzzi@unicz.it

Academic Editor: Andrea Scribante

Introduction. Vitamin D deficiency and periodontitis are common diseases among people. These conditions interact with each other and worsen the patient's health. Modern dentistry aims to rehabilitate oral health and bring it back to the original state or even improve aesthetics. Without analysing the general health conditions of patients and without a multidisciplinary approach, it is sometimes not possible to solve a case such as we describe. This study shows how a vitamin D deficit can influence the choice of dental treatment. The patient, a 40-year-old woman, in generally good health, came to our observation complaining about pain during mastication, and profuse bleeding during home hygiene maneuvers. She wished to solve this situation. *Materials and Methods*. Since the patient did not respond well to the initial periodontal therapy, we carried out some accurate research concerning the patient's previous clinical history, and as we suspected that a vitamin D deficit might be involved, a chemical test for vitamin D was carried out and the results confirmed our suspicions. The team programmed the following therapeutical plan: Phase 1—rehabilitation of normal values of vitamin D with the support of an endocrinologist; Phase 2—full mouth disinfection; Phase 3—periodontal surgical restorative therapy; and Phase 4—orthodontic therapy and fixed prosthetics rehabilitation. *Results*. The results for this clinical case were extremely satisfying; we were able to bring the periodontal illness under control; resolve the orthodontic problems; and rehabilitate the patient both functionally and aesthetically. *Conclusion*. Thanks to the collaboration and communication between specialists from different sectors of medicine and dentistry, the clinical case was solved with absolutely satisfactory results.

1. Introduction

Vitamin D deficit is very common in the population and it is becoming more predominant in the groups of older and elderly people [1–3].

A vitamin D deficit leads to inadequate absorption of calcium and phosphate. This consequently gives rise to a reduction in the levels of calcium in the blood plasma, thus stimulating the parathyroid hormone, which acts to realign the calcium levels in the blood at the expense of the bones.

Periodontitis is a very common disease affecting over 50% of adults and a significant percentage of this group suffers from a very severe form [4, 5].

Periodontitis is a multifactorial disease primarily caused by plaque microorganisms, modified by the immune inflammatory response to chronic infection, which leads to the destruction of periodontal tissues in a susceptible host.

It is very well known that vitamin D plays a vital role in bone homeostasis and immunity. There is a biological rationale to suspect that vitamin D deficiency could negatively affect the periodontium [6–8].

When considering the periodontal area, normal levels of vitamin D reduce the expression of interleukin-8 and interleukin-6, reducing the virulence of *Porphyromonas gingivalis* [9].

Other natural substances, such as probiotics, could play a similar role since these seem to contribute to the maintenance of tissue homeostasis [10–13].

The two conditions, which are epidemiologically relevant, seem to interact empirically; vitamin D deficits are correlated to a higher prevalence of periodontitis and

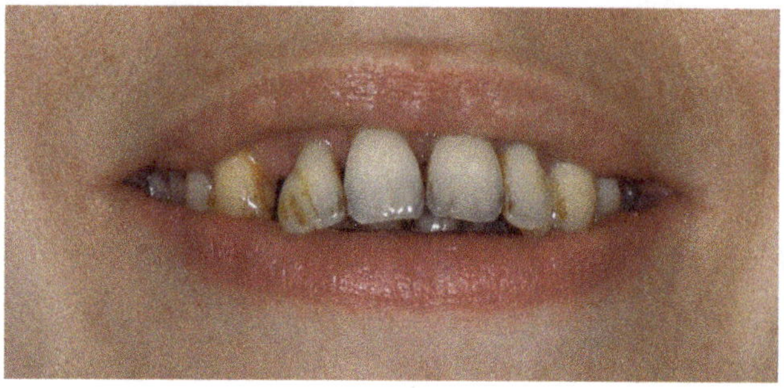

Figure 1: Clinical case: frontal view.

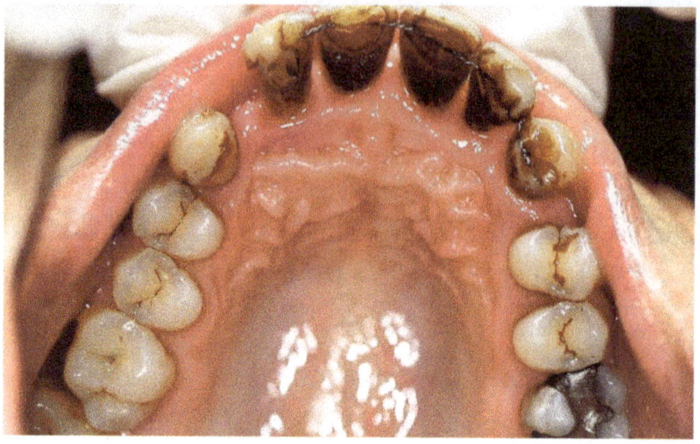

Figure 2: Clinical case: occlusal view, lower jaw.

periodontopathic patients show lower levels of this vitamin [14, 15].

Vitamin D could play a role in the treatment of periodontitis [16–18].

Moreover, it seems that polymorphisms of vitamin D receptors are involved in the etiopathogenesis of periodontitis, but this point is controversial [19–21].

Today's dentistry is not only carried out to restore the functionality of the stomatognathic apparatus but also aims to improve the general health of the patient and to restore and/or improve the aesthetics of the patient; therefore, it is advisable that clinicians become familiar with all the disciplines that make up dentistry to guarantee an adequate performance [22].

The objective of this study is to demonstrate how the patient's general health influences oral health, and especially the periodontium, and that an improvement in general health can sometimes be an effective way forward to achieving a satisfactory resolution, using multidisciplinary treatment, and thus obtaining an aesthetical and functional rehabilitation of the patient.

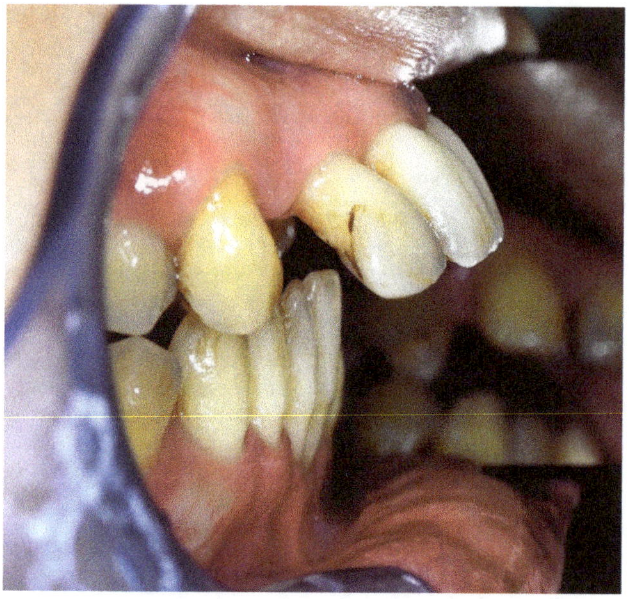

Figure 3: Clinical case: lateral view.

2. Materials and Methods

2.1. The Clinical Case. When the patient came to our notice, they presented a severe impairment of the entire stomatognathic apparatus with hyperaemic, oedemic gums, and severe functional and aesthetic problems, severely impaired dental arches, serious malocclusion, and diastema [12, 13].

The patient presented with an increased overjet due to a significant proclination of the upper incisors and a deviation of the upper midline to the left. This situation was probably due to a horizontal bone reabsorption associated with labial interposition (Figures 1–3).

The patient told us that they had undergone a number of periodontal therapies (scaling and root planing and non-surgical periodontal therapy) in the past but that they had never obtained satisfactory results.

After carrying out the anamnesis, the patient underwent a clinical check-up, X-rays (Figure 4), and a periodontal scan.

The patient's periodontal values (Figure 5) were followed and measured before the rehabilitation therapy (and again at 6 and 12 months after completion of the therapy):

(i) Plaque index presence/absence of visible plaque in 6 points of each tooth [23].

(ii) Bleeding on probing (BoP) presence/absence of bleeding when using probes in 6 points for each tooth [24].

(iii) Full mouth plaque score (FMPS) expressed as a percentage [25].

(iv) Full mouth bleeding score (FMBS) for BoP expressed as a percentage.

(v) Probing depth registered in millimetres in 6 points for each tooth [26, 27].

Both microbiological tests (biomolecular diagnostics) and genetic tests (genetical periodontic screening) were carried out (Figures 6 and 7).

Hematochemical tests were prescribed and, in particular, the one to test vitamin D levels.

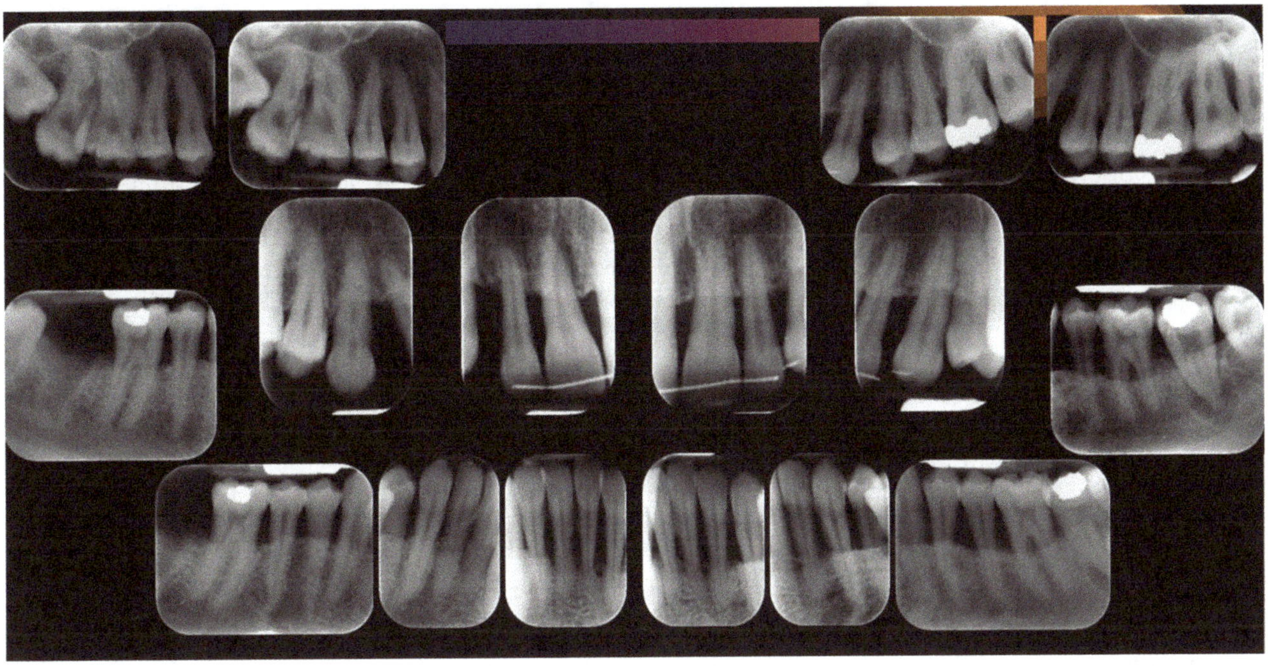

Figure 4: Rx full endoral clinical case: Rx.

The exam of the levels of vitamin D in the plasma were outside the normal levels.

The patient suffered from a severe vitamin D absorption deficit (Figure 8).

The patient underwent a bone densitometry exam on the femur.

Computerised bone mineralometry confirmed the low bone mineralisation levels.

2.2. The Therapeutical Plan. From the results of the clinical visit, the X-rays, the microbiological tests, the genetic test which showed an alteration of interleukin L1, and the laboratory tests, the following therapeutic plan (based on scientific evidence) was drawn up [28–32].

(i) Phase 1: rehabilitation of normal values of vitamin D with the support of an endocrinologist; A vitamin D supplementation protocol made it possible to re-establish the normal systemic homeostasis of the organism:

(ii) 1,25-OH vitamin D: 45.1 pg/ml.

(iii) 25-OH-vitamin D: 26.3 pg/ml.

(iv) Phase 2: full mouth disinfection.

(v) Phase 3: periodontal surgical restorative therapy.

(vi) Phase 4: orthodontic therapy and fixed prosthetics rehabilitation.

The dental treatment methods are described in detail as follows:

(i) Instruction and motivation.

(ii) Causal periodontal therapy associated with pharmacological antibiotic and antiseptic therapy using chlorhexidine 0.2%.

Full mouth disinfection with pharmacological antibiotic therapy using tetracillin chloridate 250 mg 3 times a day every 8 hours (Ambramicina Scharper SpA, Milan, Italy) and amoxicillin with clavulanic acid (Augmentin, Glaxosmithkline SpA, Verona, Italy) 1 g per day for 8 days. Chlorexidine 0.2% mouthwash (Cliadent 0.2% Budetta Farma s.r.l., Salerno, Italy) 2 rinses for 1 minute each per day for 10 days.

The periodontal parameters were normal throughout the period of the study (6 months), the FMPS and the FMBS were less than 20% before the prosthetic therapy and at 6 months from the definitive cementation (Figure 4).

(i) Splinting from 33 to 43 associated with stripping.

(ii) Devitalisation of 37.

(iii) Splinting of 35, 36, and 37.

(iv) Extraction of 28 and 38.

(v) Grafting with biomaterial followed by an implant on 47.

(vi) Fixed orthodontic therapy.

When the tissues were stabilised, the orthodontic therapy was initialised using a fixed multibracket and aesthetic orthodontic therapy according to the prescription of Prof.

	18	17	16	15	14	13	12	11	21	22	23	24	25	26	27	28
Mobilità		0	0	0	0	0	0	0	0	0	0	0	0	0	1	
Impianto																
Forcazione																
Sanguinamento al sondaggio		■	■ ■	■ ■	■			■	■ ■ ■	■ ■ ■		■	■	■ ■ ■	■ ■	
Placca																
Margine gengivale		-2 -2 -2	-2 -1 0	0 0 0	0 0 0	-1 -3 -1	-3 -4 -3	-2 -1 -1	-1 -1 -1	-1 -1 -1	-1 -2 -1	0 -1 0	0 -1 0	-2 -2 -3	-3 -3 -3	
Profondità di sondaggio		7 3 4	6 3 3	3 2 4	3 2 5	3 2 5	5 2 4	4 2 5	5 2 4	3 2 7	5 2 5	5 2 4	7 3 5	6 3 6	6 5 5	

Buccale

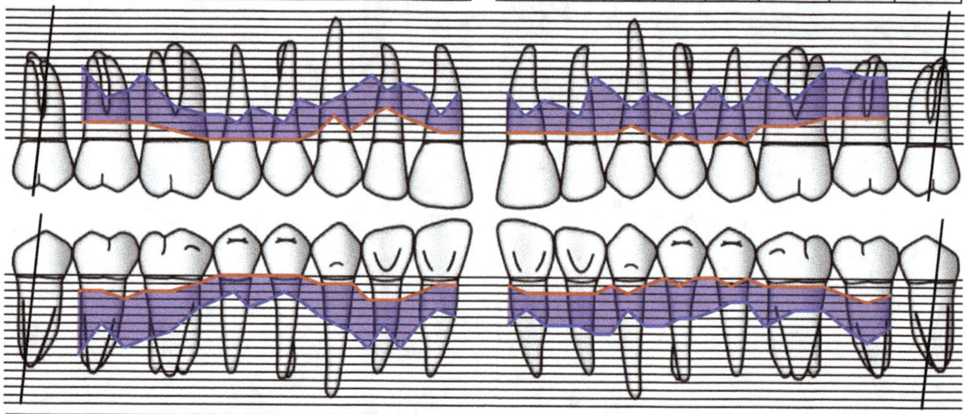

Linguale

	18	17	16	15	14	13	12	11	21	22	23	24	25	26	27	28
Margine gengivale		-2 -2 -3	-2 -2 -1	0 0 0	0 0 0	-1 -1 -1	-3 -3 -3	-2 -1 -1	-1 -2 -2	-2 -2 -2	-1 -2 -1	0 -1 0	0 -1 0	-1 -1 -1	-2 -3 -2	
Profondità di sondaggio		8 4 6	6 5 3	3 2 4	3 2 3	4 5 6	6 3 6	4 3 4	5 2 4	4 4 5	6 2 5	6 4 5	4 2 3	5 3 3	4 5 4	
Placca																
Sanguinamento al sondaggio		■ ■ ■	■ ■ ■	■ ■ ■	■ ■	■ ■	■ ■	■ ■ ■	■ ■	■ ■ ■	■ ■	■ ■	■ ■ ■	■ ■ ■	■	
Forcazione	|	|	|		|							|		|	|	|
Note							SPLINT	SPLINT	SPLINT	SPLINT	SPLINT					

Media prof. di sondaggio = 4 mm Media livello di attacco = −6 mm 0% Placca 59% Sanguinamento al sondaggio

	48	47	46	45	44	43	42	41	31	32	33	34	35	36	37	38
Note						SPLINT	SPLINT	SPLINT	SPLINT	SPLINT	SPLINT		SPLINT	SPLINT	SPLINT	
Forcazione																
Sanguinamento al sondaggio				■	■	■ ■ ■	■ ■ ■	■ ■ ■	■ ■ ■	■ ■	■ ■ ■	■	■ ■ ■	■ ■	■ ■	
Placca																
Margine gengivale			-2 -2 -1	-1 -2 -2	-1 -2 -2	-1 -2 -2	-3 -3 -4	-5 -4 -4	-4 -5 -5	-5 -3 -4	-3 -3 -2	-3 -3 -4	-3 -4 -3	-4 -4 -3	-4 -3 -3	
Profondità di sondaggio			4 3 5	5 2 5	5 3 5	4 3 2	2 3 4	2 3 5	4 2 4	5 3 4	3 3 4	3 3 4	4 3 4	5 4 4	5 4 7	

Lingual

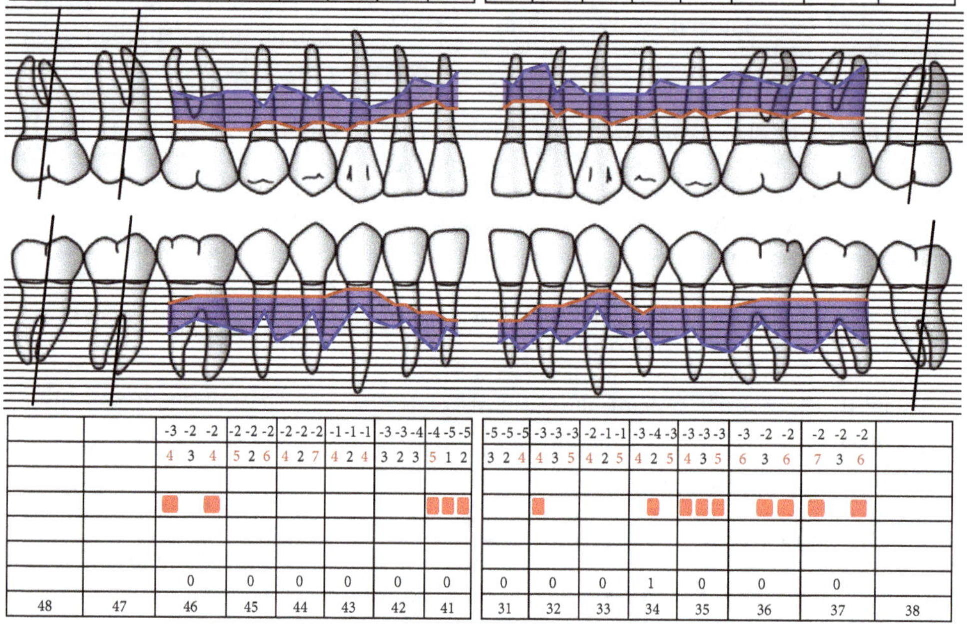

Buccale

	48	47	46	45	44	43	42	41	31	32	33	34	35	36	37	38
Margine gengivale			-3 -2 -2	-2 -2 -2	-2 -2 -2	-1 -1 -1	-3 -3 -4	-4 -5 -5	-5 -5 -5	-3 -3 -3	-2 -1 -1	-3 -4 -3	-3 -3 -3	-3 -2 -2	-2 -2 -2	
Profondità di sondaggio			4 3 4	5 2 6	4 2 7	4 2 4	3 2 3	5 1 2	3 2 4	4 3 5	4 2 5	4 2 5	4 3 5	6 3 6	7 3 6	
Placca																
Sanguinamento al sondaggio			■ ■					■ ■ ■		■		■	■ ■ ■	■ ■	■ ■	
Forcazione																
Impianto																
Mobilità			0	0	0	0	0	0	0	0	0	1	0	0	0	

FIGURE 5: Probing with periodontal indices.

DENTE	SITO	PPD	REC	BOP	PUS	PROVETTA
26	MP	8 mm	1 mm	SI	SI	BIANCA
16	DP	8 mm	2 mm	SI	SI	BIANCA
46	ML	7 mm	2 mm	SI	NO	BIANCA
36	MV	8 mm	3 mm	SI	SI	BIANCA
22	DP	6 mm	4 mm	SI	SI	BIANCA

NOME BATTERIO	CONTA BATTERICA	*	% RELATIVA
Aggregatibacter actinomycetemcomitans	< 1.00 * 10^2		0.0000
Porphytomonas gingivalis	< 1.00 * 10^2		0.0000
Tennerella forsythensys	1.18 * 10^5	+++	3.1635
Treponema denticola	2.93 * 10^3	++	0.0786
Peptostreptococcus micros	7.03 * 10^2	+	0.0188
Prevotella intermedia	4.31 * 10^2	+	0.0116
Fusobacterium nucleatum ssp	4.30 * 10^4	++	1.1528
Campylobacter rectus	7.60 * 10^4	++	2.0375
Eikonella corrodens	5.06 * 10^3	++	0.1357
Carica batterica totale	3.73 * 10^5		100

10^2 10^3 10^4 10^5 10^6 10^7 10^8

Genotipo Aggregatibacter actinomycetemcomitans:
Genotipo JP2 maggiore patogenicità rispetto 652-

Genotipo Porphyromonas Gingivalis FimA:
FimA Tipo I: Scarsa patogenicità. FimA Tipo II-IV: Altà patogenicità

*LEGENDA:
+ Batterio Individuato
++ Batterio presente in quantità elevata
+++ Batterio presente in quantità molto elevata

Carica batterica elevata richiede eventuale terapia

Figure 6: Microbiological test results.

IL-1a (-889); IL-1b (+3954); IL-1RN (+2018)	Modesta alterazione della risposta infiammatoria
IL-10 (-1082CoA, -819C>T, -592C>A)	ACC\GCC
IL-6 (-174G/C)	CG
COX-2 (-765G/C)	CG
Vitamin D Receptor (VDR TaqI)	TT
FUMO	SI (10 /die)
GRAVIDANZA	NO

In rosso i risultati associati alla malattia parodontale.

Valutazione del rischio individuale: Basso | Medio | **Alto** | Molto Alto

Figure 7: Genetic test results.

1,25-Diidrossi Vitamina D (metodo RIA)	68,5	pg/mL	20,0-67,0
25-Idrossi Vitamina D (metodo ECLIA)	15,2	ng/mL	< 30 ridotte riserve < 30 valori desiderabili

FIGURE 8: Laboratory test results related to vitamin D: vitamin D values.

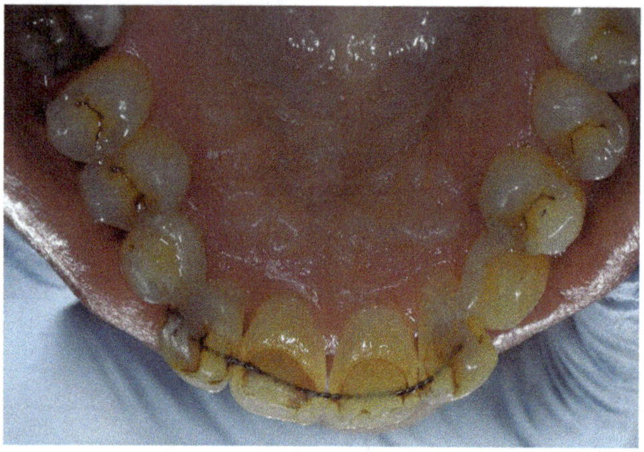

FIGURE 9: Clinical case: occlusal view, lower jaw, orthodontic therapy.

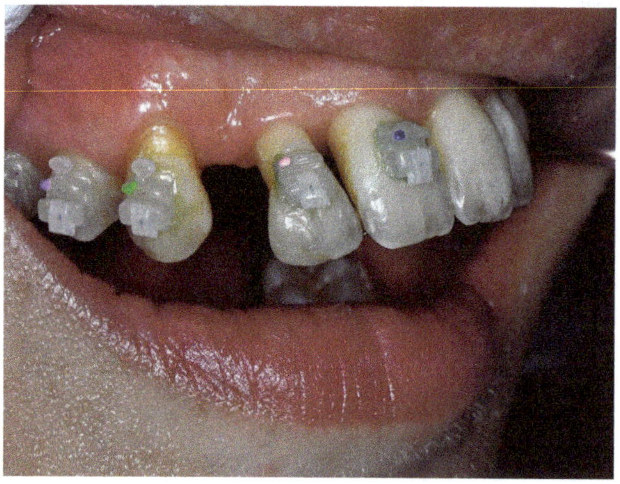

FIGURE 10: Clinical case: 3/4 view, orthodontic therapy.

W. Roth. Over the timespan of six months the orthodontic treatment was carried out with a sequence of standard arches (0.014 niti, 0.016 niti, 0.017 × 0.025 niti, 0.019 × 0.025 niti, e 0.019 × 0.025 ss plus an elastic chain) with the aim of retroclininig the upper incisors and resolving the position of the midline (Figures 9 and 10).

(i) Functional prosthetic and aesthetic rehabilitation

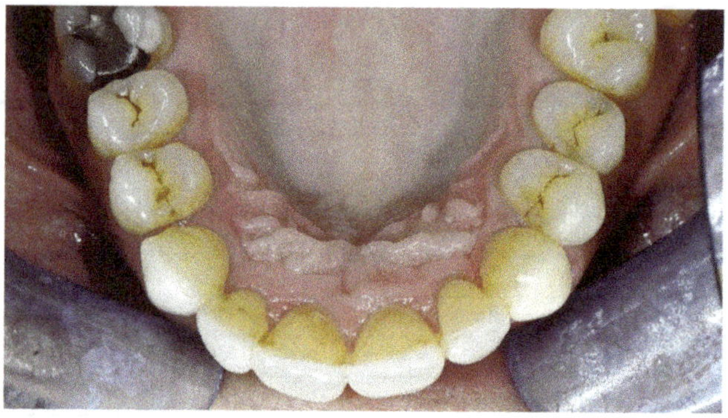

FIGURE 11: Clinical case: occlusal view, lower jaw, prosthetic therapy.

(ii) After completing the orthodontic therapy (Figure 11) prosthetic rehabilitation was carried out.

3. Results

We were able to:

(i) Bring the periodontal illness under control.

(ii) Take the FMBS and the FMPS down to zero.

(iii) Resolve the orthodontic problems.

(iv) Rehabilitate the patient both functionally and aesthetically (Figures 12–14).

4. Discussion

This work aims at explaining how a well-considered and multidisciplinary approach, based on a rigorous scientific method, which considers the organism's high reparative potential, can resolve a highly compromised situation in a patient with severe periodontitis associated with a vitamin D deficit, malocclusions, and diastemas. In today's interdisciplinary world, treatment planning must start with well-defined aesthetic goals.

By starting with aesthetics and considering the impact on function, structure, and biology, the clinician will be able to use the various disciplines of dentistry to deliver the highest level of dental care to each patient.

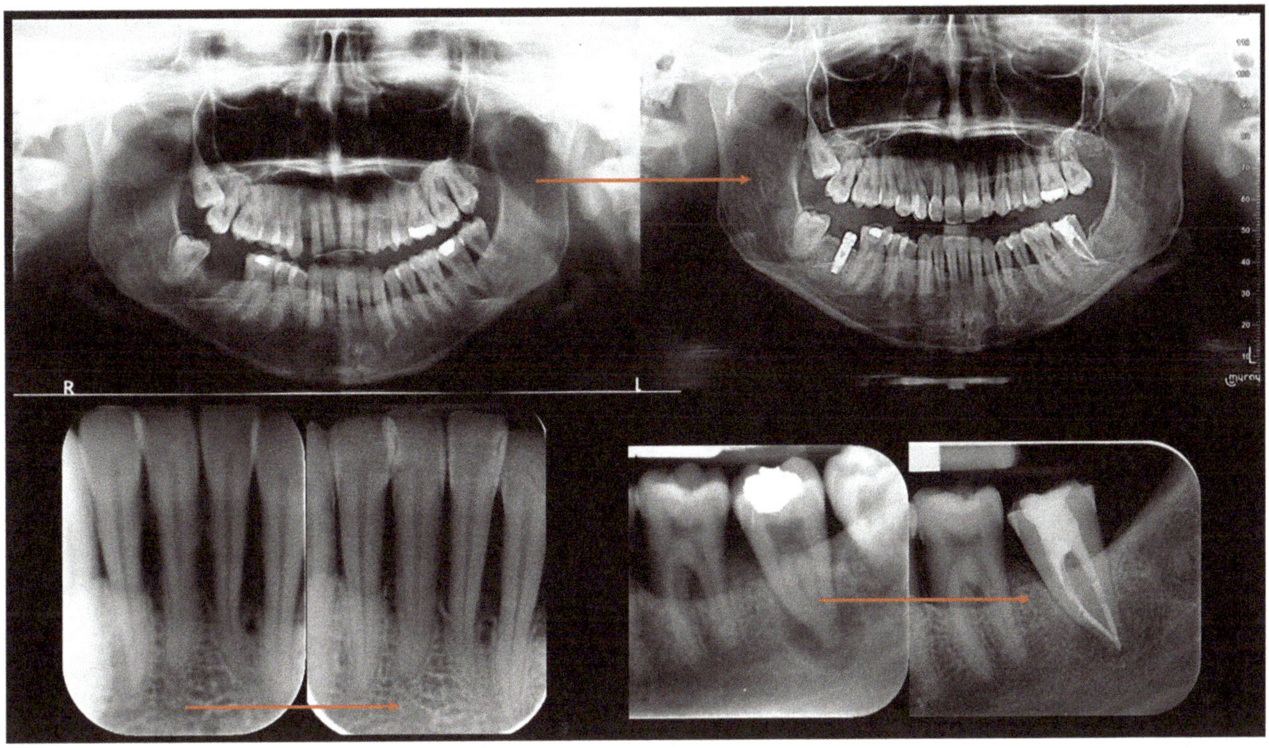

FIGURE 12: Clinical case: Rx pre- and post-treatment.

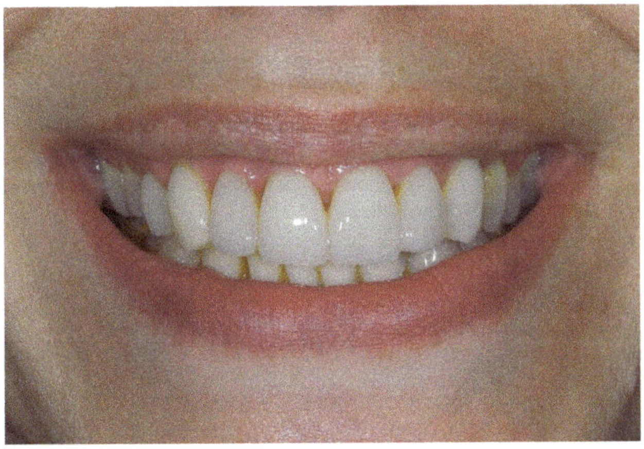

FIGURE 13: Clinical case: frontal view, at the end of the treatment.

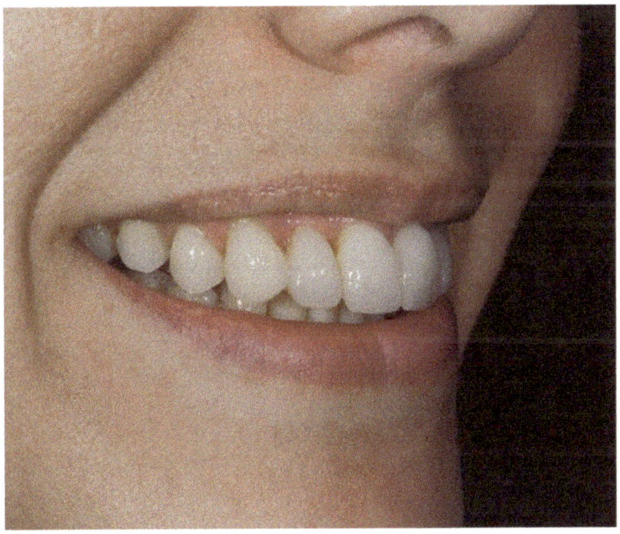

FIGURE 14: Clinical case: 3/4 view, at the end of the treatment.

Several dentists worked on the same case, each acting in their own specific field of action but with constant communication and synergy of intent.

Furthermore, this study highlights how important it is to consider other health parameters as the case was solved thanks to the intuition of the possibility of a vitamin D deficit with the relative confirmation from laboratory analyses.

Few cases of this type are reported in literature and therefore this study will serve as a guide to solving similarly complex cases. Correlation of vitamin D with periodontitis is an interesting topic, according to literature [7, 15], which requires more study to be clarified. This study, in particular, is yet another piece of evidence showing that, in our opinion, adequate serum levels of vitamin D could be essential in some cases for the control of periodontal disease.

The application of postbiotic gels to activate a proactive phase in combination with vitamin D treatment could be useful [33].

5. Conclusion

Once again, the importance of knowing and evaluating the patient's general state of health must be emphasized in order to be able to identify any systemic causes of a periodontal problem; in this case, it was important to identify the vitamin D deficiency, a widely spread condition among the population.

We believe that, today, a multidisciplinary approach to solving such complicated clinical cases is essential. Even if the literature is not exhaustive on the topic, we believe that vitamin D deficiency should be suspected, investigated, and eventually treated, in the case of periodontal situations that do not improve after conventional treatment. We sincerely hope that this topic will be further researched in the near future, producing new studies that could consider, for example, the use of other support molecules, such as postbiotics.

References

[1] M. F. Holick, "High prevalence of vitamin D inadequacy and implications for health," *Mayo Clinic Proceedings*, vol. 81, no. 3, pp. 353–373, 2006.

[2] M. C. Chapuy, P. Preziosi, M. Maamer et al., "Prevalence of vitamin D insufficiency in an adult normal population," *Osteoporosis International*, vol. 7, no. 5, pp. 439–443, 1997.

[3] C. M. Gordon, K. C. DePeter, H. A. Feldman, E. Grace, and S. J. Emans, "Prevalence of vitamin D deficiency among healthy adolescents," *Archives of Pediatrics & Adolescent Medicine*, vol. 158, no. 6, pp. 531–537, 2004.

[4] P. I. Eke, L. Wei, W. S. Borgnakke et al., "Periodontitis prevalence in adults ≥65 years of age, in the USA," *Periodontology 2000*, vol. 72, no. 1, pp. 76–95, 2016, PMCID: PMC8223257.

[5] P. I. Eke, G. O. Thornton-Evans, L. Wei, W. S. Borgnakke, B. A. Dye, and R. J. Genco, "Periodontitis in US adults: National Health and Nutrition Examination Survey 2009–2014," *Journal of the American Dental Association (1939)*, vol. 149, no. 7, pp. 576.e6–588.e6, 2018, PMCID: PMC8094373.

[6] V. Machado, S. Lobo, L. Proença, J. J. Mendes, and J. Botelho, "Vitamin D and periodontitis: a systematic review and meta-analysis," *Nutrients*, vol. 12, no. 8, p. 2177, 2020, PMCID: PMC7468917.

[7] E. Jagelavičienė, I. Vaitkevičienė, D. Šilingaitė, E. Šinkūnaitė, and G. Daugėlaitė, "The relationship between vitamin D and periodontal pathology," *Medicina*, vol. 54, no. 3, p. 45, 2018, PMCID: PMC6122115.

[8] S. H. Stein, R. Livada, and D. A. Tipton, "Re-evaluating the role of vitamin D in the periodontium," *Journal of Periodontal Research*, vol. 49, no. 5, pp. 545–553, 2014, Epub 2013 Nov 21.

[9] X. Tang, Y. Pan, and Y. Zhao, "Vitamin D inhibits the expression of interleukin-8 in human periodontal ligament cells stimulated with *Porphyromonas gingivalis*," *Archives of Oral Biology*, vol. 58, no. 4, pp. 397–407, 2013, Epub 2012 Oct 17.

[10] A. Butera, S. Gallo, C. Maiorani et al., "Probiotic alternative to chlorhexidine in periodontal therapy: evaluation of clinical and microbiological parameters," *Microorganisms*, vol. 9, no. 1, p. 69, 2021.

[11] A. Butera, S. Gallo, C. Maiorani et al., "Management of gingival bleeding in periodontal patients with domiciliary use of toothpastes containing hyaluronic acid, lactoferrin, or paraprobiotics: a randomized controlled clinical trial," *Applied Sciences*, vol. 11, no. 18, p. 8586, 2021.

[12] A. Butera, S. Gallo, M. Pascadopoli et al., "Paraprobiotics in non-surgical periodontal therapy: clinical and microbiological aspects in a 6-month follow-up domiciliary protocol for oral hygiene," *Microorganisms*, vol. 10, no. 2, p. 337, 2022.

[13] A. Scribante, A. Butera, and M. Alovisi, "Customized minimally invasive protocols for the clinical and microbiological management of the oral microbiota," *Microorganisms*, vol. 10, no. 4, p. 675, 2022.

[14] J. Botelho, V. Machado, L. Proença, A. S. Delgado, and J. J. Mendes, "Vitamin D deficiency and oral health: a comprehensive review," *Nutrients*, vol. 12, no. 5, p. 1471, 2020, PMCID: PMC7285165.

[15] A. Bhargava, P. Rastogi, N. Lal, R. Singhal, S. Khatoon, and M. A. Ali, "Relationship between vitamin D and chronic periodontitis," *Journal of Oral Biology and Craniofacial Research*, vol. 9, no. 2, pp. 177–179, 2019, Epub 2018 Jul 9, PMCID: PMC6561900.

[16] G. Brock and I. L. Chapple, "The potential impact of essential nutrients vitamins C and D upon periodontal disease pathogenesis and therapeutic outcomes," *Current Oral Health Reports*, vol. 3, no. 4, pp. 337–346, 2016.

[17] J. Perayil, K. S. Menon, S. Kurup et al., "Influence of vitamin D & calcium supplementation in the management of periodontitis," *Journal of Clinical and Diagnostic Research*, vol. 9, no. 6, pp. ZC35–ZC38, 2015, Epub 2015 Jun 1, PMCID: PMC4525604.

[18] W. Gao, H. Tang, D. Wang, X. Zhou, Y. Song, and Z. Wang, "Effect of short-term vitamin D supplementation after nonsurgical periodontal treatment: a randomized, double-masked, placebo-controlled clinical trial," *Journal of Periodontal Research*, vol. 55, no. 3, pp. 354–362, 2020, Epub 2020 Jan 20.

[19] K. Murthykumar, R. Arjunkumar, and V. P. Jayaseelan, "Association of vitamin D receptor gene polymorphism (rs10735810) and chronic periodontitis," *Journal of Investigative and Clinical Dentistry*, vol. 10, no. 4, article e12440, 2019, Epub 2019 Jul 19.

[20] H. X. Guo, J. Pan, H. B. Pan, S. J. Cui, and C. Y. Fang, "Correlation of vitamin D receptor gene (ApaI) polymorphism with periodontitis: a meta-analysis of Chinese population," *Food Science & Nutrition*, vol. 7, no. 11, pp. 3607–3612, 2019, PMCID: PMC6848803.

[21] T. Cai, Z. Y. Yang, L. Nie, J. X. Zhen, L. Deng, and Z. Zhou, "Association between vitamin D receptor BsmI gene polymorphism and periodontitis: a meta-analysis in a single ethnic group," *Cellular and Molecular Biology*, vol. 63, no. 11, pp. 1–4, 2017.

[22] F. M. Spear and V. G. Kokich, "A multidisciplinary approach to esthetic dentistry," *Dental Clinics of North America*, vol. 51, no. 2, pp. 487–505, 2007, x–xi.

[23] A. Tsamtsouris, G. E. White, and R. E. Clark, "A comparison between the plaque indices of Silness-Loe and Greene-Vermillion," *The Journal of Pedodontics*, vol. 5, no. 1, pp. 51–61, 1980.

[24] A. Joss, R. Adler, and N. P. Lang, "Bleeding on probing. A parameter for monitoring periodontal conditions in clinical practice," *Journal of Clinical Periodontology*, vol. 21, no. 6, pp. 402–408, 1994.

[25] J. S. Holtzman, K. A. Atchison, M. D. Macek, and D. Markovic, "Oral health literacy and measures of periodontal disease," *Journal of Periodontology*, vol. 88, no. 1, pp. 78–88, 2017, Epub 2016 Aug 13. PMID, PMCID: PMC5557021.

[26] S. Khan and L. L. Cabanilla, "Periodontal probing depth measurement: a review," *The Compendium of Continuing Education in Dentistry*, vol. 30, no. 1, pp. 12–14, 2009, 16, 18–21; quiz 22, 36.

[27] M. A. Listgarten, "Periodontal probing: what does it mean?," *Journal of Clinical Periodontology*, vol. 7, no. 3, pp. 165–176, 1980, 7000852.

[28] D1. Edelhoff and J. A. Sorensen, "Tooth structure removal associated with various preparation designs for anterior teeth," *The Journal of Prosthetic Dentistry*, vol. 87, no. 5, pp. 503–509, 2002.

[29] J. Y. Chai and J. W. Steege, "Effects of labial margin design on stress distribution of a porcelain-fused-to-metal crown," *Journal of Prosthodontics*, vol. 1, no. 1, pp. 18–23, 1992.

[30] L. Cho, J. Choi, Y. J. Yi, and C. J. Park, "Effect of finish line variants on marginal accuracy and fracture strength of ceramic optimized polymer/fiber-reinforced composite crowns," *The Journal of Prosthetic Dentistry*, vol. 91, no. 6, pp. 554–560, 2004.

[31] J. R. Gavelis, J. D. Morency, E. D. Riley, and R. B. Sozio, "The effect of various finish line preparations on the marginal seal and occlusal seat of full crown preparations," *The Journal of Prosthetic Dentistry*, vol. 45, no. 2, pp. 138–145, 1981.

[32] R. Ed, "The social solution-denture esthetics, phonetics and function," *Journal of Prosthodontics*, vol. 18, no. 2, pp. 112–115, 2009.

[33] A. Butera, S. Gallo, M. Pascadopoli, D. Taccardi, and A. Scribante, "Home oral care of periodontal patients using antimicrobial gel with postbiotics, lactoferrin, and aloe barbadensis leaf juice powder vs conventional chlorhexidine gel: a split-mouth randomized clinical trial," *Antibiotics*, vol. 11, p. 118, 2022.

28

Periodontal Manifestation in a Patient with Kindler Syndrome

Aysegul Sari[1] **and Salih Celik**[2]

[1]*Faculty of Dentistry, Department of Periodontology, Hatay Mustafa Kemal University, Hatay, Turkey*
[2]*Department of Oral and Maxillofacial Surgery, TDC Dental Clinic, Antalya, Turkey*

Correspondence should be addressed to Aysegul Sari; aysegulsari@mku.edu.tr

Academic Editor: Sukumaran Anil

Kindler syndrome is a rare subtype of inherited epidermolysis bullosa. A 42-year-old female patient was admitted to our clinic with a complaint of tooth mobility. Multiple hypo- and hyperpigmented macules dissipated all over her body, prominent poikilodermatous changes, xerosis of the skin, and atrophy were seen in the clinical extraoral examination. Intraoral examination showed atrophy of the buccal mucosa, limited oral opening, epidermal tissue easily separated from the connective tissue, painful ulcers of the hard palate, severe periodontitis, and keratosis of the lips. All of the teeth showed mobility. After dermatologist consultation, the diagnosis of the patient was clinically identified as "Kindler syndrome." All of her teeth were extracted due to her progressive periodontal disease and late admission to our clinic. Periodontal treatment might be effective in treating and controlling oral symptoms related to the syndrome and in improving the patient's quality of life.

1. Introduction

Kindler syndrome (KS) is defined as a rare autosomal recessive genodermatosis disease. Progressive poikiloderma, the presence of trauma-induced blisters, diffuse cutaneous atrophy, abnormal pigmentation, varying degrees of photosensitivity, and skin fragility are prominent clinical characteristics of the syndrome. Theresa Kindler described the syndrome for the first time in a 14-year-old girl with acral blistering since childhood who subsequently developed photosensitivity and poikiloderma in 1954 [1].

The genetic origin of the syndrome was first defined in 2003, with the identification of loss-of-function mutations in the gene KIND1 held on chromosome 20p12.3 [2]. More than 25 mutations have been revealed in this gene. Gene KIDIN 1 encodes kindlin-1 protein, which is one of the components of focal contacts in keratinocytes expressed particularly in the basal keratinocytes located in the epidermis. Abnormal skin fragility with defects in the actinextracellular matrix linkage is caused by loss of this protein [3, 4].

Histopathological examination of the cutaneous biopsy in KS reported a presence of pigmentary incontinence, degeneration of focal vacuole in the basal layer accompanied by subepidermal cleft, dilatation of blood vessels in the upper dermis, and epidermal atrophy [5, 6].

Other clinical symptoms of KS include nail dystrophy; acral hyperkeratosis [7]; webbing and contractures of toes and fingers [6]; alopecia [8]; actinic changes [9]; mucosal involvement including esophageal [6], oral commissure [10], vaginal [6], and urethral [8] stenosis; ectropion of the eyelids [10]; pigmentation of the lips [8]; and onychodystrophy [6].

The present case reported periodontal management of a 42-year-old female patient KS.

2. Case Report

A 42-year-old female patient presented to Hatay Mustafa Kemal University, Faculty of Dentistry, Periodontology Department, with complaints of tooth mobility in February 2016. Multiple hypo- and hyperpigmented macules dissipated all over her body, prominent poikilodermatous changes, xerosis of the skin, alopecia, and atrophy were seen in the clinical extraoral examination. There was a distinct

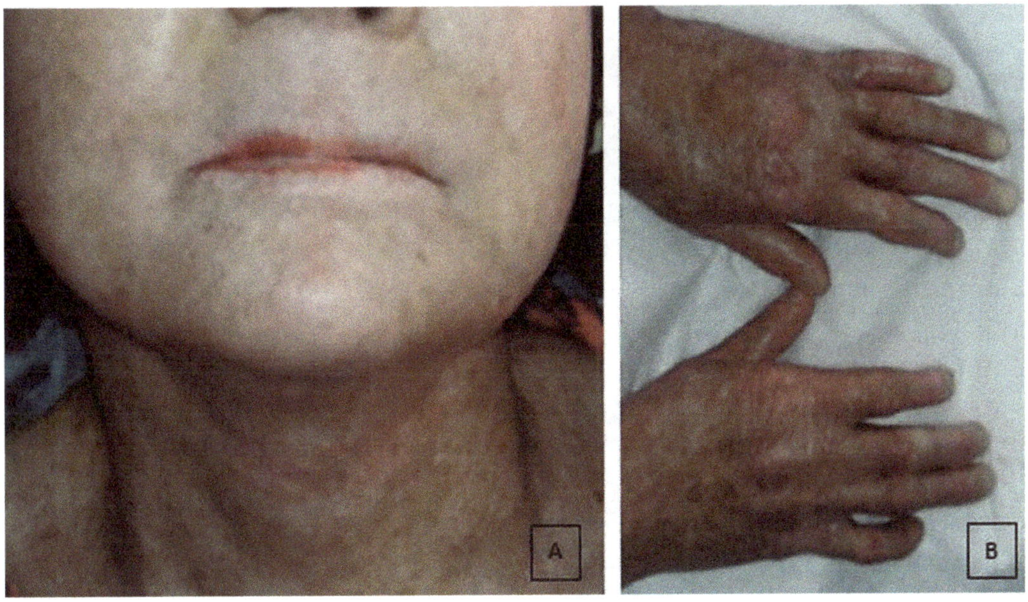

FIGURE 1: (a) The image showing multiple hypo- and hyperpigmented macules, prominent poikilodermatous changes, xerosis, alopecia, and atrophy of the skin. (b) The image showing cigarette paper-like wrinkling on the dorsum of the feet and hands. Atrophy and adhesions were detected in the fingers.

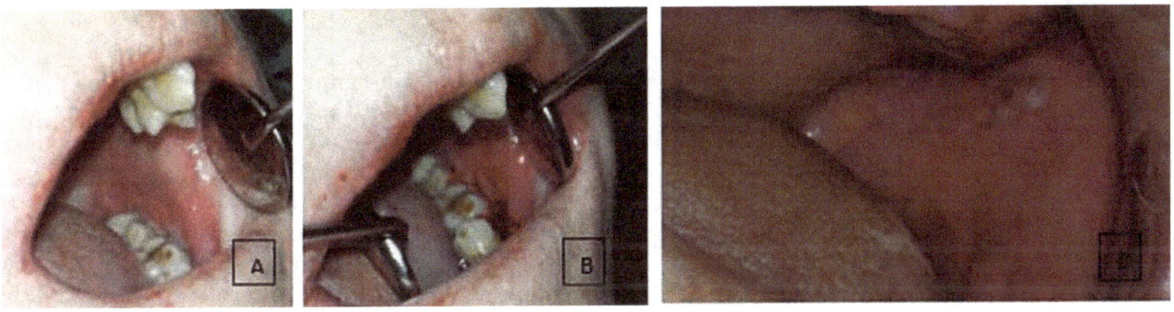

FIGURE 2: (a) The image showing atrophy of the lip, painful ulcers of the buccal mucosa, and keratosis of the lips. (b) It was clinically detected that the oral epidermal tissue easily separated from the connective tissue. (c) Leukoplakia-like lesions were observed in the buccal mucosa.

cigarette paper-like wrinkling on the dorsum of the feet and hands. Atrophy and adhesions were present in the fingers (Figure 1). Her mental and motor statuses were normal.

Intraoral examination showed atrophy of the buccal mucosa, limited oral opening, epidermal tissue easily separated from the connective tissue, painful ulcers of the hard palate, severe periodontitis, and keratosis of the lips. Also, leukoplakia-like lesions were observed in the buccal mucosa (Figure 2). Clinical attachment loss was severe in the periodontal tissue. There were few teeth in the mouth. All of the teeth showed mobility. The gingiva was thin and fragile. Bleeding, swelling, atrophy, and floppy were observed in the gingival tissue (Figure 3).

The patient stated that she had a syndrome in her anamnesis; however, she would not give to us sufficient information about her disorder. Hospital records of the patient could not be reached. The patient was referred to the dermatology department for a definitive diagnosis. The patient's disorder was diagnosed as "Kindler syndrome" by the dermatologist. All of her teeth were extracted due to her progressive periodontal disease and late admission to our clinic. Furthermore, floppy gingival tissue was removed with gingivectomy for tissue modeling (Figure 4). She was prescribed 0.2% chlorhexidine gluconate for mouth rinsing (2x1, during 14 days), in addition to tetracaine chlorhydrate (0.5 mg) and hexamidine isethionate (1 mg) solution for relieving the oral symptoms.

Conservative treatment was preferred since the results of surgical and dental implant treatments to the patient were not predictable. The patient was referred to the prosthodontics department for the prosthetic process and maintained under clinical follow-up.

3. Discussion

Kindler syndrome is a rare heritable skin disorder with a complex phenotype and poorly understood pathogenesis [11, 12]. The current case reported the oral findings of a 42-year-old female patient with KS who applied to our clinic when her periodontal prognosis had advanced.

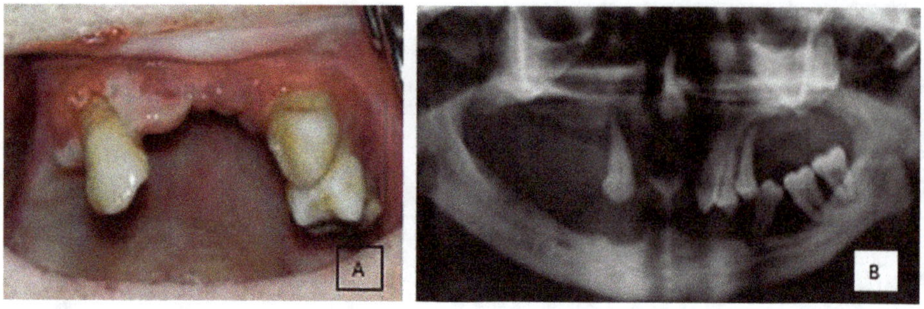

Figure 3: (a) The image showing that the clinical attachment loss was severe in the periodontal tissue. Bleeding, swelling, atrophy, and floppy were observed in the gingival tissue. (b) The panoramic radiography image of the patient.

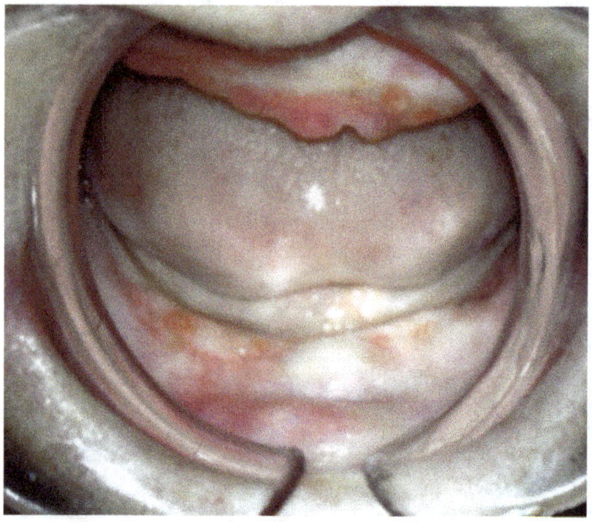

Figure 4: The image showing six-week postoperative healing after medicine treatment and gingivectomy.

KS has various clinical symptoms such as acral skin blisters, progressive poikiloderma [1], alopecia, nail dystrophy, acral hyperkeratosis [7], contractures and webbing of toes and fingers [6], photosensitivity [1], and actinic changes [9]. In addition, oral symptoms are very common in this disorder. It was reported that oral manifestations often include severe periodontitis which begins with permanent teeth eruption and progresses rapidly, poor dentition with premature loss of teeth, erosive areas in the labial and buccal mucosa and gingiva, spontaneous bleeding, desquamative gingivitis, angular cheilitis, leukokeratosis of the lips, caries, halitosis, and xerostomia [13]. Clinical and oral manifestations of the present case were similar to those reported in previous studies.

Oral ulcerations and rapidly progressing periodontitis are conditions that should be considered in terms of periodontal health in patients with KS. Kindlin-1 mutations can cause these symptoms [14]. Kindler syndrome is a genetic disorder that occurs as a result of mutations in the fermitin family homolog 1 gene that encodes the kindlin-1 protein which plays a role in cell adhesion, spreading, and migration [15]. It has been reported that kindlin-1 has a basic role in actin-dependent keratinocyte cell adhesion, which is necessary for epidermal and periodontal health. Lack of this protein in keratinocytes results in reduction of cell spreading, proliferation, and migration rate [16]. Larjava et al. indicated that rapid progression of periodontal disease can be caused by deficiency of integrin activation in the junctional epithelium which can be caused by kindlin-1 mutations [17].

There are few studies evaluating periodontal condition in patients with KS. Wiebe et al. [18] reported that in a case report, by periodontal therapy and long-term follow-up, many teeth were maintained for >10 years despite the rapid prognosis of periodontal disease in patients with KS. Siegel et al. suggested that periodontitis progression was rapid in patients with KD compared to healthy controls [19]. Also, Wiab et al. indicated that kindler subjects exhibited largely similar patterns of periodontal destruction on both sides of the mouth [20]. In accordance with previous data, periodontal disease prognosis was very advanced in the present case. The patient's admission for treatment was in the late period, which limited the periodontal treatment. Since all the teeth had serious mobility and almost all periodontal attachments were lost, all of the teeth were extracted. It can be considered that periodontal disease process could have been accelerated because the patient had never received periodontal treatment before.

4. Conclusion

Management of patients with Kindler syndrome requires a multidisciplinary approach. Periodontal treatment might be effective in treating and controlling oral symptoms related to the syndrome and in improving the patient's quality of life.

Authors' Contributions

The authors contributed to the conception and design of the case report. Treatment and follow-up of the case were performed by Aysegul Sari and Salih Celik. The draft of the manuscript was written by Aysegul SARI. All the authors commented on the previous versions of the manuscript. All the authors read and approved the final manuscript.

Acknowledgments

The author would like to thank Ebru Celik, Assist. Prof., from Hatay Mustafa Kemal University, Medical Faculty, Dermatology Department, for medical diagnosis.

References

[1] E. de la Rosa-Garcia and A. Mosqueda-Taylor, "Leiomyomatous hamartoma of the anterior tongue: report of a case and review of the literature," *International Journal of Paediatric Dentistry*, vol. 9, no. 2, pp. 129–132, 1999.

[2] M. Nava-Villalba, F. Ocampo-Acosta, A. Seamanduras-Pacheco, and B. C. Aldape-Barrios, "Leiomyomatous hamartoma: report of two cases and review of the literature," *Oral Surgery, Oral Medicine, Oral Pathology, Oral Radiology, and Endodontics*, vol. 105, no. 4, pp. e39–e45, 2008.

[3] H. S. McGuff, A. C. Jones, J. Heim-Hall, and T. A. Keller, "Case of the month. Leiomyomatous hamartoma," *Texas Dental Journal*, vol. 126, pp. 544-545, 2009.

[4] K. H. Ng, C. H. Siar, and H. Abdul Latif, "Leiomyoma of the incisive papilla region: a case report," *Annals of Dentistry*, vol. 51, no. 1, pp. 29–31, 1992.

[5] L. Mendes, L. Nogueira, V. Vilasboas, C. Talhari, S. Talhari, and M. Santos, "Kindler syndrome: report of two cases," *Anais Brasileiros de Dermatologia*, vol. 87, no. 5, pp. 779–781, 2012.

[6] H. Shimizu, M. Sato, M. Ban et al., "Immunohistochemical, ultrastructural, and molecular features of Kindler syndrome distinguish it from dystrophic epidermolysis bullosa," *Archives of Dermatology*, vol. 133, no. 9, pp. 1111–1117, 1997.

[7] S. Hacham-Zadeh, A. A. Garfunkel, J. M. Opitz, and J. F. Reynolds, "Kindler syndrome in two related Kurdish families," *American Journal of Medical Genetics*, vol. 20, no. 1, pp. 43–48, 1985.

[8] A. Y. Kapasi, U. Khopkar, S. Raj, and S. L. Wadhwa, "Weary-Kindler syndrome with multiple seborrheic keratoses," *International Journal of Dermatology*, vol. 32, no. 6, pp. 444-445, 1993.

[9] R. M. Haber and W. M. Hanna, "Kindler syndrome. Clinical and ultrastructural findings," *Archives of Dermatology*, vol. 132, no. 12, pp. 1487–1490, 1996.

[10] D. N. Ricketts, C. L. Morgan, J. M. McGregor, and P. R. Morgan, "Kindler syndrome: a rare cause of desquamative lesions of the gingiva," *Oral Surgery, Oral Medicine, Oral Pathology, Oral Radiology, and Endodontics*, vol. 84, no. 5, pp. 488–491, 1997.

[11] M. Lotem, M. Raben, R. Zeltser et al., "Kindler syndrome complicated by squamous cell carcinoma of the hard palate: successful treatment with high-dose radiation therapy and granulocyte-macrophage colony-stimulating factor," *The British Journal of Dermatology*, vol. 144, no. 6, pp. 1284–1286, 2001.

[12] F. Jobard, B. Bouadjar, F. Caux et al., "Identification of mutations in a new gene encoding a FERM family protein with a pleckstrin homology domain in Kindler syndrome," *Human Molecular Genetics*, vol. 12, no. 8, pp. 925–935, 2003.

[13] N. M. Barbosa, F. Visioli, M. D. Martins, M. A. Martins, and M. C. Munerato, "Oral manifestations in Kindler syndrome: case report and discussion of literature findings," *Special Care in Dentistry*, vol. 36, no. 4, pp. 223–230, 2016.

[14] J. M. Albandar, C. Susin, and F. J. Hughes, "Manifestations of systemic diseases and conditions that affect the periodontal attachment apparatus: case definitions and diagnostic considerations," *Journal of Clinical Periodontology*, vol. 89, Supplement 20, pp. S183–S203, 2018.

[15] E. Rognoni, R. Ruppert, and R. Fassler, "The kindlin family: functions, signaling properties and implications for human disease," *Journal of Cell Science*, vol. 129, no. 1, pp. 17–27, 2016.

[16] G. Petricca, M. Leppilampi, G. Jiang et al., "Localization and potential function of kindlin-1 in periodontal tissues," *European Journal of Oral Sciences*, vol. 117, no. 5, pp. 518–527, 2009.

[17] H. Larjava, L. Koivisto, J. Heino, and L. Hakkinen, "Integrins in periodontal disease," *Experimental Cell Research*, vol. 325, no. 2, pp. 104–110, 2014.

[18] C. B. Wiebe, G. Petricca, L. Hakkinen, G. Jiang, C. Wu, and H. S. Larjava, "Kindler syndrome and periodontal disease: review of the literature and a 12-year follow-up case," *Journal of Periodontology*, vol. 79, no. 5, pp. 961–966, 2008.

[19] D. H. Siegel, G. H. Ashton, H. G. Penagos et al., "Loss of Kindlin-1, a Human Homolog of the _Caenorhabditis elegans_ Actin -Extracellular-Matrix Linker Protein UNC-112, Causes Kindler Syndrome," *American Journal of Human Genetics*, vol. 73, no. 1, pp. 174–187, 2003.

[20] C. B. Wiebe, H. Penagos, N. Luong et al., "Clinical and microbiologic study of periodontitis associated with Kindler syndrome," *Journal of Periodontology*, vol. 74, no. 1, pp. 25–31, 2003.

29

Resolution of Abfraction-Associated Gingival Fenestration Utilizing Connective Tissue Grafting

Braydon Haskell, J. Kobi Stern, Jordan Ghiassi, Andrew Kurialacherry, Sadja Gaud-Quintana, and Mark E. Peacock

The Dental College of Georgia at Augusta University, Augusta, GA, USA

Correspondence should be addressed to Andrew Kurialacherry; akurialacherry@augusta.edu

Academic Editor: Mine Dündar

Introduction. Gingival fenestration (GF) is a distinct clinical entity of uncertain etiology that is seldom documented in the literature. It has been associated mainly with submucosal mechanical irritants such as calculus that subsequently create an opening in the oral soft tissue, usually at facial anterior sites. Surgical correction may be indicated to address functional and/or esthetic concerns. *Case Presentation.* The patient, a 74-year-old male, presented to the clinic with a chief complaint of "something is poking through my gum." Clinical exam revealed a gingival fenestration on the facial of tooth #11, associated with what appeared to be a pronounced noncarious cervical lesion (NCCL). Surgical treatment consisted of a connective tissue graft and odontoplasty of the sharp protruding edge of the root surface. Healing was uneventful with excellent closure of the fenestration and no evidence of recurrence after 18 months of follow-up. *Conclusion.* GF is a perforation of the mucosa typically associated with underlying sharp mechanical etiology. This report describes a fenestration that developed from a probable abfractive lesion, which later was successfully closed and exhibits long-term stability.

1. Introduction

Gingival fenestration is an opening through oral keratinized mucosa that is reported infrequently, possibly due to lack of symptoms and/or patient unawareness [1]. Unlike fenestrations, the gingival margin for a dehiscence is noncontinuous and apically positioned. Although previously mentioned in the literature, Lane in 1977 was the first to describe it as a distinct pathologic entity [2]. The etiological basis for GF has not been completely elucidated but is probably multifactorial.

Local factors that have been reported to be associated with GF include plaque/calculus [1–4], cervical enamel projections (CEP) [5], tooth malpositioning [1, 2], trauma [3], chewing habits/foreign body (gutka) [6], occlusal factors [7], and implant fixture threads [8]. Anatomic factors associated with noncarious cervical lesions (abfraction, abrasion) could possibly lead to sharp irregular cervical "notching," [9] resulting in a soft tissue fenestration [10]. Almost all reported cases of GF occurred on the facial surfaces of incisor teeth.

Soft tissue fenestrations linked with NCCLs are almost never documented. NCCLs may have very rough and serrated line angles that could lead to GF. A strong relationship between NCCLs and occlusal overload (bruxism, grinding) has been reported [11], and patients with group function can have NCCLs occurring six times more frequently than those with cuspid-protected occlusion [12]. The theoretical concept of abfraction, described by Lee and Eakle [13], is controversial, but this phenomenon is still supported by a multitude of practitioners.

Most gingival fenestrations described have occurred on the facial surfaces of thin unattached gingiva and are associated with heavy calculus deposits. This case report documents a GF linked to a subgingival NCCL, along with its surgical treatment and follow-up.

2. Case Report

A 74-year-old Caucasian male was referred to the Periodontics Clinic of the Dental College of Georgia, Augusta

University, Augusta, Georgia, in May of 2015, with a chief complaint of "something has poked through my gum." The patient had been on a routine three-month maintenance cycle and reported no previous incidence of the condition, which had been present approximately six months. The medical history review was remarkable for hypertension, hyperlipidemia, and implanted artificial pacemaker and noncontributory social history (no use of gutka products). Current medications included metoprolol, amlodipine, losartan, ezetimibe/simvastatin, and aspirin daily. Clinical examination revealed a $3 \times 5\,mm$ fenestration through the facial gingiva at tooth #11 (Figure 1). Patient reported daily brushing and flossing using an extra soft toothbrush that was routinely changed at each hygiene appointment. Oral hygiene instructions were reinforced and reviewed at each appointment, and through demonstration, the patient exhibited proper brushing and flossing technique. All gingival probings were ≤3 mm with no mobility, no suppuration or swelling present, and no decay detected, but there was a sharp, pointy edge of what appeared to be the coronal border of a NCCL (abfraction). Evidence of previous occlusal trauma to #11 was visible with blunted cusp tip and craze line; similarly, tooth #10 displayed a wear facet. The patient does not present with cuspid-protected occlusion. The tooth tested vital, and the lesion was asymptomatic, except for the noticeable perforation of the gingiva. A radiograph taken showed only mild interproximal horizontal bone loss (Figure 2).

Various treatment options were discussed with the patient including no treatment, gingivectomy and direct restoration, gingival flap and odontoplasty, or connective tissue grafting (CTG) with odontoplasty, along with limited occlusal adjustment. The patient was thoroughly informed of all aspects of the treatment for this unique association between NCCL and GF. CTG was preferred to improve upon the patient's thin phenotype in order to address the patient's chief complaint. He was counseled and consented to surgical treatment to correct the soft tissue defect and odontoplasty of the root surface irregularity.

Occlusal adjustment was made on #11 cuspid until light occlusal contacts evenly distributed bilaterally. Under local anesthesia with 2% lidocaine and 1 : 100,00 epinephrine, a facial sulcular-modified papilla preservation incision was made from #10 to #12, and a mucoperiosteal flap reflected revealing a NCCL with prominent sharp edges at #11 (Figure 3). The root prominence of the NCCL was reduced with high speed rotary instrumentation (Figure 4), and the site prepared for soft tissue grafting. A connective tissue graft was taken from the left maxillary tuberosity region, and closure was obtained with 5-0 PTFE monofilament sutures after copious irrigation of the surgical site (Figure 5).

The surgical site healed without complication. Figure 6 shows healing at 2 months with correction of the gingival perforation evident. An 18-month follow-up (Figure 7) reveals mature healing of the defect, and the patient has had no complaints. Noticeable from the 2-month to the 18-month postop is approximately 1 mm coronal gingival migration by "creeping attachment," a phenomenon described by Goldman and Cohen [14].

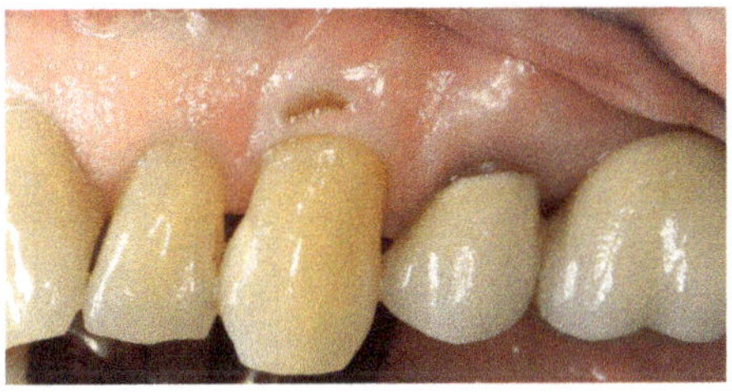

Figure 1: Fenestration on facial gingiva #11.

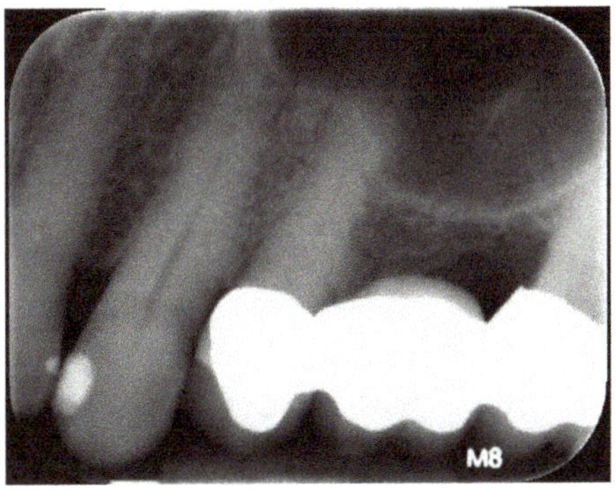

Figure 2: Periapical radiograph #11.

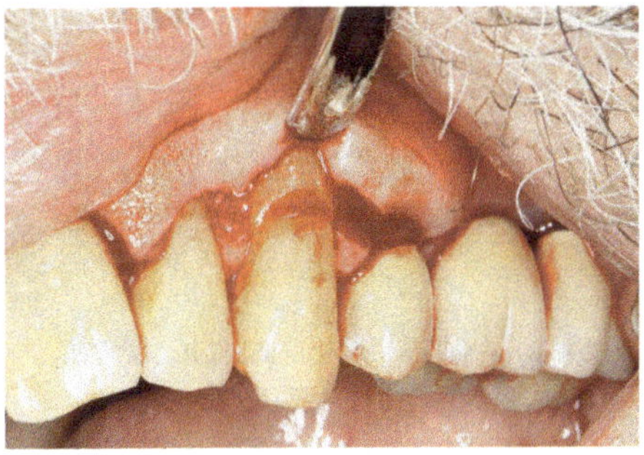

Figure 3: Prominent edge of NCCL #11.

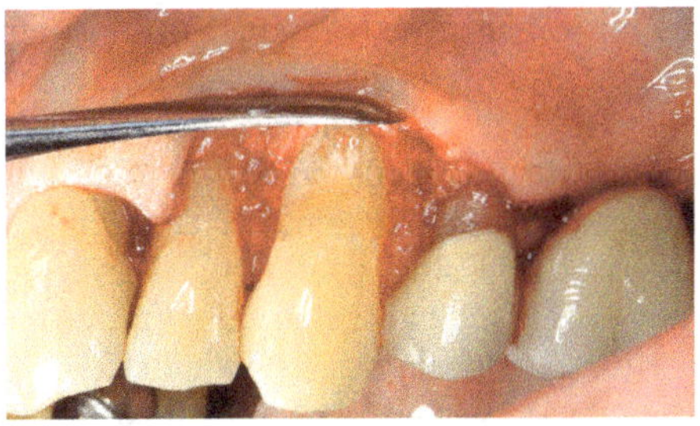

Figure 4: Postodontoplasty #11.

3. Discussion

Documented gingival fenestration lesions are uncommon, though the prevalence could be higher due to underreporting. The pathogenesis of GF is uncertain; however, it has been

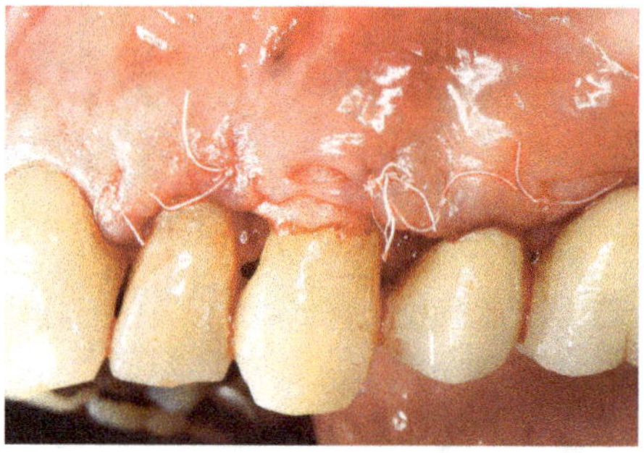

Figure 5: Closure of surgical graft site.

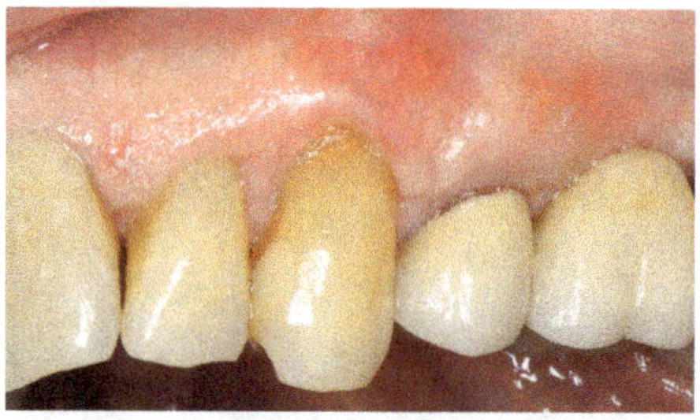

Figure 6: 2-month postop healing.

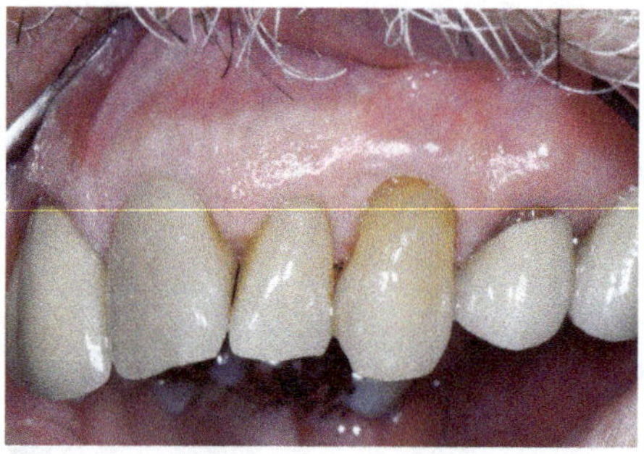

Figure 7: 18-month follow-up.

proposed that it is a transient stage in gingival cleft formation from a combination of thin tissue and subgingival irritants [2]. Because these lesions are often asymptomatic, the perceived need for treatment to many patients is minimal.

Most scientific reports reveal calculus to be the most common irritant that results in a soft tissue fenestration. Davies et al.'s review on management of NCCLs is the only other documentation in the literature describing a cervical cavity (abfraction) causing a GF [10]. They suggest that because the overlying gingiva exerted a "protective" effect, the lesion etiology was abfraction without any abrasive or erosive element. As is in the case presented here, abrasion and/or erosion would probably have produced recession versus a protrusion through the gingiva.

Most documented accounts of GF occurred on the facial of anterior teeth (maxillary and mandibular). Comparably, almost all NCCLs also occur on the facial, with only 2% of them reported to exist on the lingual or palatal surface [15]. Excessive occlusal forces producing stress near the cementoenamel junction (CEJ), combined with mechanical abrasion, may predispose a patient to gingival recession. However, as can be seen in this case, a fenestration in the gingiva may occasionally form which will not revert to a recession defect. This rare defect was successfully closed by surgical treatment, with long-term verified follow-up.

Surgical rationale for utilizing an autogenous CTG versus acellular dermal matrix stems from historic success as the gold standard for long-term stability, tissue thickening, and ability to remain exposed [16]. Access to the lesion was a critical component to the surgical intervention; thus, reflection of a mucoperiosteal flap provided adequate visual and surgical field to perform odontoplasty.

4. Conclusion

Gingival fenestration is a perforation of the mucosa typically associated with underlying sharp mechanical etiology. This report describes a fenestration that developed from a probable abfractive lesion, which later was successfully closed and exhibits long-term stability. Further research and follow-up would provide more evidence to support the results of this case report.

Additional Points

Summary. This case documents an infrequently reported soft tissue lesion, the gingival fenestration, and the accompanying probable etiology, a prominent subgingival abfraction.

References

[1] M. E. Peacock, D. A. Mott, M. F. Cuenin, S. D. Hokett, and E. B. Fowler, "Periodontal plastic surgical technique for gingival fenestration closure," *General Dentistry*, vol. 49, no. 4, pp. 393–395, 2001.

[2] J. J. Lane, "Gingival fenestration," *Journal of Periodontology*, vol. 48, no. 4, pp. 225–227, 1977.

[3] A. Dilsiz, "Gingival fenestrations due to poor oral hygiene in children and adolescents: report of two cases," *JSM Dental Surgery*, vol. 2, no. 2, p. 1018, 2017.

[4] S. Balasubramanian, V. Singh, G. S. Bhat, S. R. Acharya, V. Nidambur Ballal, and D. Vinayachanan, "Isolated mucosal fenestration with localized gingival recession: closure with an acellular dermal graft. A rare case report with two years' follow-up," *Quintessence International*, vol. 47, no. 5, pp. 425–431, 2016.

[5] B. G. Askenas, H. R. Fry, and J. W. Davis, "Cervical enamel projection with gingival fenestration in a maxillary central incisor: report of a case," *Quintessence International*, vol. 23, no. 2, pp. 103–107, 1992.

[6] S. Pendor, V. Baliga, A. Muthukumaraswamy, P. V. Dhadse, K. K. Ganji, and K. Thakare, "Coverage of gingival fenestration using modified pouch and tunnel technique: a novel approach," *Case Reports in Dentistry*, vol. 2013, Article ID 902585, 5 pages, 2013.

[7] A. M. Geiger, "Malocclusion as an etiologic factor in periodontal disease: a retrospective essay," *American Journal of Orthodontics and Dentofacial Orthopedics*, vol. 120, no. 2, pp. 112–115, 2001.

[8] L. G. Breault, R. C. Brentson, E. B. Fowler, and F. C. Bisch, "Repair of a gingival fenestration using an acellular dermal matrix allograft," *US Army Medical Department Journal*, vol. 1, pp. 81–85, 2016.

[9] W. D. Sneed, "Noncarious cervical lesions: why on the facial? A theory," *Journal of Esthetic and Restorative Dentistry*, vol. 23, no. 4, pp. 197–200, 2011.

[10] S. J. Davies, R. J. M. Gray, and A. J. E. Qualtrough, "Management of tooth surface loss," *British Dental Journal*, vol. 192, no. 1, pp. 11–23, 2002.

[11] D. A. Brandini, C. L. Trevisan, S. R. Panzarini, and D. Pedrini, "Clinical evaluation of the association between noncarious cervical lesions and occlusal forces," *The Journal of Prosthetic Dentistry*, vol. 108, no. 5, pp. 298–303, 2012.

[12] L. R. Marion, S. C. Bayne, D. A. Shugars et al., "Effects of occlusion type and wear on cervical lesion frequency," *Journal of Dental Research*, vol. 76, p. 2364, 1997.

[13] W. C. Lee and W. S. Eakle, "Possible role of tensile stress in the etiology of cervical erosive lesions of teeth," *The Journal of Prosthetic Dentistry*, vol. 52, no. 3, pp. 374–380, 1984.

[14] H. M. Goldman and D. W. Cohen, *Periodontal Therapy*, CV Mosby Company, 1973.

[15] F. Khan, W. G. Young, S. Shahabi, and T. J. Daley, "Dental cervical lesions associated with occlusal erosion and attrition," *Australian Dental Journal*, vol. 44, no. 3, pp. 176–186, 1999.

[16] C. G. Hutton, G. K. Johnson, C. A. Barwacz, V. Allareddy, and G. Avila-Ortiz, "Comparison of two different surgical approaches to increase peri-implant mucosal thickness: a randomized controlled clinical trial," *Journal of Periodontology*, vol. 89, no. 7, pp. 807–814, 2018.

30

Restoring Teeth with an Advanced Lithium Disilicate Ceramic: A Case Report and 1-Year Follow-Up

Felicitas Hölken and Helmut Dietrich

Department of Prosthodontics and Materials Science, University Medical Center of University of Mainz, Augustusplatz 2, 55131 Mainz, Germany

Correspondence should be addressed to Felicitas Hölken; felicitas.hoelken@unimedizin-mainz.de

Academic Editor: Asja Celebic

Advancements in materials science and bonding protocols as well as new manufacturing methods foster the development of novel ceramic materials to meet the increased demands for highly aesthetic, biocompatible, and long-lasting restorations in fixed prosthodontics. This case report highlights the minimally invasive rehabilitation with a new advanced lithium disilicate (ALD) ceramic block. It is reinforced with virgilite crystals in managing esthetic demand of patient besides having a high flexural strength. According to the manufacturer, the material provides a biaxial strength measured at >700 MPa and improved optical properties. The remarkable speed sintering time of approx. 4.5 minutes makes processing very fast. Time efficiency, predictability, and economically interesting treatment options are of great importance in current dentistry and can be well implemented in CAD/CAM dentistry. The newly introduced ALD ceramic for the "Chairside Economical Restoration of Esthetic Ceramics"/ "CEramic REConstruction" (CEREC) system produces an esthetically pleasing and clinically excellent restoration. The shorter processing time combined with high flexural strength will optimize the chairside workflow. New treatment indication options for lithium disilicate ceramics will expand. Although more evidence from long-term clinical studies is needed to verify the clinical performance and manufacturer recommendations regarding indication, preparation and cementation must be followed very strictly. In the present case report, restorations were indicated for seven posterior teeth, which were prepared, scanned, designed with CEREC-Primescan SW 5.1.3, and fabricated with MCX5. The monolithic restorations were placed adhesively. The rehabilitation with the ALD blocks resulted in an aesthetically pleasing, functional outcome that improved overall treatment time and increased patient and practitioner satisfaction, which remained stable over a one-year follow-up period.

1. Introduction

Everybody is talking about digitalization today. It impacts not only social life but also the way dentistry is performed. The advent of computerized technologies in restorative dentistry has led to an enormous change for dentists and dental technicians. Indirect restorations can now be made in dental practices (chairside), laboratories, or even production centers [1, 2]. The use of digitally generated data sets, computer-aided design, and numerical control (NC) technology for processing silicate and oxide ceramics allows us to work with new, industrially prefabricated and almost defect-free restorative materials [1]. Dental ceramics are known for their high esthetics and biocompatibility. Because of these properties and the patients' demand for materials that are as lifelike as possible, ceramics are widely used in present-day dentistry. While in the past almost exclusively manual techniques, such as layering or pressing, were used to produce ceramic restorations, computer-aided design and computer-aided manufacturing (CAD/CAM) technology now help us to process completely new materials, which are unfit for manual processing. In the 1990s, the first oxide ceramic crowns and bridges were made, thanks to new computer-aided grinding and milling systems and polycrystalline crystals reinforced with 5.35% by weight of yttrium oxide [3]. As a viable alternative to metal-based restorations, featuring a high esthetic potential and excellent biocompatibility, these ceramics have become very popular and have

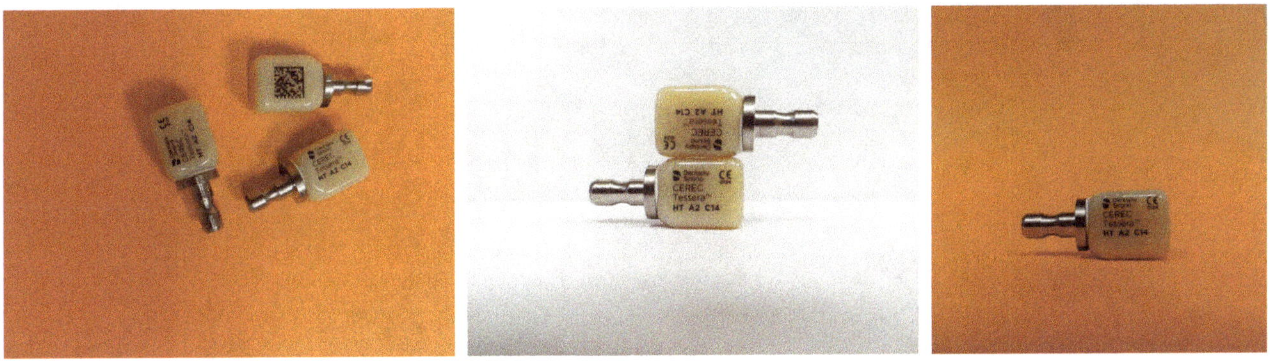

FIGURE 1: CEREC tessera blocks.

replaced metals in a variety of indications [4–6]. After numerous improvements, we can now distinguish between five generations of modern zirconia restoratives. Users should be aware of the indications and limitations of these different ceramics. Just like silicate ceramics, they differ greatly in their optical and mechanical properties [5]. Technique sensitivity in the processing steps, chipping of veneering materials, or even fracturing of zirconia frameworks gave rise to criticism in the past [4, 6–10].

In recent years, there has been a trend toward the use of monolithic restorations to avoid any chipping of veneering ceramics on oxide ceramic frameworks [5, 11, 12].

Monolithic crowns can be made of silicate or oxide ceramics. Ultimately, the users of CEREC systems were the ones who demanded industrially prefabricated ceramics with clearly defined properties, suitable for chairside grinding in one appointment. These industrial ceramic blocks are characterized by a controlled, uniform structural quality. This is important when using ceramics, because every pore, every irregularity, may cause cracking and lead to the failure of a restoration. Because of the benefits of adhesive bonding, short production times and high esthetics, numerous CEREC users prefer glass ceramic blocks. High success and survival rates of chairside fabricated restorations have been described [3, 10, 13–15]. Lithium disilicate (LS2) ceramics are the most frequently used materials in chairside processing and is particularly proven in terms of esthetics and strength and therefore widely accepted and used (e.g., CEREC Tessera, Dentsply Sirona, Charlotte, USA; IPS e.max CAD, Ivoclar Vivadent, Schaan, Liechtenstein) [15, 16]. A relatively high glass content also allows users to adhesively bond restorations after etching with hydrofluoric acid, and thanks to their higher strength of more than 350 MPa (3-point flexural strength), as compared to other glass ceramics, LS2 ceramics requires less tooth structure reduction in the preparation step. This opens the doors to defect-oriented, nonretentive preparation designs. In this combination, it is suitable for a large variety of indications, including single-tooth crowns, partial crowns, veneers, inlays, onlays, or implant-supported restorations. Even according to the manufacturers' information, 3-unit fixed partial dentures (FPDs) up to the first premolar can be fabricated (e.g., IPS e.max CAD, Ivoclar Vivadent, Schaan, Liechtenstein). A prerequisite for this is compliance with the minimum material thickness of 1.0 mm and the demanding adhesive bonding [17, 18]. Following the trend toward monolithic restorations [5], LS2 ceramics can even be used in esthetically demanding cases without additional veneering, thanks to its translucency [15, 19].

The following case report demonstrates the fabrication of seven monolithic single-tooth restorations by using a novel advanced lithium disilicate (ALD) ceramic (CEREC Tessera, Dentsply Sirona, Charlotte, USA) fabricated with the CEREC system (Primescan and MC X5, Dentsply Sirona, Charlotte, USA) (Figure 1). The material is a tooth-colored block but needs a mandatory firing to reach its final strength. This ALD ceramic features a special microstructure. According to the manufacturer, it consists of LS2 and virgilite, i.e., lithium aluminum silicate, embedded in a glass matrix enriched with zirconia. During firing, more virgilite crystals are formed. On the one hand, the rod-shaped LS2 crystals create high tensile strength, counteracting crack propagation, and on the other hand, the small virgilite crystals formed during firing substantially contribute to the high biaxial flexural strength of >700 MPa by increasing precompression stress.

2. Case History

A patient presented in the Prosthodontic Department of the Dental Clinic of the University Mainz, Germany. Teeth 16-14 and 44-47 had been restored with large composite fillings. Parts of these restorations had fractured shortly after placement and had been repeatedly repaired. Teeth 16, 45, and 46 had also been endodontically treated several years ago. The X-ray diagnostics revealed a sufficient endodontic treatment ad-apex without apical findings and the patient was pain-free. Teeth 16 and 46 showed minor discolorations of the tooth structure. The other vital teeth showed insufficient restoration margins and carious lesions (Figures 2 and 3). The patient chewed only on the left side, for fear of losing her fillings again, and wished to finally receive durable restorations. In addition to an improvement in her functional situation, esthetics mattered to the patient. An open edge-to-edge bite in the region of teeth 16, 46 and a cross bite in the region of teeth 15, 45 were diagnosed. No additional temporomandibular disorders were found.

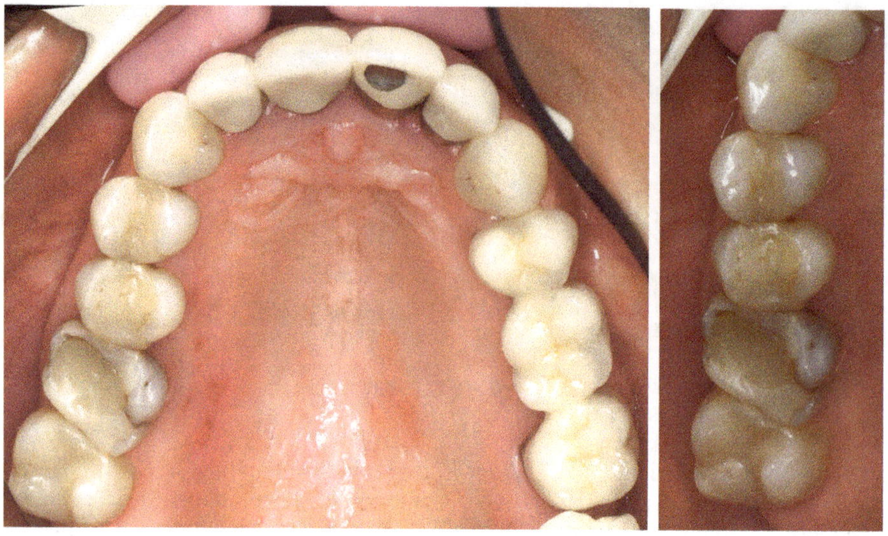

Figure 2: Initial situation of the maxilla: teeth 16-14 insufficient composite restorations; tooth 16 endodontically treated.

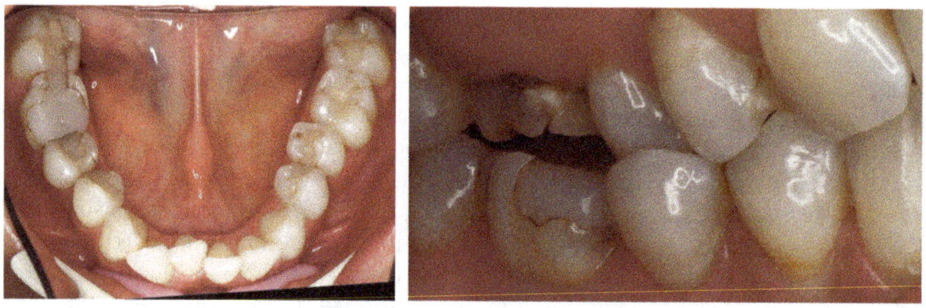

Figure 3: Initial situation in the mandible: teeth 44-47 insufficient composite restorations; tooth 45, 46 endodontically treated; lateral view: open edge-to-edge bite in the region of teeth 16, 46 and a cross bite in the region of teeth 15, 45.

2.1. Material Selection. Seven restorations were made using the CEREC system. To simplify the complexity of the bite, the fourth quadrant (44-47) was treated first. Depending on defect size, teeth 47 and 44 received inlays, tooth 45 received an onlay, and tooth 46 received a partial crown. Adhesively bonded restorations have frequently proven to be a successful alternative to traditional crowning [20]. For a tooth affected by an extensive intracoronal lesion, like tooth 46 in this case, a crown is often preferred as the treatment of choice. However, a crown preparation will usually weaken the residual tooth structure even further when there is such a large defect [21]. An adhesively bonded partial ceramic crown can be an alternative in this situation. It is less invasive, because of its defect-oriented preparation design [22–24]. To preserve as much tooth structure as possible, a material which, thanks to high flexural strength, helps to minimize the height of the restoration while still meeting high esthetic requirements was selected. After completing the restorations of the mandibular teeth, the maxillary teeth (14–16) were treated. Due to the root canal treatment and the loss of substance, the tooth 16 received a partial crown. With regard to the defect size and as much preservation of tooth structure as possible, tooth 15 received an onlay, and tooth 14 an inlay; all restorations were adhesively bonded.

2.2. Preparation and Digital Workflow. Shade selection using a conventional shade guide (Vitapan classic, Vita Zahnfabrik, Bad Säckingen, Germany) was performed. Following the removal of the existing composites from teeth 44-47 and caries excavation, cavity bases were placed to cover the root canal fillings and cavity floors (Clearfil DC core plus, Dentin, Kuraray Noritake Dental Inc., Tokyo, Japan) (Figure 4). Subsequent preparations had to meet the material-specific requirements of CAD/CAM milled ceramics [25]. For defect-oriented partial crown preparation, minimum wall thicknesses recommended by the manufacturer (1.5 mm for occlusal and 1.0 axial walls) were strictly adhered to and internal line angles were rounded (4562.314, Komet Dental, Lemgo, Germany). The occlusal design from the partial crowns (teeth 16 and 46) were prepared with a rhombic (8899.314.027, Komet Dental, Lemgo, Germany) and a bud-shaped instrument (8368.314.016, Komet Dental, Lemgo, Germany) [25, 26]. The inlay preparation (1.0 mm occlusal minimal width and height) was free of undercuts, all line angles were rounded, a taper of approx. 6°–10° relative to the occlusal surface was prepared, and the margins were not located in occlusal contact points (8863.204.012 and 4562.314, Komet Dental, Lemgo, Germany). Sharp line angles should be avoided, especially when using CAM inlays, because they may create problems during production and placement [25].

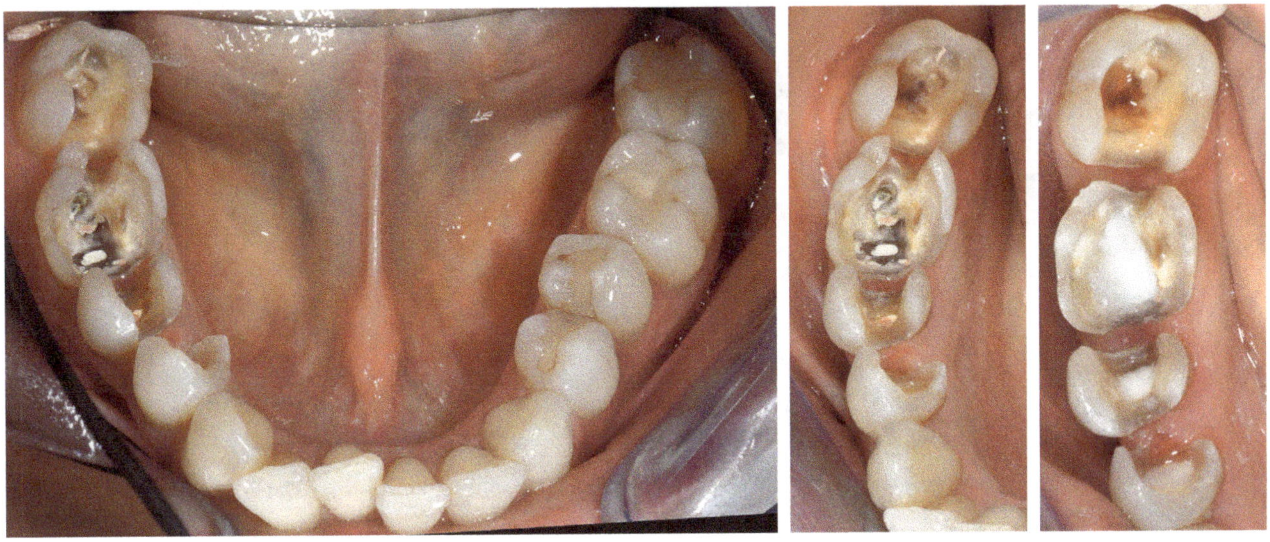

FIGURE 4: Cavity preparations and bases in the mandible.

The quadrant, the opposite jaw, and a lateral bite registration were intraorally scanned (CEREC Primescan AC SW 5.1.3, Dentsply Sirona, Charlotte, USA). The automatically determined restoration proposals have improved immensely with new software updates that deliver reliable restorations that hardly need to be modified. Due to the number of restorations, the decision was made in this case to set the model axis, enter the preparation margin, and define the insertion axis oneself. The software used in the biogeneric individual mode presented a restoration design for the missing occlusal surfaces. Various tools can be used to easily customize this design (Figures 5 and 6). A modification of the restoration design was only necessary by adjusting the occlusal and proximal contacts. Digital scanning was followed by the placement of temporary restorations. The chairside restorations were not placed in this appointment, considering the scope of this work, the cross bite, and the need to individually stain the ceramic.

After initial shade determination, CEREC Tessera blocks in size C14 (18 × 14 × 12 mm) were selected in shade MT A2 for teeth 46 and 47, and in shade HT A2 for the other teeth. The blocks come in a variety of shades and in two translucencies, and differ in fluorescence depending on the shade. HT (High Translucency) blocks are suitable for the production of inlays, onlays, or anterior restorations, which should be highly translucent. Medium translucency (MT) blocks are more opaque and therefore preferably used for posterior restorations masking discolored tooth structure or cast post and cores. After grinding in the CEREC MC X5 production unit, the retention pin of the crown was removed, and the connecting area was finished with a fine-grid diamond instrument (Figure 7). The restorations were checked for accuracy of fit and occlusal contacts on a printed model (SolFlex, W2P, Vienna, Austria) and adjusted where necessary (Figure 8). Then the restorations were individually stained and glazed for furnace firing (DS Body Stain S1, DS Incisal Stain S1, DS Mahogany, Dentsply Sirona, Charlotte, USA). The stains should be thoroughly mixed with a non-metallic spatula and diluted on a glass slab as desired before application. The restorations should be clean and free of grease. The restorations were placed on a firing tray with a firing pad (DeguDent, Hanau-Wolfgang, Germany) and fired at 760°C (Figure 9). The restorations should

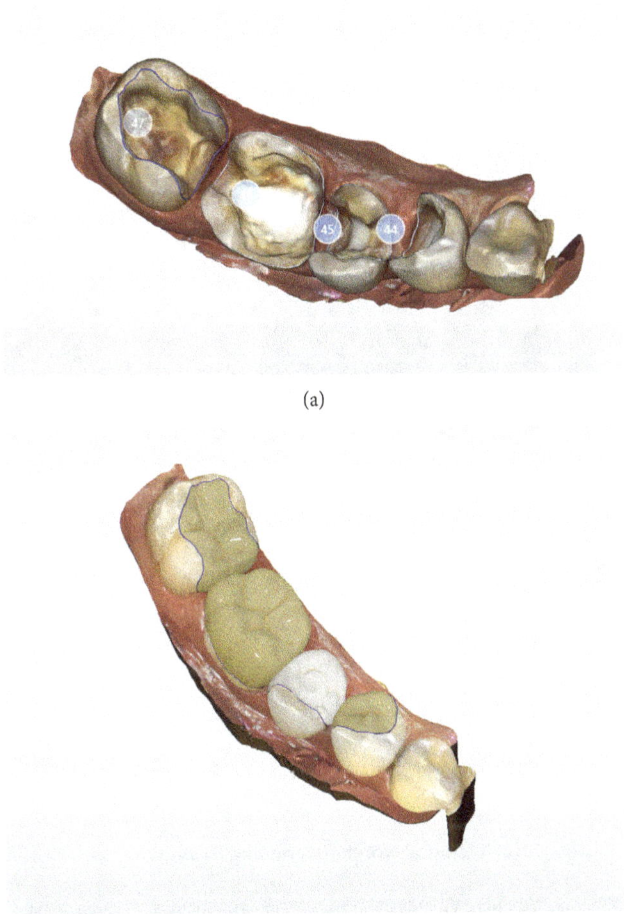

(a)

(b)

FIGURE 5: Digital design for teeth 44, 45, 46, and 47; CEREC SW 5.1.3.

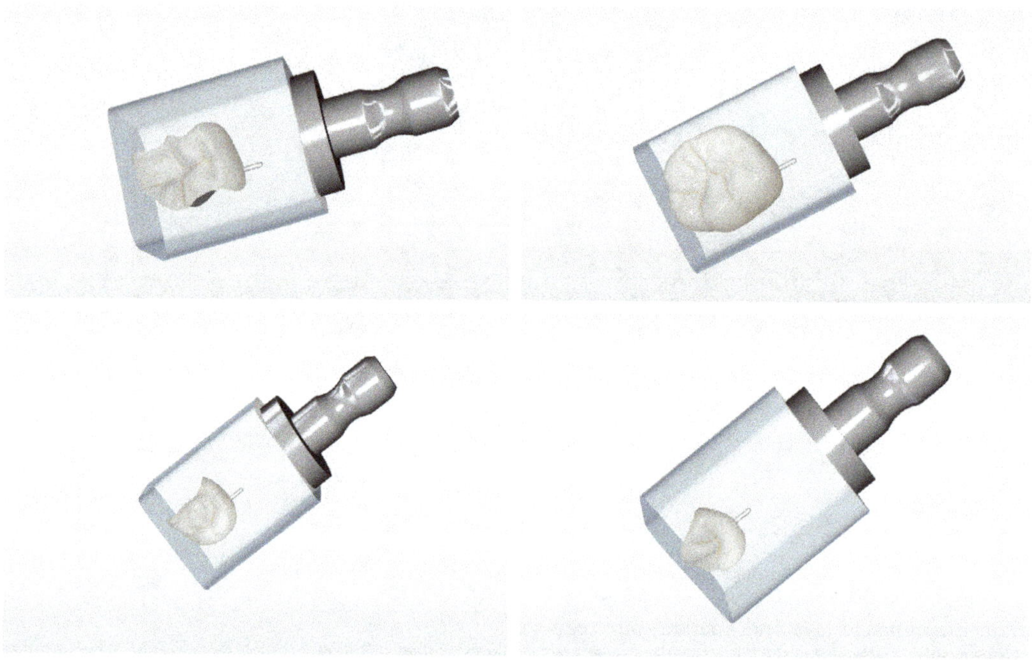

Figure 6: Restorations designed for teeth 47, 46, 45, and 44, ready for grinding.

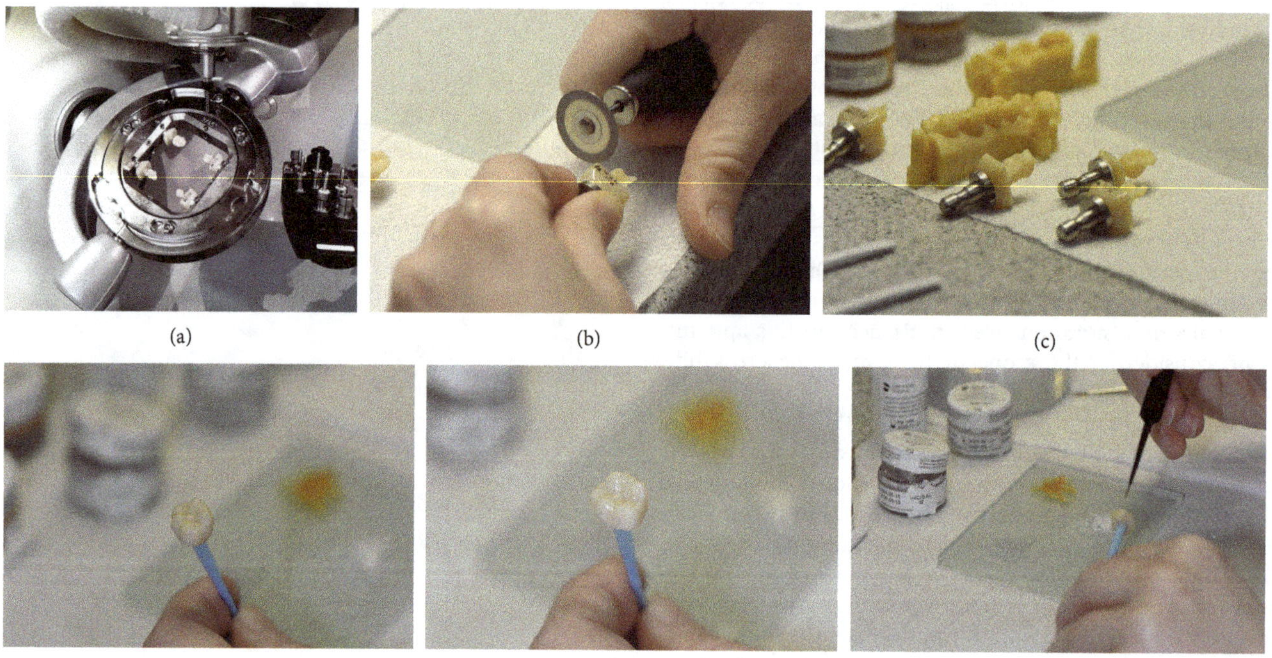

(a) (b) (c)

(d) (e) (f)

Figure 7: (a) Technical workflow: grinding restorations with MC X5; (b) & (c) handling preparations (d)–(f) staining and glazing restorations.

be positioned in the center to ensure they are exposed to the correct temperature. The firing is indispensable to achieving the high final strength of this ceramic; firing for individual characterization with stains is optional. Polishing alone will not lead to high final strength, in contrast to other (glass) ceramics (e.g., IPS e.max CAD, Ivoclar Vivadent, Schaan, Liechtenstein; Celtra duo, Dentsply Sirona, Charlotte, USA). Any conventional ceramic furnace will allow users to easily set the right firing parameters. Using a SpeedFire furnace (Dentsply Sirona, Charlotte, USA), however, the firing time of CEREC Tessera restorations can be reduced to 4.5 minutes. Prior to speed firing in this furnace, only spray glaze needs to be applied to the ceramic. Finally, the restoration was high-shine polished with a diamond polishing paste (Fegupol 8059, Feguramed, Buchen, Germany) (Figure 9.

2.3. Placement. The restorations were checked for marginal and interproximal fit. They all fitted accurately without any

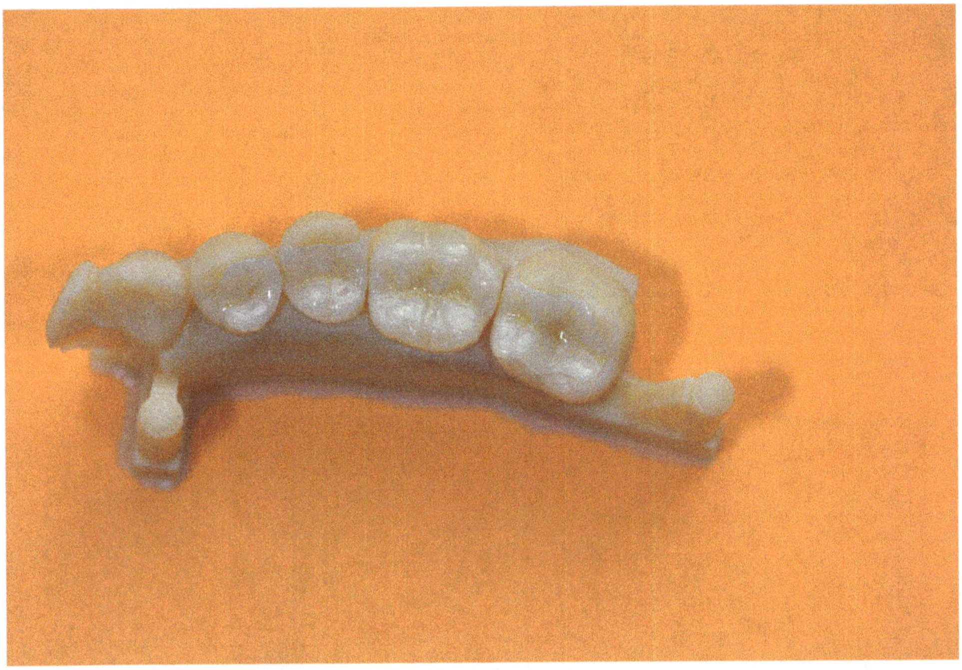

FIGURE 8: Finalization of the restorations 47, 46, 45, and 44 on a printed model.

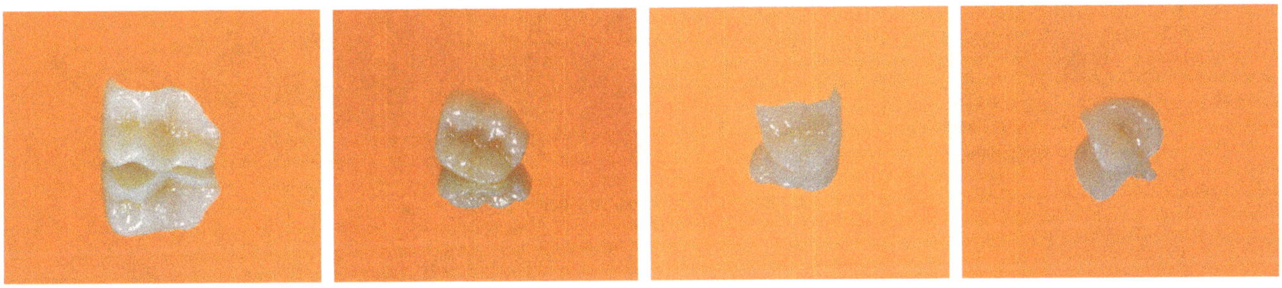

FIGURE 9: Final restorations of the teeth 47, 46, 45, and 44.

looseness or gaps. Then the order in which the restorations would be placed was determined. The ceramic was cleaned with alcohol, and the inner surfaces were etched with 5% hydrofluoric acid gel (IPS Ceramic Etching Gel, Ivoclar Vivadent, Schaan, Liechtenstein). After etching for 30 seconds, the surfaces were cleaned, first in a water beaker and then with air/water spray. The dried restoration surfaces were coated with a silane coupling agent (Calibra silane, Dentsply Sirona, Charlotte, USA) for 60 seconds, and then surplus was removed by strong air stream. The enamel surfaces were selectively etched with 37% phosphoric acid gel, rinsed with water spray, and carefully air-dried. Then a universal adhesive (Prime & Bond active, Dentsply Sirona, Charlotte, USA) was applied to the dry tooth structure for 20 seconds and light-cured after solvent evaporation. The restorations were luted using adhesive resin cement (Calibra Ceram, Dentsply Sirona, Charlotte, USA). Gross excess cement was removed with foam pellets, and interproximal areas were cleaned with dental floss. This was followed by tack-curing to easily remove the remaining excess cement in a gel state with a scaler. Then, each surface was light-cured for at least 20 seconds, and the margins were polished if necessary, followed by polishing with a three-step ceramic polisher set (New Technology Instruments, P30032A, Kahla, Germany). Static and dynamic occlusions were checked. The restoration proved to be a good color match with the adjacent teeth (Figure 10). After placing the mandibular restorations, the maxillary teeth (16-14) were prepared, and a digital impression was taken, in the same appointment (Figures 11 and 12). The restorations were produced as described above (Figures 13, 14, and 15) and placed in another appointment (Figure 16). At the follow-up visit, the patient was very satisfied with the esthetic results of the treatment and dared to bite normally again. To prevent excessive stressing of the restorations, a relaxation splint to be worn at night was made. The esthetics, functional occlusion, and gingival tissue remained stable over a follow-up period of 6 months and 1 year. No signs of fractures within the restorations were observed.

2.4. Discussion. CAD/CAM is a promising technology and has been employed in the chairside fabrication of all-ceramic restorations [27, 28]. The advance of this science and a high demand for metal-free restorations have led to

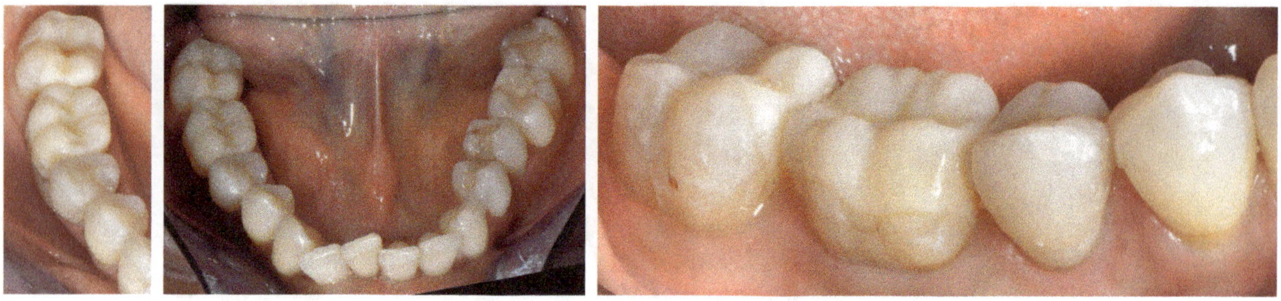

Figure 10: Restorations placed on teeth 44, 45, 46, and 47.

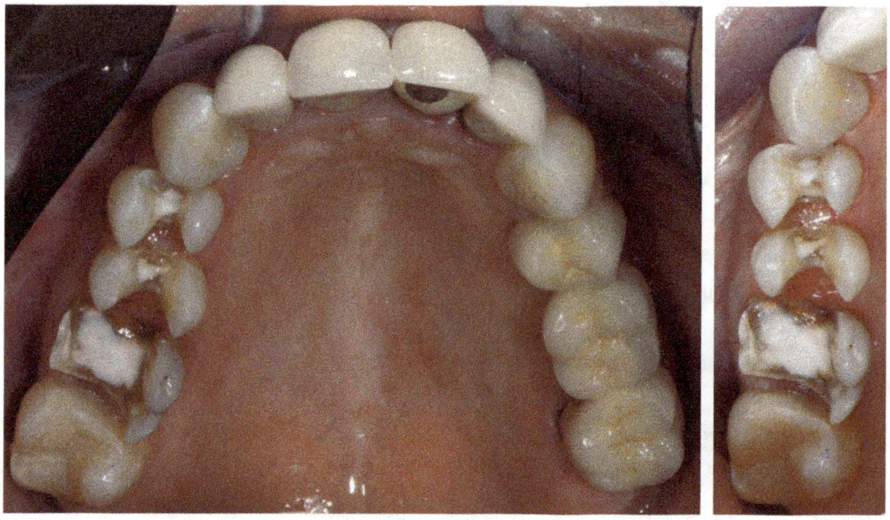

Figure 11: Cavity preparations and bases in the maxilla.

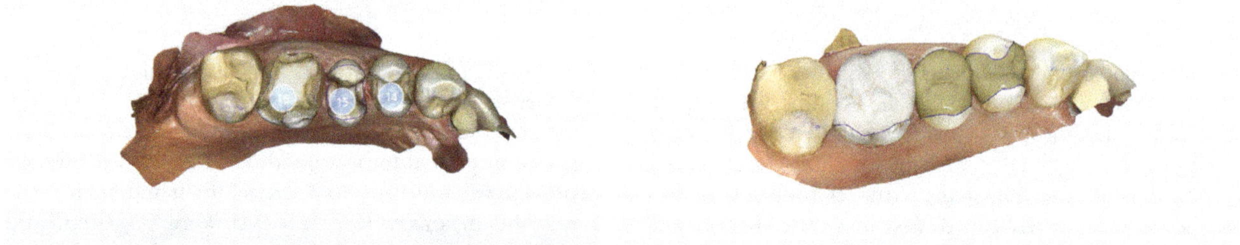

(a) (b)

Figure 12: Digital design for teeth 16, 15, and 14; CEREC SW 5.1.3.

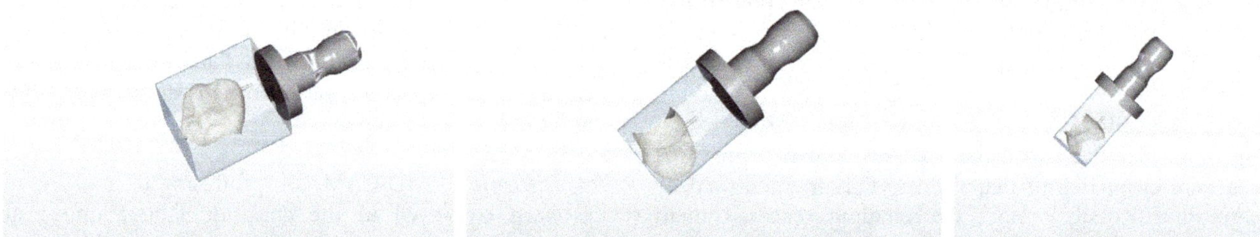

Figure 13: Restorations designed for teeth16, 15, and 14, ready for grinding.

rapid advancements in processing technologies and the development of newer restorative materials [15]. With continuous improvements in intraoral scanning technology, new software updates and material innovations, this technique is becoming increasingly widespread [29–32].

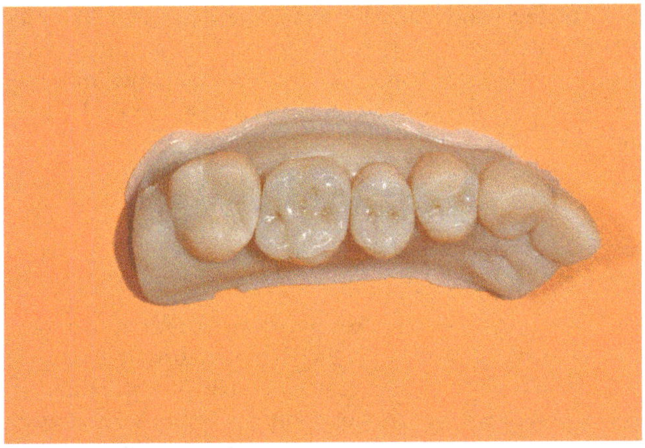

FIGURE 14: Finalization of the restorations 16, 15 and 14 on a printed model.

Due to their high strength combined with great translucency, LS2 ceramic monolithic blocks have become the material of choice for chairside dentistry [15, 16].

This case report describes the fabrication of seven monolithic restorations with a novel ALD ceramic. On account of the number of restorations, the restorations were milled with the CEREC MCX5. Taking the path of chairside production, the CEREC Primemill in the superfast mode would have reduced the grinding time compared to previous chairside milling processes (CEREC MCXL) [18, 28, 33].

Due to the constant development of the software (CEREC SW 5, Dentsply Sirona, Charlotte, USA) the design process has become simpler and more intuitive [31, 34, 35]. The current software offers practical design proposals that mainly only need minor adjustments at the occlusal and proximal contact points [17], which leads to a significant reduction in time [18].

As one major advantage of the digital workflow, the time needed for occlusal and internal adjustments is shorter than for restorations fabricated in the conventional workflow [27, 31, 34].

The optional speed-sintering process reduces the fabrication time significantly. While the influence of the speed-sintering process on the mechanical and optical properties

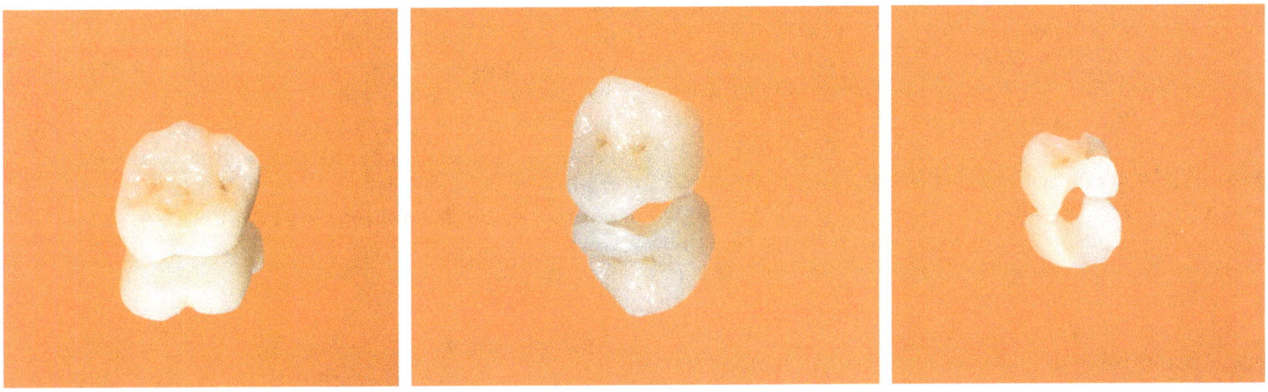

FIGURE 15: Final restorations for teeth 16, 15 and 14.

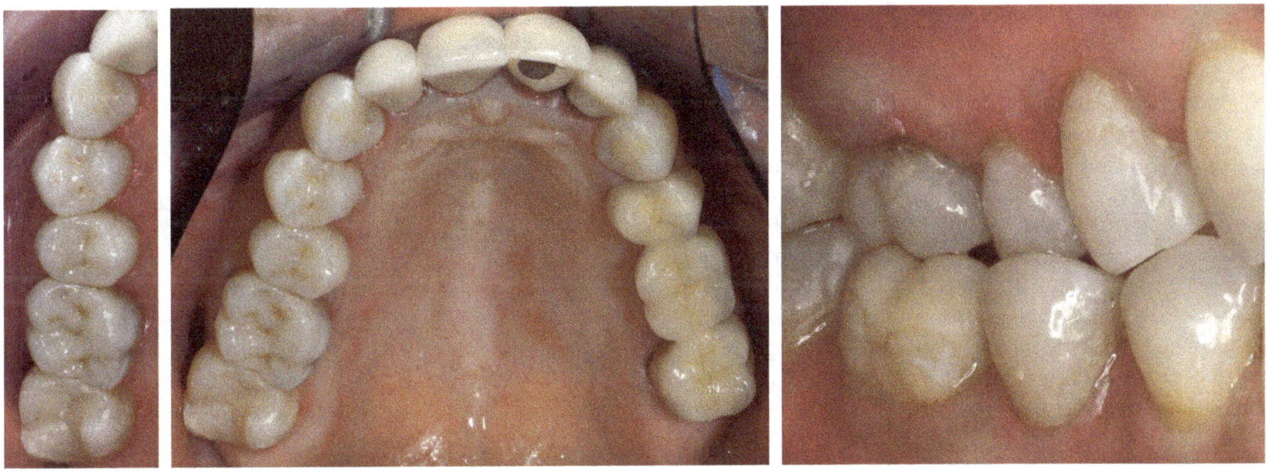

FIGURE 16: Restorations placed on teeth 16, 15 and 14 with final lateral view.

of zirconia ceramics has been investigated in several in vitro studies [36–39], further studies of this relatively new processing technique on ALD ceramics would be necessary.

The high flexural strength of ALD ceramics present an advantage of this new material in comparison to other LS2 ceramics and might expand the range of indications for restorations exposed to high stress areas. Compared to zirconia ceramics the processing of ALD is easier, faster, and practicable for chairside use.

Flexural strength is a critical material property, evaluated in standardized tests. The value of >700 MPa indicated by the manufacturer was achieved in biaxial flexural tests. As there are different testing methods, such as three-point, four-point or biaxial flexural tests, measurements are difficult to compare [40]. The flexural strength of the ALD ceramic considerably exceeds that of other silicate ceramics. This is why it can be both adhesively bonded and conventionally cemented, the latter only if retentive preparation is carried out and the manufacturer's instructions have been followed (minimum wall thicknesses of full crowns for conventional cementation: occlusal and axial walls 1.5 mm each; for adhesive bonding: occlusal and axial walls 1.0 mm each for all indications except onlays, which need 1,5 mm occlusal thickness). And you can count on the material's strength even at wall thicknesses down to 1.0 mm, giving you greater flexibility in your restoration designs. A study on LS2 ceramics showed a significant increasing strength of the restoration when an adhesive cement is used rather than a conventional one [41]. Whereas the adhesive bond of glass-ceramics with low flexural strength (e.g., feldspar or leucite ceramics) is necessary for mechanical strength of the restoration [42]. In the present case report, the ALD ceramic was conditioned by an etching process with 5% hydrofluoric acid for 30 seconds. This pretreatment ensures a bonding strength comparable to the well examined LS2 ceramics in combination with dual curing composite cements and self-adhesive cements [43]. A recently published in vitro study showed that there is only a minor effect of cementation technique (adhesive resin, glass-ionomer cement, and hybrid glass-ionomer cement) of the ALD ceramic on durability during in vitro mastication and fracture force [44]. The same study showed a significantly lower wear of ALD and a tendency toward lower antagonist wear than LS2 [44]. Further long-term clinical trials are needed here to confirm this.

According to the manufacturer, the crystal sizes of 500–700 nm correspond to the wavelengths of visible light; this is intended to lead to an increased light diffusion effect that is independent of wavelengths. High light transmission and diffusion create a chameleon effect, so that restorations blend in with the natural tooth structure. The translucent properties of LS2 ceramics are a major advantage compared to zirconia ceramics. Also the ALD ceramics deliver the tooth-like esthetics of glass ceramics which can be confirmed in the present case report. The blocks are currently only available in monochromatic color and can be stained for individual characterization. Especially for the production of crowns and partial crowns a multilayer block with a prefabricated color gradient could facilitate the staining process and could be a further time-saving innovation.

An alternative treatment option for the case presented would have been the fabrication of restorations made from a high-strength glass-ceramics (e.g., IPS e.max CAD, Ivoclar Vivadent, Schaan, Liechtenstein). Due to the remaining walls of the endodontically treated teeth, a post build-up was not necessary [45]. Nevertheless, it is a limitation of these new materials that data from clinical studies are missing. Therefore, the manufacturer's instructions must be carefully observed.

3. Conclusion

Chairside restorations are becoming more and more important in dental practice. Industrially prefabricated ceramic blocks allow dentists to produce monolithic restorations in one appointment with optional finalization in a laboratory. The ALD ceramic combines a high biaxial flexural strength of >700 MPa and esthetically pleasing results. Beside to the wide range of indications for chairside fabrication, the high flexural strength also allows restorations to be made in load-bearing areas. In addition to the benefits of ease of use and good material properties, time efficiency plays a crucial role in dental practice. The time saving speed-sintering process of approx. 4.5 minutes makes processing very fast. Therefore, this ceramic is an interesting material for monolithic restorations produced in a digital workflow. Results from additional clinical studies are required to validate the positive results from these initial clinical experiences.

Abbreviations

ALD:	Advanced lithium disilicate
CEREC:	Chairside economical restoration of Esthetic ceramics/CEramic REConstruction
NC:	Numerical control
CAD/CAM:	Computer-aided design/computer-aided manufacturing
LS2:	Lithium disilicate
FPDs:	Fixed partial dentures
HT:	High translucency
MT:	Medium translucency
CAD/CAM:	Computer-aided design and computer-aided manufacturing.

Consent

Written informed consent for publication of photographs and radiographs was obtained from the patient.

Acknowledgments

The authors wish to thank our MDT Manuela Meereis for dental laboratory work. The study was funded by the Department of Prosthodontics and Materials Science, University Medical Center of University of Mainz, Augustusplatz 2, 55131 Mainz, Germany.

References

[1] F. Beuer, J. Schweiger, and D. Edelhoff, "Digital dentistry: an overview of recent developments for CAD/CAM generated restorations," *British Dental Journal*, vol. 204, no. 9, pp. 505–511, 2008.

[2] A. Mehl, "Digitaltechnik dringt weiter vor," *ZWP Spezial*, vol. 8, no. 4, p. 3, 2008.

[3] F. Zarone, M. I. Di Mauro, P. Ausiello, G. Ruggiero, and R. Sorrentino, "Current status on lithium disilicate and zirconia: a narrative review," *BMC Oral Health*, vol. 19, no. 1, p. 134, 2019.

[4] A. J. Raigrodski, G. J. Chiche, N. Potiket et al., "The efficacy of posterior three-unit zirconium-oxide-based ceramic fixed partial dental prostheses: a prospective clinical pilot study," *The Journal of Prosthetic Dentistry*, vol. 96, no. 4, pp. 237–244, 2006.

[5] J. F. S. B. Güth, D. Edelhoff, and A. Liebermann, "Zirkonoxid ist nicht gleich Zirkonoxid—Was muss ich als Praktiker wissen?," *Quintessenz Zahntechnik*, vol. 6, pp. 620–629, 2020.

[6] I. Sailer, M. Balmer, J. Husler, C. H. F. Hammerle, S. Kanel, and D. S. Thoma, "10-year randomized trial (RCT) of zirconia-ceramic and metal-ceramic fixed dental prostheses," *Journal of Dentistry*, vol. 76, pp. 32–39, 2018.

[7] J. Tinschert, K. A. Schulze, G. Natt, P. Latzke, N. Heussen, and H. Spiekermann, "Clinical behavior of zirconia-based fixed partial dentures made of DC-Zirkon: 3-year results," *The International Journal of Prosthodontics*, vol. 21, no. 3, pp. 217–222, 2008.

[8] F. Beuer, M. Stimmelmayr, J. F. Gueth, D. Edelhoff, and M. Naumann, "In vitro performance of full-contour zirconia single crowns," *Dental Materials*, vol. 28, no. 4, pp. 449–456, 2012.

[9] I. Sailer, A. Feher, F. Filser, H. Luthy, L. J. Gauckler, P. Scharer et al., "Prospective clinical study of zirconia posterior fixed partial dentures: 3-year follow-up," *Quintessence International*, vol. 37, no. 9, pp. 685–693, 2006.

[10] R. E. Matta, C. Motel, E. Kirchner et al., "Wear of feldspathic-ceramic-veneered zirconia posterior FPDs after 10 years," *BMC Oral Health*, vol. 20, no. 1, p. 345, 2020.

[11] B. E. Pjetursson, I. Sailer, A. Latyshev, K. Rabel, R. J. Kohal, and D. Karasan, "A systematic review and meta-analysis evaluating the survival, the failure, and the complication rates of veneered and monolithic all-ceramic implant-supported single crowns," *Clinical Oral Implants Research*, vol. 32, Suppl 21, pp. 254–288, 2021.

[12] C. Leitao, G. V. O. Fernandes, L. P. P. Azevedo, F. M. Araujo, H. Donato, and A. R. M. Correia, "Clinical performance of monolithic CAD/CAM tooth-supported zirconia restorations: systematic review and meta-analysis," *Journal of Prosthodontic Research*, 2021.

[13] L. Fu, H. Engqvist, and W. Xia, "Glass–ceramics in dentistry: a review glass-ceramics in dentistry," *Materials*, vol. 13, no. 5, p. 1049, 2020.

[14] A. Rauch, S. Reich, L. Dalchau, and O. Schierz, "Clinical survival of chair-side generated monolithic lithium disilicate crowns: 10-year results," *Clinical Oral Investigations*, vol. 22, no. 4, pp. 1763–1769, 2018.

[15] A. Aziz, O. El-Mowafy, and S. Paredes, "Clinical outcomes of lithium disilicate glass-ceramic crowns fabricated with CAD/CAM technology: a systematic review," *Dental and Medical Problems*, vol. 57, no. 2, pp. 197–206, 2020.

[16] N. Bustamante-Hernandez, J. M. Montiel-Company, C. Bellot-Arcis, J. F. Manes-Ferrer, M. F. Sola-Ruiz, R. Agustin-Panadero et al., "Clinical behavior of ceramic, hybrid and composite onlays: a systematic review and meta-analysis," *International Journal of Environmental Research and Public Health*, vol. 17, no. 20, 2020.

[17] S. Rinke, A. K. Pabel, M. Rodiger, and D. Ziebolz, "Chairside fabrication of an all-ceramic partial crown using a zirconia-reinforced lithium silicate ceramic," *Case Reports in Dentistry*, vol. 2016, 2016.

[18] G. Marchesi, A. Camurri Piloni, V. Nicolin, G. Turco, and R. Di Lenarda, "Chairside CAD/CAM materials: current trends of clinical uses," *Biology*, vol. 10, no. 11, 2021.

[19] P. Baldissara, V. F. Wandscher, A. M. E. Marchionatti, C. Parisi, C. Monaco, and L. Ciocca, "Translucency of IPS e.max and cubic zirconia monolithic crowns," *The Journal of Prosthetic Dentistry*, vol. 120, no. 2, pp. 269–275, 2018.

[20] P. Magne, "Immediate dentin sealing: a fundamental procedure for indirect bonded restorations," *Journal of Esthetic and Restorative Dentistry*, vol. 17, no. 3, pp. 144–54; discussion 155, 2005, discussion 55.

[21] M. T. B. Federlin and G. Schmalz, "Teilkronen aus Keramik – ein Therapiekonzept im Fluss," *ZWP*, 2011.

[22] R. R. C. Frankenberger, M. J. Roggendorf, and N. Krämer, "Direkte oder indirekte Restaurationen im Seitenzahnbereich? Erfahrungen aus klinischen Studien mit Komposit und Keramik," *Die Quintessenz*, vol. 61, pp. 575–579, 2010.

[23] A. McDonald, "Preparation guidelines for full and partial coverage ceramic restorations," *Dental Update*, vol. 28, no. 2, pp. 84–90, 2001.

[24] U. S. Beier, I. Kapferer, and H. Dumfahrt, "Clinical long-term evaluation and failure characteristics of 1,335 all-ceramic restorations," *The International Journal of Prosthodontics*, vol. 25, no. 1, pp. 70–78, 2012.

[25] M. Ahlers, G. Mörig, U. Blunck, J. Hajtó, L. Pröbstere, and R. Frankenberger, "Guidelines for the preparation of CAD/CAM ceramic inlays and partial crowns," *International Journal of Computerized Dentistry*, vol. 12, no. 4, pp. 309–325, 2009.

[26] D. Edelhoff and M. O. Ahlers, "Occlusal onlays as a modern treatment concept for the reconstruction of severely worn occlusal surfaces," *Quintessence International*, vol. 49, no. 7, pp. 521–533, 2018.

[27] D. Fasbinder, "Using digital technology to enhance restorative dentistry," *The Compendium of Continuing Education in Dentistry*, vol. 33, no. 9, pp. 666–668, 2012, 70, 72 passim.

[28] M. J. Skramstad, "Welcome to cerec primescan AC," *International Journal of Computerized Dentistry*, vol. 22, no. 1, pp. 69–78, 2019.

[29] T. A. Sulaiman, "Materials in digital dentistry—A review," *Journal of Esthetic and Restorative Dentistry*, vol. 32, no. 2, pp. 171–181, 2020.

[30] M. B. Blatz and J. Conejo, "The current state of chairside digital dentistry and materials," *Dental Clinics of North America*, vol. 63, no. 2, pp. 175–197, 2019.

[31] K. Baroudi and S. N. Ibraheem, "Assessment of chair-side computer-aided design and computer-aided manufacturing restorations: a review of the literature," *Journal of International Oral Health*, vol. 7, no. 4, pp. 96–104, 2015.

[32] R. Kallala, M. H. Chaouch, K. Nasr, and T. Courset, "Step-by-step Esthetic rehabilitation with chairside system," *Case Reports in Dentistry*, vol. 2021, 2021.

[33] M. J. Skramstad, "A new milling unit for an efficient workflow," *International Journal of Computerized Dentistry*, vol. 23, no. 1, pp. 83–91, 2020.

[34] S. Ting-Shu and S. Jian, "Intraoral digital impression technique: a review," *Journal of Prosthodontics*, vol. 24, no. 4, pp. 313–321, 2015.

[35] D. J. Poticny and J. Klim, "CAD/CAM in-office technology," *Journal of the American Dental Association*, vol. 141, Suppl 2, pp. 5S–9S, 2010.

[36] H. Liu, M. Inokoshi, K. Nozaki, M. Shimizubata, H. Nakai, T. D. Cho Too et al., "Influence of high-speed sintering protocols on translucency, mechanical properties, microstructure, crystallography, and low-temperature degradation of highly translucent zirconia," *Dental Materials*, vol. 38, no. 2, pp. 451–468, 2022.

[37] J. U. Jansen, N. Lumkemann, I. Letz, R. Pfefferle, B. Sener, and B. Stawarczyk, "Impact of high-speed sintering on translucency, phase content, grain sizes, and flexural strength of 3Y-TZP and 4Y-TZP zirconia materials," *The Journal of Prosthetic Dentistry*, vol. 122, no. 4, pp. 396–403, 2019.

[38] F. Mayinger, R. Pfefferle, A. Reichert, and B. Stawarczyk, "Impact of high-speed sintering of three-unit 3Y-TZP and 4Y-TZP fixed dental prostheses on fracture load with and without artificial aging," *The International Journal of Prosthodontics*, vol. 34, no. 1, pp. 47–53, 2021.

[39] S. M. Cokic, J. Vleugels, B. Van Meerbeek, B. Camargo, E. Willems, M. Li et al., "Mechanical properties, aging stability and translucency of speed-sintered zirconia for chairside restorations," *Dental Materials*, vol. 36, no. 7, pp. 959–972, 2020.

[40] P. T. J. Pospiech and A. Raigrodski, *Ein Kompendium für die keramikgerechte Anwendung vollkeramischer Systeme in der Zahnmedizin*, 3M ESPE, 2004.

[41] A. Bindl, H. Luthy, and W. H. Mormann, "Thin-wall ceramic CAD/CAM crown copings: strength and fracture pattern," *Journal of Oral Rehabilitation*, vol. 33, no. 7, pp. 520–528, 2006.

[42] W. S. Oh, "Cement type (adhesive vs. conventional) may not affect clinical Performance of zirconia and lithium disilicate tooth-supported crowns," *Journal of Evidence-Based Dental Practice*, vol. 20, no. 2, p. 101415, 2020.

[43] R. Frankenberger, V. E. Hartmann, M. Krech, N. Kramer, S. Reich, A. Braun et al., "Adhesive luting of new CAD/CAM materials," *International Journal of Computerized Dentistry*, vol. 18, no. 1, pp. 9–20, 2015.

[44] M. Rosentritt, A. Schmid, C. Huber, and T. Strasser, "In vitro mastication simulation and wear test of virgilite and advanced lithium disilicate ceramics," *The International Journal of Prosthodontics*, 2022.

[45] M. Naumann, M. Schmitter, and G. Krastl, "Postendodontic restoration: endodontic post-and-core or no post at all?," *The Journal of Adhesive Dentistry*, 2018.

Permissions

All chapters in this book were first published by Hindawi Publishing Corporation; hereby published with permission under the Creative Commons Attribution License or equivalent. Every chapter published in this book has been scrutinized by our experts. Their significance has been extensively debated. The topics covered herein carry significant findings which will fuel the growth of the discipline. They may even be implemented as practical applications or may be referred to as a beginning point for another development.

The contributors of this book come from diverse backgrounds, making this book a truly international effort. This book will bring forth new frontiers with its revolutionizing research information and detailed analysis of the nascent developments around the world.

We would like to thank all the contributing authors for lending their expertise to make the book truly unique. They have played a crucial role in the development of this book. Without their invaluable contributions this book wouldn't have been possible. They have made vital efforts to compile up to date information on the varied aspects of this subject to make this book a valuable addition to the collection of many professionals and students.

This book was conceptualized with the vision of imparting up-to-date information and advanced data in this field. To ensure the same, a matchless editorial board was set up. Every individual on the board went through rigorous rounds of assessment to prove their worth. After which they invested a large part of their time researching and compiling the most relevant data for our readers.

The editorial board has been involved in producing this book since its inception. They have spent rigorous hours researching and exploring the diverse topics which have resulted in the successful publishing of this book. They have passed on their knowledge of decades through this book. To expedite this challenging task, the publisher supported the team at every step. A small team of assistant editors was also appointed to further simplify the editing procedure and attain best results for the readers.

Apart from the editorial board, the designing team has also invested a significant amount of their time in understanding the subject and creating the most relevant covers. They scrutinized every image to scout for the most suitable representation of the subject and create an appropriate cover for the book.

The publishing team has been an ardent support to the editorial, designing and production team. Their endless efforts to recruit the best for this project, has resulted in the accomplishment of this book. They are a veteran in the field of academics and their pool of knowledge is as vast as their experience in printing. Their expertise and guidance has proved useful at every step. Their uncompromising quality standards have made this book an exceptional effort. Their encouragement from time to time has been an inspiration for everyone.

The publisher and the editorial board hope that this book will prove to be a valuable piece of knowledge for researchers, students, practitioners and scholars across the globe.

List of Contributors

Carmen Lucia Mueller Storrer, Leonardo Luiz Muller, Janes Francio Pissaia, Carla Frehner Andrade, Claudia Roberta Tenório Trevisani and Tatiana Miranda Deliberador
School of Health Science, Universidade Positivo, Curitiba, Paraná, Brazil

Hadeel Alqatami
Pediatric Dental Department, Hamad Dental Centre, Doha, Qatar

Khalid N. Said
Department of Dentistry, Oral Health Institute, Al Wakra Hospital, Hamad Medical Corporation, Doha, Qatar
College of Dental Medicine, Qatar University, Doha, Qatar

Adham A. Ammar
Surrey and Sussex Health care Trust, Surrey, UK

Hani Nazzal
Pediatric Dental Department, Hamad Dental Centre, Doha, Qatar
College of Dental Medicine, Qatar University, Doha, Qatar

Marc El Hage and Mark Bischof
Ardentis Clinique Dentaire Lausanne, Swiss Dental Clinics Group, Voie du Chariot 6, 1003 Lausanne, Switzerland

Nathalie Nurdin and Rabah Nedir
Ardentis Clinique Dentaire Vevey, Swiss Dental Clinics Group, Rue du Collège 3, 1800 Vevey, Switzerland

Alberto De Biase, Giulia Mazzucchi, Dario Di Nardo, Marco Lollobrigida, Giorgio Serafini and Luca Testarelli
Department of Oral and Maxillo-Facial Sciences, Sapienza University of Rome, Italy

Alvaro Francisco Bosco and Juliano Milanezi de Almeida
Department of Surgery and Integrated Clinic, School of Dentistry, São Paulo State University, Araçatuba, São Paulo, Brazil

Belén Retamal-Valdes and Renata Tavares
Department of Periodontology, Dental Research Division, Guarulhos University, Guarulhos, São Paulo, Brazil

Jessica M. Latimer
Department of Oral Medicine, Infection, and Immunity, Harvard School of Dental Medicine, Boston, MA, USA

Diego Messina, Matheus Henke, Laura Gantes Rodrigues Dias and Thiago Marchi Martins
Department of Semiology and Clinic, Periodontology Discipline, Federal University of Pelotas, Pelotas, Rio Grande do Sul, Brazil

Carlo Maiorana, Paola Polacco and Pier Paolo Poli
Implant Centre for Edentulism and Jawbone Atrophies, Maxillofacial Surgery and Odontostomatology Unit, Fondazione IRCCS Cà Granda Ospedale Maggiore Policlinico, University of Milan, Milan, Italy

Dario Andreoni
Private Practice, Via Milano 19, 20871 Vimercate, Monza Brianza, Italy

Arun Sadasivan, Elizabeth Koshi and Ashna Mariya Benny
Department of Periodontics, Sree Mookambika Institute of Dental Sciences, Kulashekaram, Tamil Nadu, India

K. Rakul Nambiar
Sree Mookambika Cancer Centre, Kulasekharam, Tamil Nadu 629161, India

Deepu George Mathew
Department of Oral and Maxillofacial Pathology, Annoor Dental College, Muvatupuzha, Kerala, India

Roshni Ramesh
Department of Periodontics, Government Dental College, Trivandrum, Kerala, India

Dler Ali Khursheed and Faraedon Mostafa Zardawi
Department of Periodontics, University of Sulaimani, Sulaymaniyah, Kurdistan Region, Iraq

Yashodeep Chauhan, Shaleen Khetarpal, Madhu Singh Ratre and Manish Varma
Department of Periodontology, Govt. College of Dentistry, Indore, M.P., India

R. Varsha and P. S. Manoharan
Department of Prosthodontics, Indira Gandhi Institute of Dental Sciences, Sri Balaji Vidyapeeth Deemed-to-Be University, Pillaiyarkuppam, Puducherry 607 402, India

Vigneshvar Chandrasekaran
Department of Psychiatry, Mahatma Gandhi Medical College and Research Institute, Sri Balaji Vidyapeeth, Deemed-to-Be University, Pillaiyarkuppam, Puducherry 607 402, India

K. Savitha
Department of Prosthodontics, Mahatma Gandhi Postgraduate Institute of Dental Sciences, Kalaivaanar Nagar, Puducherry 605006, India

Luca Francetti, Stefano Corbella and Nicolò Cavalli
Department of Biomedical, Surgical and Dental Sciences, Università degli Studi di Milano, via L. Mangiagalli 31, 20133 Milan, Italy
IRCCS Istituto Ortopedico Galeazzi, Via R. Galeazzi, 4, 20161 Milan, Italy

Claudia Dellavia and Elena Canciani
Department of Biomedical, Surgical and Dental Sciences, Università degli Studi di Milano, via L. Mangiagalli 31, 20133 Milan, Italy

Claudia Moscheni
Department of Biomedical and Clinical Sciences "L. Sacco", Università degli Studi di Milano, via G.B. Grassi 74, 20157 Milan, Italy

Nicoletta Gagliano
Department of Biomedical Sciences for Health, Università degli Studi di Milano, via L. Mangiagalli 31, 20133 Milan, Italy

Diana Mostafa
Clinical Periodontology Department, Faculty of Dentistry, Alexandria University, Alexandria, Egypt

Shaden M. Alotaibi
Preventive Dental Sciences, Vision colleges for dentistry and Nursing, Riyadh, Saudi Arabia

Michele Perelli and Roberto Abundo
Indipendent Researcher, Turin, Italy
Private Practice, Turin, Italy

Giuseppe Corrente
Private Practice, Turin, Italy
Department of Periodontology, University of Pennsylvania, PA, USA

Paolo Giacomo Arduino
Department of Surgical Sciences, CIR-Dental School, University of Turin, Turin, Italy

Mario Semenza
Indipendent Researcher, Sant'Angelo Lodigiano, Italy

Hector Sarmiento
Indipendent Researcher, New York City, USA

Marah Damdoum
Department of Clinical Sciences, College of Dentistry, Ajman University, Ajman, UAE

Sudhir Rama Varma and Mohamed A. Jaber
Department of Clinical Sciences, College of Dentistry, Ajman University, Ajman, UAE
Centre of Medical and Biomedical Allied Health Sciences Research, Ajman University, Ajman, UAE

Manjusha Nambiar
Department of Periodontics, Sri Rajiv Gandhi College of Dental Sciences and Hospital, Banguluru, Karnataka State 560032, India

P. L. Ravishankar, Preethikaa Guruprasath, Padmaja Vangipuram, Jasmine Vaidya and G. Visithiriyan
Department of Periodontics, SRM Kattankulathur Dental College, Potheri, 603203, Tamil Nadu, India

A. Thirumal Raj
Department of Oral Pathology and Microbiology, Sri Venkateswara Dental College and Hospital, Chennai 600130, India

Shilpa Bhandi
Department of Restorative Dental Science, Division of Operative Dentistry, College of Dentistry, Jazan University, Jazan 45142, Saudi Arabia

Shankargouda Patil
Department of Maxillofacial Surgery and Diagnostic Sciences, Division of Oral Pathology, College of Dentistry, Jazan University, Jazan 45142, Saudi Arabia

Snehashish Ghosh
Department of Oral Pathology, College of Medical Sciences, Bharatpur, Nepal

Sundar Ramalingam
Department of Oral and Maxillofacial Surgery, College of Dentistry, King Saud University, Riyadh 11545, Saudi Arabia

Yasser Fahad Alrayyes and Khalid Buayjan Almutairi
Dental University Hospital, College of Dentistry, King Saud University, Riyadh 11545, Saudi Arabia

Ibrahim O. Bello
Department of Oral Medicine and Diagnostic Sciences, College of Dentistry, King Saud University, Riyadh 11545, Saudi Arabia

Abdulhameed Alsarraf
Ministry of Health, Kuwait

Kunj Mehta
Private Practice, Perth 6000 Western Australia, Australia

Nabil Khzam
NK Perio & Implants, Perth 6172 Western Australia, Australia

Johannes Müller
Department of Prosthodontics and Biomaterials, Danube Private University, Krems, Austria
Deputy Medical Director, Danube Private University, Krems, Austria

Rüdiger Junker
Department of Prosthodontics and Biomaterials, Danube Private University, Krems, Austria

Karim Chebbi, Khaoula Bouaziz, Oumaima Tayari, Azza Berkaoui, Mohamed Ali Bouzidi and Jamila Jaouadi
Complete Removable Prosthodontic Department, Research Laboratory LR12ES11, Faculty of Dental Medicine, University of Monastir, Monastir, Tunisia

T. Raut, S. Keshwar and A. Shrestha
Department of Oral Pathology, College of Dental Surgery, BP Koirala Institute of Health Sciences, Dharan, Nepal

M. R. Jaisani
Department of Oral and Maxillofacial Surgery, College of Dental Surgery, BP Koirala Institute of Health Sciences, Dharan, Nepal

Roshni Ramesh
Department of Periodontics, Government Dental College, Thrissur, Kerala, India

Deepu George Mathew
Department of Oral and Maxillofacial Pathology, Annoor Dental College, Muvattupuzha, Kerala, India

Dhanushka Leuke Bandara and Ruwan Duminda Jayasinghe
Department of Oral Medicine & Periodontology, Faculty of Dental Sciences, University of Peradeniya, Peradeniya 20400, Sri Lanka

Primali Rukmal Jayasooriya
Department of Oral Pathology, Faculty of Dental Sciences, University of Peradeniya, Peradeniya 20400, Sri Lanka
Department of Periodontology, University of Pennsylvania, PA, USA

Paolo Giacomo Arduino
Department of Surgical Sciences, CIR-Dental School, University of Turin, Turin, Italy

Moody Kaldas
Private Practice, Oetwil am See, Switzerland
Clinic of Conservative and Preventive Dentistry, Center of Dental Medicine, University of Zurich, Switzerland

André Barghorn
Institute of Pathology Medica, Zurich, Switzerland

Patrick R. Schmidlin
Clinic of Conservative and Preventive Dentistry, Center of Dental Medicine, University of Zurich, Switzerland

Alexei Bolyachin and Takhir Teberdiev
Iceberg Dental Trauma Center, Moscow, Russia

Zurab Khabadze and Oleg Mordanov
RUDN University (People's Friendship University of Russia), Moscow, Russia

Magomed Gasbanov
Iceberg Dental Trauma Center, Moscow, Russia
RUDN University (People's Friendship University of Russia), Moscow, Russia

Arjun Hari Rijal
Department of Periodontology and Oral Implantology, Kathmandu University School of Medical Sciences, Dhulikhel, Kavrepalanchok, Nepal

Bhageshwar Dhami
Department of Periodontology and Oral Implantology, Kantipur Dental College and Hospital, Basundhara, Kathmandu, Nepal

Pratistha Ghimire
Dental Department, Methinkot Hospital, Kavrepalanchok, Nepal

Figliuzzi Michele Mario, Parentela Luca, Aiello Domenico and Altilia Simone
Department of Health Sciences, "Magna Graecia" University, Catanzaro 88100, Italy

Aysegul Sari
Faculty of Dentistry, Department of Periodontology, Hatay Mustafa Kemal University, Hatay, Turkey

Salih Celik
Department of Oral and Maxillofacial Surgery, TDC Dental Clinic, Antalya, Turkey

Braydon Haskell, J. Kobi Stern, Jordan Ghiassi, Andrew Kurialacherry, Sadja Gaud-Quintana and Mark E. Peacock
The Dental College of Georgia at Augusta University, Augusta, GA, USA

Felicitas Hölken and Helmut Dietrich
Department of Prosthodontics and Materials Science, University Medical Center of University of Mainz, Augustusplatz 2, 55131 Mainz, Germany

Index

A
Actinomycosis, 151-152, 155-157
Adenoid, 128-132
Advanced Lithium Disilicate, 188-189, 196, 198
Aggregatibacter Actinomycetemcomitans, 175
Anterior Maxilla, 97
Apical Periodontitis, 158
Autologous Graft, 16, 20

B
Bisphosphonates, 108-109, 117, 120-121
Bone Augmentation, 35, 108, 118-120, 122
Bone Regeneration, 32-33, 35, 37, 92-93, 97-98, 100, 103-104, 108, 111, 120, 122, 164
Bovine Colostrum, 92-96

C
Cell Gingivitis, 53, 57
Cells, 4-5, 7-10, 19, 37, 39-41, 43-46, 49, 53-54, 62, 64, 67, 69, 71-73, 75, 77, 89-90, 96-98, 100-102, 108, 120, 129-131, 135, 141-144,148, 152, 154, 168, 178
Cementum-enamel Junction, 145-146
Chronic Periodontitis, 38, 46, 106, 155, 159, 178
Cone Beam, 40, 45, 99-100, 119, 160, 162
Connective Tissue, 1, 5, 23-27, 30-31, 37, 40, 43, 48-51, 53-54, 62-63, 65-67, 69-71, 76, 79, 81-82, 84, 86, 101, 130, 135, 137, 145, 148-149, 180-181, 184-185
Cystic Cavity, 97, 100, 103
Cytokeratin, 40, 44-45

D
Dentin Autologous Graft, 16, 20

E
Emphysema, 11-15

F
Filamentous Bacteria, 151, 154
Fluorodeoxyglucose, 41, 45

G
Gene Mutation, 139
Gingival Enlargements, 91, 133-134, 138-139
Gingival Fenestration, 184-187
Gingival Index, 16-17, 37, 73
Gingival Overgrowth, 44, 62, 65, 69-71, 85-91
Gingival Recession, 1-5, 23, 25-27, 29-31, 48, 51-52, 59, 76, 79-80, 84, 145-146, 149, 186

H
Hyperkeratosis, 89-90, 106, 180, 182

I
Intra-oral Plasmacytosis, 6, 10

K
Kindler Syndrome, 180-183

L
Lateral Periodontal Cyst, 97, 100, 103-104
Laterally Positioned Flap, 23-27
Leukoplakia, 141, 143-144, 181
Lichen Planus, 53, 96, 105, 107
Ligneous Conjunctivitis, 133-134, 136, 139-140
Ligneous Periodontitis, 133-134, 136-137, 139
Lipids, 117
Lithium Disilicate, 188-189, 196-198
Lymph Node, 92, 123-124, 130

M
Mandibular Canine, 97, 99-101, 103
Metastatic Carcinoma, 39, 46
Mucoepidermoid Carcinoma, 123, 131

N
Noonan Syndrome, 10

O
Oestrogen Receptor, 45
Oral Cavity, 36, 39-40, 42-43, 45-47, 73, 96, 105, 107, 118, 124-125, 129-132, 141, 156, 160-161
Oral Hygiene, 5-6, 10-11, 24, 36, 48, 51, 57, 73-74, 80, 85-89, 94, 96, 105-107, 109, 111, 116, 125, 143, 146, 152-153, 185-186
Oral Leukoplakia, 141, 144
Oral Lichen Planus, 96, 105, 107
Oral Rehabilitation, 32, 37, 198

P
Palatogingival Groove, 163, 169-170
Periodic Acid-schiff, 130-131, 139
Periodontal Cyst, 97, 100, 103-104
Periodontal Disease, 8, 10, 21, 30, 32-33, 36, 38, 43, 63, 92, 94, 105, 107, 121, 133-134, 139, 160, 162, 169, 177-178, 180-183, 187
Periodontal Manifestation, 180
Periodontal Tissues, 21, 27, 97, 103, 120, 136, 158, 160, 171, 183
Periodontitis, 6, 9-10, 32, 36-38, 43, 46, 48,

58-60, 86, 91-93, 98, 106, 109, 118, 120-121, 133-134, 136-137, 139-140, 151-152, 155-159, 161-162, 166, 170-172, 176-178, 180-183
Plaque Index, 16-17, 92, 109, 172
Plasma Cell, 8-10, 53-54, 56-57, 89, 91
Plasma Cell Gingivitis, 53, 57
Plasminogen, 133-140
Platelet-rich Fibrin, 21, 77, 119, 163, 167, 170
Porphyromonas Gingivalis, 92, 171, 175, 178
Positron Emission, 40, 45
Posterior Mandible, 108-109, 111
Probing Pocket Depth, 16-17
Proliferative Verrucous Leukoplakia, 141, 144
Proteins, 45, 62, 64, 69, 117, 134-135, 137, 152, 168
Pseudo Glandular, 129-131

S

Soft Tissue, 6, 8, 10, 14, 20, 29-30, 32, 36-38, 41, 44-45, 48, 62-63, 76, 79-84, 89, 97, 100, 108, 126, 130, 135, 145, 148-149, 151-152, 156, 184-186
Squamous Cell Carcinoma, 44, 123-124, 129-132, 144, 183
Surgical Excision, 86, 88, 123, 127, 137, 141
Surgical Extraction, 16-17, 21

T

Thyroid Transcription, 41, 45
Titanium Mesh, 108, 110-114, 117-120, 122
Tumour Cells, 40-41, 43-45

U

Ulcerative Gingivitis, 85, 89-90

V

Verrucous Leukoplakia, 141, 144
Vertical Osseous, 92-93

www.ingramcontent.com/pod-product-compliance
Lightning Source LLC
LaVergne TN
LVHW082231200926
848484LV00008B/2337
* 9 7 9 8 8 8 7 4 0 6 5 3 4 *

www.ingramcontent.com/pod-product-compliance
Lightning Source LLC
LaVergne TN
LVHW082233200926
848484LV00008B/2349